The Excellent Board

The Excellent Board

Practical Solutions
for Health Care Trustees and CEOs

Karen Gardner

Editor

Foreword by Richard J. Umbdenstock

Health Forum, Inc.
An American Hospital Association Company
CHICAGO

AHA
press

Cover design by Tim Kaage

Library of Congress Cataloging-in-Publication Data

The excellent board: practical solutions for health care trustees and CEOs / Karen
   Gardner, editor; foreword by Richard J. Umbdenstock.
       p. cm.
    Includes index.
    Collection of 48 articles originally published in Trustee.
    ISBN 1-55648-309-0 (pbk.)
       1. Hospital trustees. 2. Hospitals—Administration. 3. Health facilities—Administration. 4.
    Chief executive officers. I. Gardner, Karen. II. Umbdenstock, Richard J.

RA971.E9865 2003
362.1'1'068—dc21   2003045266

ISBN: 1-55648-309-0   Item Number: 196125

Contents

About the Editor

Karen Gardner has been a health care editor for more than 20 years—as editor of *Trustee* magazine since 1989 and, prior to that, as executive editor of periodicals for the Joint Commission on Accreditation of Healthcare Organizations (JCAHO). Before entering the health care field, Gardner edited several legal publications.

Gardner writes a monthly column in *Trustee,* has published numerous articles in the magazine, and is the editor of a book on quality in hospice care published by the JCAHO.

Gardner shepherded a major redesign of *Trustee* in 1995, and under her editorial direction, the magazine has won a number of editorial and graphic awards—from the Society of National Association Publications (including a Gold Award for General Excellence), from the American Society of Business Press Editors, and from the American Society of Healthcare Publication Editors.

Gardner received a master of arts in teaching (M.A.T.) English from the University of Chicago, and before entering the editorial field, taught English at the high school and middle school levels in Chicago.

Foreword

A friend taught me years ago that mission "is the point of intersection between an organization's founding principles and its current environment." The value of this insight increases each year as we face growing challenges.

For the 25 years that I have observed, served on, and staffed voluntary health care boards, their primary focus has always been the organization's mission—how to define it, how to pursue it, how to accomplish it, how to hold management accountable for it, and how to keep it viable. What has changed, is changing as you read this, and will continue to change, is the "current environment."

The relentless torrent of changes for health care organizations is staggering—from regulations to reimbursement rates, medical advances to niche providers, aging populations to educated consumers. There is one constant, however, and that is our commitment to mission. For 2003 and beyond, the reason for that commitment is quite clear—across communities, more people with more challenges need access to care more than ever. Trustees understand, both intellectually and personally, that this is no time to lose sight of our mission.

How should boards approach their responsibilities today? Although those in the health care field might agree that governance requires the same formula of skills and attributes that it always has, no one can deny that the dosages of those skills have gone up. Never before has such a premium been placed on vision, leadership, business acumen, risk management, collaboration, diplomacy, and mental agility. Never before have boards been in such need of educated, informed, experienced, wise, compassionate, and conscientious trustees.

If health care organizations are going to succeed, our current environment requires trustees and CEOs to reassess their understanding of the board's accountability to its community; its composition and structure; its strategic plan; its responsibilities for clinical quality, patient safety, finances, patient satisfaction, and community benefit; and its ability to assess the recommendations and performance of executive management.

Whether in my executive role or my community volunteer role, I continue to apply another lesson I learned long ago: "Every board meeting is really a referendum on only two questions—do we have the right plan, and do we have the right leadership, board, and CEO to achieve our plan?" The pressures of the health care environment and the risks they apply to mission require a dispassionate reality check of such a referendum.

If you've been exploring effective governance for as long as I have, you have appreciated the insight, assistance, and educational quality of *Trustee* over the decades. Just like the times, *Trustee* has changed, from pamphlet to respected magazine. Now "the magazine for health care governance" has compiled a collective resource for those intent on preserving the mission of volunteer governance and improving performance in the boardroom.

I hope you will reread and rediscover these thoughtful selections. I know that many articles will provide timely insights, and others will refresh prior learnings. This collection speaks to the mission of health care governance as well as to the mission of *Trustee*.

Richard J. Umbdenstock
President and CEO
Providence Services
Spokane, Washington

Preface

Timing is everything. As editors and journalists, we at *Trustee* magazine usually try to publish articles that address the issues our readers will soon be confronting. There is an inherent problem with this approach, however—if your board or your part of the country or your particular market hasn't yet had to deal with an issue, you're likely to put the magazine aside and forget about it. Then, when you're ready for an article, the magazine has moved on. We may not revisit that topic for another six, nine, or twelve months; and it is certain that we won't revisit it in the same way. And since few readers have the physical space or inclination to save their magazine back issues, the opportunity to get the information they need when they need it has come and gone.

That's why we decided to collect 48 of *Trustee*'s best articles published over the past few years, covering the topics with which boards continue to wrestle—board composition, the governance process and trustee education, board/CEO relations, board work, finance, quality, patient safety, and strategic planning. These topics comprise the eight parts of the book.

The parts on board composition and governance come first in order to give the reader a sound context within which to work. Trying to understand and improve your relationship with the hospital's or system's CEO won't make a lot of sense if you don't first know who should be sitting on your board and why. In the same way, learning about the complexities of patient safety and the board's role in effecting change will only be confusing and confounding unless you first have a firm grasp of what comprises a health care trustee's fundamental roles and responsibilities.

The articles collected here will give both new and experienced trustees, as well as board and committee chairs, a firm grounding in what it takes to be an excellent board member and how to reach the level of excellence health care organizations must achieve. Not only has the learning curve for boards contracted significantly in the past decade, but with more attention being paid to public governance in the wake of recent business scandals, the not-for-profit sector is feeling the deflected heat.

Although boards have always had a fiduciary duty to their communities for finance, quality, and patient safety, developments and revelations in those fields have upped the ante and put more pressure on boards. Reduced reimbursement; higher prices for technology, pharmaceuticals, malpractice insurance, and staffing; and increasing numbers of uninsured patients have put hospitals' bottom lines in serious jeopardy. Boards must somehow find the resources to invest in more quality and patient safety initiatives on a tighter budget.

The combination of articles included in *The Excellent Board* will give you a thorough understanding of these issues and the practical guidance and tools you need to undertake your job. And the final section on strategic planning will show you how to plan your future in the most direct and efficient manner possible.

All the articles in this book were selected with the following criteria in mind:

- They are as timely today as when they were published.
- They are balanced and provide different perspectives on the issue.
- They are practical and provide information you can use immediately.
- They are straightforward.

And, best of all, in the tradition of *Trustee*, they are interesting, well written, and engaging. We hope this book will make the work you have chosen to do for your communities, your organizations, and the nation's health care system easier and more rewarding.

Acknowledgments: First, I would like to thank all the authors of the articles included in *The Excellent Board*, both professional and volunteer. Their articles were great when they were originally published, and they have stood the test of time.

A major thank you is due to Richard Hill, editor of *Health Forum Journal* and editorial director for AHA Press. Rick not only guided the process of putting this book together but also lent his considerable expertise to the final product.

And finally, Peggy DuMais, assistant manager for production at Health Forum, was responsible for shaping this book into its present format.

PART ONE

Board Composition

Wanted:
A Few Good Trustees

Boards Must Use New Techniques
and Look in New Places
to Recruit the Best Members

By Michelle Blecher

Hospital trustees have always given freely of their time and energy. Most consider it an honor to serve the health care needs of their communities. And the term "trustee" says it all—these are the people that communities of all types and sizes have entrusted to guard their most trusted possession, their health. Where would communities be without hospitals and medical professionals? But trustees know all of this. They've already made the sacrifice, spending hours at meetings or burning the midnight oil to bone up on hospital matters. Finding new, qualified board members to join their ranks isn't easy in any business these days. "I'm not sure it's not any harder than it would be for a bank or an HMO or any other company to get good trustees," says Errol Biggs, co-author of *Practical Governance* and director of graduate programs in health administration at the University of Colorado, Denver.

But what is particular to hospitals and their mounting difficulty in recruiting trustees is the increasing complexity of the health care field, and, as a result, the time it takes to get up to speed on a multitude of

---

Michelle Blecher is a Chicago-based writer.

complex issues may be daunting to even the most well-intentioned and qualified citizen.

"Boards simply have to do a lot more to be informed and to go through oversight and deliberative processes," says Barry S. Bader, governance consultant and president of Bader and Associates in Potomac, Maryland. "It's a lot more work and a lot more responsibility."

Decisions to open, close, or expand services; a new awareness of patient safety and medical errors; an understanding of government regulations and reimbursement; and a renewed emphasis on quality improvement are all issues with "a steep ramp-up curve in terms of the board's understanding and decisionmaking," Bader says.

The pool of qualified candidates is also narrowing as hospital boards increasingly seek board members who have specific skills and reflect diversity. Others also may be dissuaded because some key local decisions, such as approving budgets and hiring a CEO, may now be assumed by the system-level board.

Ratchet that difficulty up another notch for hospitals enduring turbulent times. It's more difficult to find strong individuals in those circumstances willing to enter the fray, says governance expert J. Larry Tyler, president and CEO of Tyler & Company in Atlanta. "Organizations that are doing very well usually don't have as hard a problem recruiting their board members as others that are in turmoil, or losing money, or at war with physicians," says Tyler, who coauthored *Practical Governance* (Health Administration Press) with Biggs.

Recruiting challenges haven't gotten so bad that seats are left vacant for long, but they are bothersome, experts say. "It's a frustration on the part of governance and nominating committees," explains Bader. "It's just harder coming up with potential names of people to talk to."

Michael Fay, a trustee of Fairview Health Services in Minneapolis, who used to sit on one of the local hospital boards, sees the difficulties firsthand. Right now [as of this writing in December 2001], there are two out of seven seats open on the University Medical Center board that will need to be filled by the first of the year.

"Generally they find someone, but to be honest with you, when you add geography [i.e., trustees representing different communities in the service area] to diversifying . . . I hate to say it, but there are times we end up with a board representative somewhat by default—it's not our first or second choice, but we've got to fill it."

Ditto for Ted McKinney, a board member and past chair of Lincoln Health System's Lincoln General Hospital in Ruston, Louisiana, who says two trustees in the past year and a half resigned because of time demands. "If they're willing to learn and don't have conflicts of interest and time restraints, then you have a pretty narrow selection of people to draw from," he says.

So what options does a board have?

The Price of Service

Biggs and Tyler advocate compensating trustees as a way to improve board recruitment, as well as a psychological incentive to take the job seriously and put in the time it takes. Biggs estimates that more than 20 percent of hospital boards pay trustees "in the $5,000 range," but compensation also may include deferred insurance and deferred income.

"Even if you only pay a small amount, you open up a different category of people who wouldn't normally volunteer their time . . . and you have an opportunity to go outside the community and bring in people with a skill set you wouldn't normally get," Tyler says.

But others disagree. "People are doing this [serving on hospital boards] because they're committed to it, period, not because of what the reimbursement is, and my feeling is that you get a better quality person for that reason," says Fay.

Bader says it depends on the organization. "I talk about compensation with most of the boards I work with, and, generally, it's much more applicable at the parent board level of a larger system [where the issues and decisions may be more complex]," he says. But even there, Bader notes, some boards react violently to the idea. "They simply feel that it would destroy the culture and collegiality and basic values that they stand for . . . and until it becomes a problem for them to recruit top-caliber people, they probably aren't going to come to it."

Some boards have opted to pay only the chair because this work "is so above and beyond the demands of every other board member," Bader says. "On some boards the responsibilities of that [hospital] chairperson have really grown to the equivalent of being either the chair or lead director on a major corporate board."

William Mason, a current trustee and former chair of Baptist Health System in Jacksonville, Florida, says that local hospital board members receive a stipend of about $300 per month. But he says the system probably will discontinue the stipend because it hasn't improved recruitment or performance on the board as the system originally thought it would.

"If we really wanted to recruit a very busy chief executive and chairman of some large corporation, $300 a month isn't going to be very much of an incentive to a guy like that who is serving on other paid boards for $50,000," says Mason, adding that most board members donate their stipend to the foundation anyway.

"I don't think that we have had any difficulty recruiting the people we need for our local health ministries, because the kind of people we're interested in having on those boards are committed to that kind of service anyway and committed to a not-for-profit," he says. "They think it's a privilege and an honor to be asked to serve."

Looking Outside the Neighborhood

Biggs recommends that boards also look outside their communities for prospective trustees—a hospital CEO or physician from another system, for instance—that fit the experience and talents they need. Besides providing a wider pool of candidates, he says these individ-

---

Recruiting Tips from the Pros

Health care consultants offered these do's and don'ts for snagging quality trustees:

- Define your selection criteria and stick to them. What are the competencies, talents, and demographics that best fit your hospital's needs and strategic goals?
- Widen your traditional network for potential candidates, including expanding your search beyond your community.
- Don't sugarcoat the job specifications. Be frank with candidates about the demands and limits on their decision-making authority.
- Don't undersell the time commitment. Be honest about the hours the job takes.
- Don't overlook retention. It's not enough just to bring new trustees through the door. Make sure you've adopted an orientation program and ongoing trustee education.

uals often can be more objective than community members. "They're not so close to a tough decision," he says.

Mason believes that bringing on David Hitt, then-CEO of Baylor Health System in Dallas, "was a godsend." Hitt commuted by air to attend board meetings at Jacksonville, Florida's Baptist Medical Center's board in the 1980s as it tackled growth and expansion to become what is now a five-hospital health system. Hitt still serves on the system board.

"We were looking for somebody to bring an additional perspective from the national scene," says Mason. Hitt was also active on the American Hospital Association board and helped write the Medicare laws in the '60s. "He was probably one of the wisest and most knowledgeable of the senior health care executives in America in those days. To find somebody that wise and that mature [who had] that much ability to think through issues rationally . . . that was very fortunate for us," says Mason.

Besides providing the global thinking that has been invaluable to the system board, Hitt was also a major help to the local board, which recruited him originally, especially in working with physicians on facilities, equipment, and technology issues, Mason adds. The board paid Hitt a stipend plus travel expenses.

"The medical staff appreciated having a different perspective because they knew that David didn't have any political ax to grind," Mason says. "He was really looking at things from a very rational perspective, and he brought a great deal of wisdom and experience from a different medical staff and medical center."

Who's Right for the Job?

It's not enough anymore to base an invitation to serve on the hospital board simply on whether a candidate plays golf with the trustees and is known as "a good guy," says governance consultant Pamela R. Knecht, vice-president of Accord Limited in Chicago. Instead, she advises boards to "create and use your selection criteria."

How do you develop those criteria? It's different for every organization, and it changes as the institution's goals and strategic plans change, she says. For instance, if a hospital board needs to integrate services or collaborate with physicians in new ways, a board may consider approaching a physician from a nearby community.

Tyler mentions these common characteristics for recruitment criteria:

- Commitment—"If they're prominent and committed, great, but if they're just prominent . . . I'd rather go for commitment."
- Experience—"I'd let them learn on somebody else's nickel."
- Intelligence—"I want people on the governing board to be really smart versus a community leader who might [only] be a good talker."

Bader also suggests going outside the search committee's traditional circles. He advises that designated trustees talk to a wider-than-usual circle of contacts, including governance consultants, executives of other health care organizations, nationwide business organizations, and charitable groups such as the United Way.

"Networking still remains the primary mode of identifying potential board members," says Bader, "but boards have got to widen their networks . . . because they need to have a variety of perspectives. Boards will benefit from having one or two gadflies or contrarians who are able to challenge the prevailing wisdom in a constructive manner."

George F. Longshore, vice president of leadership formation and human resources at Catholic Health East in Newton Square, Pennsylvania, says that the organization's system board plans to assist regional boards in defining the competencies they need for a well-rounded board and provide necessary support with recruitment.

Above all, look for someone who is willing to devote the time necessary to do the job, experts advise. That includes board meetings, committee meetings, preparation, and education. Knecht says that The Governance Institute in La Jolla, California, estimates that board members spend an average of 30 hours a year in education beyond meeting time.

In an effort to ease the burden on board members and streamline the decision-making process, many boards have reduced their number of meetings per year, according to the University of Colorado's Biggs. More than half of boards now meet quarterly or six times a year rather than monthly. Ideally, trustees should be spending no more than 10 to 15 hours a month at meetings, he says.

Mason attributes some of the ease with which Baptist boards can attract new members to their efficiency and professionalism. Boards and committees at Baptist work hard to limit their meetings to about an hour each month.

"I think down through the years in our organization we have developed a culture that is strict on time," he says. "We design our board agendas and [premeeting] materials in such a way that we convene our meeting at 5:00 and at 6:15 or 6:20 we're out. We don't sit there for hours on end debating things. We do all that work in the committee structure."

The Hard Sell: Been There, Done That

The days of the hard sell with all the trimmings are over. Consultants and board members say that trustees need to be frank with prospective candidates about the time involved and the responsibilities they will have.

"We're not trying to convince people anymore," says Fay. "I think our approach has been "Here's the job, look at it as a job, and the job is that you're the representative of health care in our community."

He says he knows the dangers of sugarcoating responsibilities, especially regarding time. "We've had people we thought were aware [of the commitment] who basically just had to resign from the board," he says. "People have good intentions sometimes but ultimately find out they're in over their heads, taking on too much or just not being able to do what they thought they could do."

Even if board members who feel overwhelmed don't bow out physically, says Knecht, they may bow out mentally by missing meetings or being ill-prepared.

But while trustees shouldn't undersell the time commitment to board candidates, they also shouldn't ignore citing the rewards, Bader adds. "Make the expectations clear up front, but talk about how important the work of the organization is. Busy people find ways to make time for activities that they think are important and [for organizations that] will value their contributions."

Knecht, who sits on a not-for-profit board, agrees. "It's much more effective if an organization is very clear on what it wants from its board; that it's identified me as filling that role perfectly; and if I get a personal call from the board chair saying, 'We've really thought long and hard about this, and you're the right person to fill this job, and here's why we need your skills and talents and perspectives,'" Knecht says.

Who Wants Control and How Much?

As health system boards take on some responsibilities previously held by local boards, trustees need to recognize that they could be appealing to a different type of individual than in the past—someone who may not be concerned about being the final decisionmaker but still considers the trustee role vital to the hospital's future. "The role then becomes much more one of understanding the true needs of the community and making sure those needs are being met through the hospital and ultimately the system," Knecht says.

That's how Jacquelyn Kinder, chair of the board of St. Mary's Healthcare System in Athens, Georgia, sees her job—she's a critical link between the community and the Catholic Health East organization, not a secondary player.

"I see it as a two-way street: we need to be sure that [the system board] understands the needs of our community, and we need to be sure it's getting the information it needs to do that. Then we need to trust [the system board] to act on that [information] in good faith," she says.

Indeed, Tyler says that some for-profit systems have given back control to local boards so that trustees don't feel disenfranchised. "They're trying to work with their boards to get more commitment, and the only way you can do that is by giving away some of the power."

For example, rather than calling the chair of an advisory board and saying, "Your new CEO is on his way," some system boards are taking a different tack, Tyler says. "They say, 'Okay, we're going to send our advisory board three candidates that are acceptable to us, and we'll let it choose which one it wants, and we'll live with any of them.'"

The bottom line to recruiting and maintaining a strong, committed board, according to Tyler: Give trustees meaningful authority, keep them informed, and keep meetings to a minimum. "Those things help because you're having to deal with people and how much time they have, and if it takes too much time, people just get burned out."

The Right Fit:
Recruiting for Your Board

By Shari Mycek

The idea of befriending his community's "movers and shakers" is one that John Thomas repeatedly drives home. The chief operating officer and vice president of development at Children's National Medical Center in Washington, D.C., insists that communities' powerful and influential citizens should not be feared or written off as too busy to serve on a hospital board. Instead, they should be embraced and asked to serve.

Thomas came to Children's National in 1995 following a stint at the American Red Cross where he worked closely with then-President Elizabeth Dole. "[Dole] had extraordinary access to the right people—business, clergy, entertainers, entrepreneurs, and health leaders," says Thomas. "Whatever the organization's need, she could get the best people because she could reach out, contact, and communicate with them."

When Thomas came to Children's National, the hospital's five boards—like most nationwide—comprised hard-working, committed community leaders. Still, there were holes in each board's

Shari Mycek is a contributing writer to *Trustee*.

composition—holes in the skills and capabilities necessary to move the board and organization to the next level.

For Children's Foundation Board—charged with fund-raising (a $200 million campaign is currently under way)—one of the missing links was the ability to access the big money, power, and influence available in D.C.

"We've always had people on our boards who've cared deeply about children," says Diana Goldberg, chair of the foundation board. "I'm a perfect example. I had a child treated at Children's for minor surgery and was so impressed with the medical and nursing care, even though the facility—at the time—was pretty awful and in a pretty bad part of town.

"Many board members originally became involved because they cared deeply about the hospital and about children. They contributed time, expertise, and money (though not necessarily in a major way). The need [for money] wasn't great. Fifteen years ago, we weren't dependent on philanthropy. Today, hospitals—particularly children's hospitals—depend on philanthropy. To be modern and progressive, then, they cannot do it on reimbursement alone," Goldberg emphasizes.

Thomas proposed an idea: As vacancies became available on Children's various boards, positions would be filled in a different way. Not in the "old boy, who do you know who can fill this vacancy?" philosophy historically used by hospital boards. But in more of an executive-search, "who is the best we can get?" model.

"Boards want to be—but often are not—strategic about how they recruit new members," says Thomas. "By and large, recruitment's done at the last minute. It's done with friends of friends and those whom board members know they can get. And it's done by a nominating committee. Generally speaking, nominating committees seek new people who are one notch below them in terms of skill level, capability, interest. The danger is that boards may not always be getting the right people—people whose skills and capabilities align with the immediate and future needs of the organization."

"Different boards have different missions," says Goldberg. "On our hospital board, for example, it's important to have a cross-section [of backgrounds] to reflect different areas of the city and the different ethnicities that make up the fabric of Washington. The purpose of the foundation board is . . . raising money, so you really do have to think about who the movers and shakers are, who has influence in this city, and who can help us raise the money we really need to raise."

Two of those movers and shakers include Frank Saul, a fourth-generation Washingtonian, senior vice-president of BF Saul Company, and vice-chairman of Chevy Chase Bank. And Dan Snyder, the 35-year-old owner of the Washington Redskins football team. Both have radically different governance styles.

Saul, recruited just over a year ago, has a long and generous family history—particularly from his father—of giving to charitable organizations in Washington. He's young, bright, an active participant on the foundation board and the foundation's executive committee, and was recently named to the Children's National Medical Center parent board. One of his major contributions has been financial advice.

"Health care is a complex industry and a complex operation," says Saul. "My particular strength is finance and, logically, the area on which I dial in. Children's is the primary care source for a large percentage of the population in this city, and it's critical that the hospital remain healthy, vibrant."

Like many hospitals, Children's was going through a difficult financial period recently. Saul helped to explore various—and previously unconsidered—financing options and ultimately helped the hospital secure the appropriate lines of credit.

"Frank has been absolutely fabulous in terms of financial advice," says Thomas. "These are very uneven times for hospitals in general and children's hospitals in particular. Having the help, the eye, and the ear of someone like Frank can make all the difference."

But financial advice is not Saul's only attribute.

Saul and his wife, Dawn, recently chaired the hospital's "Jazzmatazz" Leadership Committee, which recruited music enthusiasts in their 30s and 40s to purchase tables for the hospital's annual black-tie jazz gala. Chevy Chase Bank was an event sponsor and hosted the "Chevy Chase Club" featuring some of the country's top jazz musicians. Jazzmatazz raised nearly $1.2 million to benefit Children's—an increase of more than 100 percent over last year.

"Frank is very committed to bringing along the next generation—which is something we really need to think about," says Goldberg.

Dan Snyder, who was recruited by Children's about four years ago, also grew up in Washington—adoring the Redskins. Now, at age 35, his ownership of the team has been a dream come true. But Snyder also loves children, and his contributions as a member of the Children's Foundation Board have been significant—both personally and professionally.

"Connection to kids is very important to both my wife and me," says Snyder, who has two children of his own, ages two and four. "Children's Hospital is one of the most important organizations in this city, and I'm committed to helping raise funds, adding credibility—and hopefully [influencing] other business leaders to join in."

The Snyders have made very generous donations to Children's—contributing funds directly to the renovation and expansion of the hospital's new emergency department, which handles 60,000 patient visits annually. As a trustee, Snyder is an active member of the hospital's leadership gifts committee.

"Dan has been a substantial donor," says Goldberg. "He's opened his owner's box during Redskins games—which is a wonderful way to entertain potential donors. At one point, he gave a whole bunch of Redskin seats to employees of the hospital—a wonderful morale booster."

Snyder has assisted in major fund-raising events and has encouraged Redskin players to give directly to the city's children by visiting them in the hospital, which means a lot to the children, as well as to their parents and siblings.

But—brace yourself—Dan Snyder has never attended a board meeting. And he may never do so in the future either.

"A 35-year-old who owns the Washington Redskins is going to have a very different time availability than a 55-year-old attorney from a major firm in town," says Thomas. "And that's fine. If he's willing to give, participate in the leadership gifts committee, and make seats available in the owner's box during the games, then he's doing his share.

"With this [recruitment model], one size can't fit all. We're asking a lot of board members, and it's imperative on our part to have some flexibility and some gray—instead of just black or white. It's not an 'either-or' [situation]; it's an 'and'," continues Thomas. "Boards need the . . . Dan Snyders. But they also need the long-time contributors of time, energy, commitment. They need the best [of both]."

Obviously, others agree. The Children's National Medical Center board has quickly become a preferred organization to serve in Washington. And with options like the Kennedy Center, the Air and Space Museum, and many others—competition for talented directors is stiff.

So how, exactly, does Thomas's board recruitment model work? In designing his system, Thomas worked with professionals from an executive search firm. The result is an eight-step approach:

1: Put together a board development team. "Assemble those individuals responsible for the key plans of the organization—the champions for the strategic plan, operational plan, and philanthropic plan. Then add a couple of high-energy people who represent the quality, focus, and energy you're hoping to attract to the board—that's your team," says Thomas.

2: Assess your board's needs. "Identify needs as they relate to the strategic, operational, and philanthropic plans of the organization. Example: On the strategic side, you may need people who have the background and capability to develop strategy further. On the operational side, you may need someone savvy at finance. Write those needs down, create a list. From that list, create a board profile of the person [or people] you're looking for," Thomas advises.

3: Create a position profile. "Will the 'recruits' be more strategic? More philanthropic? More operational? Will they be a combination? Do you need two of those, one of another? Create a job description, a profile that ties back to the strategic, operational, and philanthropic plans of the organization—and nothing less," says Thomas.

4: Script the story. "Everyone who's doing the recruitment, who's part of the board development team, must speak the same language, tell the same story—not just the story of the board but the story of the organization—looking at its past, present, and where you want to be in the future," he says.

5: Check out various candidates. Researching where candidates have come from is a crucial next step, Thomas says. "Who are they? What kind of person are you looking for? Executive search professionals do a careful behind-the-scenes analysis not only of what's needed—but who's available, who's the best fit. The board development team must do the same. This research is extremely important. If you think of a typical [board] pyramid, the base usually comprises the friends and colleagues of current board members; the top is scattered with a few research sources. You want to reverse it—place most of your time and emphasis on recruiting the research candidates on the top rather than the friends and colleagues on the bottom. This shifts the entire emphasis from what the board has been to what it needs to be—based on the organization's strategic, operational, and philanthropic plans," Thomas says.

6: Create a third-party referral mechanism. "The third-party referral mechanism most closely parallels the role of 'headhunter' in the executive world. Assess your community. Go to the best people you can possibly find who represent the constituency you need," Thomas says. "An example: An executive search firm calls me and says, 'John, you've been in health care fund-raising for a long time. You represent the constituency. Who do you know who would be a good fit for a job I have?' They're not going to recruit me, necessarily. I'm their third-party referral source.

"You need to identify the key constituencies from whom you may get these board members. Is it business? Clergy? Entrepreneurs? High tech? Retailers? Entertainment? Who do you know, who is at the top of the heap, who represents the best? Access their knowledge and insight. Inadvertently, you may recruit them. But they know, upfront, that's not the intent of your call, so they don't get their defense mechanism up," notes Thomas.

7: Begin to contact and meet candidates. "You're not recruiting yet, just sounding them out, telling them your story, giving them an opportunity to react, to show interest. Then, bring names back to the development team and say, 'Here's the response we got . . . so-and-so seems to be a good fit.' And begin to select the best candidates from that," advises Thomas. Frank Saul is a perfect example.

"The story [of Children's National] and how important it is to this city really came across for me," says Saul. "My family has always tried to support the important institutions in this city, and it's now my turn to carry the torch. But it's important to me to spend volunteer time doing work I know will have an impact."

8: Give it time. Rome wasn't built in a day and neither is the right health care board. "Understand that because board recruitment is so securely tied to the strategic, operational, and philanthropic needs of your organization, it is a long process," says Thomas. "It could easily take two years or more to find the right candidate. Understand, too, that the process is ongoing. None of our boards is completely up to snuff in terms of numbers. And to us, that's a mark of success. We believe it's better to have a vacancy and to be hunting for the right person than to just fill a vacancy. You must replace the sense of urgency with the sense of wanting to do what's best for the long-term interests of the organization."

Be aware that the board recruitment model may lead you to unsuspected places. For example, in Washington, Diana Goldberg says there is growing recognition of a whole new high-tech community in Virginia.

"Traditionally, people in Virginia don't cross over into Washington," says Goldberg. "But northern Virginians are a major factor in the Washington economy. There is an understanding among board members that we really need to get over there, meet these people, bring some of them to the board."

As of *Trustee*'s deadline, after a long and careful courtship, an invitation had been extended to the CEO of a major Virginia company to join Children's Foundation Board. Acceptance appeared imminent. Goldberg was also hopeful that a woman from the same side of the Potomac would soon follow suit.

Putting All the Pieces Together

*The Complete Board Needs
the Right Mix of Competencies*

By Barry S. Bader and Sharon O'Malley

Five years ago, the Sisters of Charity board was all women, all Catholic, and all Kansan, even though the system stretched from Kansas City to Los Angeles. Today, 9 of the 15 board members of the Sisters of Charity of Leavenworth's (SCL's) Health Services Corp. are men, some aren't Catholic, and they hail from California, Texas, Illinois, Pennsylvania, and Colorado, as well as Kansas. Just 3 of the 15 served on the board prior to 1995.

Overall, says Sister Marie Damian Glatt, newly retired as CEO and president of SCL's Health Services Corp., the more diverse board has "a real richness" that it lacked before.

Broadening a board of religious women was a bold, culture-changing step for the sisters. But Glatt says the system, which encompasses hospitals, skilled nursing facilities, and physician

---

Barry S. Bader is a governance consultant based in Potomac, Maryland. Bader has served as a trustee of Suburban Hospital, Bethesda, Maryland. He can be reached at (301) 340-0903. Sharon O'Malley is a freelance writer specializing in health care and organizational issues. She also teaches journalism at the University of Maryland, College Park.

organizations, needed trustees with broader expertise and a more global perspective. "We looked at what was going on in the health care industry and decided that although . . . the board had served us well, we needed added expertise to become more knowledgeable and broader in scope."

To that end, the system identified areas of expertise that could better inform board decisions about strategic direction and performance. Topping the list were depth of knowledge in business, finance, mergers, managed care, information systems, and physician integration. Although prospective trustees had to support Catholic values, they didn't have to be Catholic.

Board candidates could have past governance experience with an SCL affiliate or another Catholic hospital, but they couldn't advocate a single constituency or local ministry's interests ahead of system goals. A prospective parent board member had to be a "system thinker" who could see how the actions of one institution would affect others. To further guard against representational governance, no corporate trustees could serve simultaneously on an affiliate's board.

Using explicit, competency-based criteria to move from a constituency-based board to one with a more diverse geographic and knowledge base, says Glatt, has taken conversations at the bimonthly board meetings to "a global level." It's yielded such positive results, she says, that the system is using competencies to determine how to add nontrustees to committees and is further recommending that affiliate boards use a similar approach to diversify and enhance their composition as well.

Choosing skilled trustees is hardly an original concept, but seeking out candidates who bring specific, strategically relevant qualifications is a departure from traditional recruitment methods. Several factors are motivating this selection method:

- Systems and hospitals are moving away from constituency-based boards in favor of trustees with the objectivity, commitment, and expertise to make decisions in the best interests of the entire system, its mission, and all its communities and stakeholders.
- Mergers and governance restructuring typically necessitate unseating some trustees. Competency-based criteria help nominating committees execute this sensitive task objectively.

- Heightened risks, competition, new technology, and the need to oversee new lines of business require trustees with strong business and finance skills and the ability to understand complex enterprises.

A decline in the average size of boards leaves no room for passive or nonproductive members. Large boards can afford a few members who contribute little beyond an influential name. Smaller boards need every seat taken by an active member who brings knowledge, skills, and perspective.

Changing how board members are named starts with recognizing that looking for new trustees in the same old places in the same old ways won't necessarily produce the desired results. Systems and hospitals are applying a number of practices to foster competency-driven selection:

Make It Policy

A system's governance principles, board policy, or both call for recruitment based on a prospective trustee's personal characteristics, knowledge, skills, and perspective. Trustees are re-elected only if they have actively participated and contribute a competency that's still strategically important.

For example, the board manual of Catholic Healthcare Partners, based in Cincinnati, calls for a four-step selection process:

1. Determine needs based on the system's strategic direction.
2. Actively recruit by identifying individuals who meet current and future needs.
3. Communicate the system's mission and expectations to prospective trustees in the recruitment process.
4. Carefully assess trustees eligible to serve another term.

Adopt Term Limits

A maximum limit such as no more than three or four three-year terms necessitates an ongoing recruitment process. Consequently, term limits help the board keep up with change. They encourage a board to ask how community changes, such as ethnic diversity, social problems, and new attitudes toward the consumer's role in health, should affect the makeup and skills of the board.

Choose the Nominating Committee Carefully

Often, nominating committees are small, comprising only the most senior members. Understanding institutional history is important to give context and consistency—until it reaches the point where it fosters inbreeding of ideas and excessive comfort with current strategies. Will such members be able to analyze the board's future needs objectively? Will they encourage recruitment of qualified individuals from business and professional circles different from their own? Will they choose skills over constituencies?

Nominating committees play a pivotal role when systems merge, downsize the board, or move away from constituency-based composition. How well they do their job affects how well change is accepted by other trustees and key stakeholders. For example, Boston-based CareGroup recently decided to pare its 29-member system board, which included representatives of its hospitals, to 16 trustees, none of whom would simultaneously sit on a member's hospital board. The goal was to have a more objective board to make tough decisions about system capacity and resources.

However, to demonstrate sensitivity to its diverse stakeholders as it reconstituted, CareGroup appointed a dozen members from its hospital boards to its nominating committee, which identified core competencies and recruited appropriate candidates. The result, notes CareGroup Chief of Staff Julie Foiles, is a nominating committee that "actively thinks in terms of the community at large—all of the communities served by Care Group—keeping an eye out for individuals whom we want to recruit to our board and making that a year-round activity."

Boards should include the CEO as an ex officio member of the nominating committee. The CEO typically is active in the community and a good resource for potential candidates. He or she brings insight into competencies that could inform the board's strategic work. And having the chief executive on the committee can flag potential personality conflicts that a CEO might have with a candidate. Could a CEO dominate the process, packing the board with loyalists and buddies? Sure, but most wouldn't, and the CEO's presence is balanced by an active committee.

Explicitly Identify Needed Competencies

Competencies may refer to the personal characteristics of trustees or to the knowledge, skills, and perspectives they bring. Areas of knowledge include finance, strategic and financial planning, community needs, medical and information technology, and real estate. Relevant personal characteristics might include listening, consensus building, communication, leadership, and the ability to think "outside the box."

It can be helpful to organize competencies into three categories (see Selection Guidelines, page 23):

1. **Universal competencies:** personal characteristics all members should possess, such as commitment to the mission, integrity, and the ability to make objective decisions.
2. **Collective competencies:** qualifications at least some trustees should have, such as financial and business acumen and executive-level business experience.
3. **Desirable competencies:** needs the board hopes to fill, such as greater gender and ethnic diversity, or expertise in such emerging fields as information technology and consumerism.

Use the Criteria to Assess the Board's Needs

Based on the competencies, the nominating committee assesses the present board against its ideal criteria and identifies gaps—i.e., recruiting needs—to be met as terms expire. The committee also engages in succession planning for the board chair and other leaders, ensuring future leaders are in the pipeline.

On some boards the nominating process is a black box. Trustees first hear whom the committee has chosen when the slate is presented for approval. Instead, the nominating committee should recommend its draft competencies to the board for discussion, modification, and approval. Reaching consensus on board competencies and recruiting

Selection Guidelines for the ABC Health System Board

Universal Competencies	Collective Competencies	Desirable Competencies
(Required of all trustees)	*(Should be present in the board as a whole and, therefore, be strong attributes of at least one member)*	*(Characteristics that would currently be an asset to the board, given ABC's strategic priorities)*
1. A demonstrated commitment to ABC's mission and vision and to the communities we serve	1. Knowledge about the communities served by ABC	1. Experience in marketing and public and community relations
2. A demonstrated willingness to devote the time necessary to governance, including education	2. High-level executive experience in a business	2. Experience in human resources
3. A demonstrated ability to exercise leadership, teamwork/consensus building, systems thinking, and sound judgment on difficult and complex matters	3. Financial background and expertise	3. Experience in government and public affairs
4. Personal integrity and objectivity, including no conflicts of interest that would prevent a trustee from carrying out his or her responsibilities	4. Experience in medicine and health care	4. Experience in educational leadership with a school system, college, or university
		5. Experience in information and/or medical technology
		6. Diversity of experience, ages, gender, and ethnic origin

needs turns every trustee into a recruiter and widens the search for candidates.

Cast a Wide Net

Consider candidates from nontraditional business and community circles who bring a needed competency. For hospitals and systems operating in a single market, that could mean considering potential trustees from outside the local area. For systems that traditionally choose trustees from within their ranks, as many Catholic systems have, that means recruiting outsiders with no history or allegiance to any part of the system.

Outside directors can inject fresh, objective perspectives into board work, as well as bring a hard-to-find, needed competency. For example, Clarian Health in Indianapolis went to Washington, D.C., to seek the former CEO of a major teaching hospital for its board. In one move, Clarian added executive experience in academic health centers, an individual of national stature, and racial diversity to boot.

Vet and Interview Candidates

The board would never hire an executive without a background check and interview, yet that often happens with new trustees. Many new trustees are elected based on reputation alone. Was the candidate a productive member of the other boards on his or her résumé? How was the prospect's relationship with the CEO? A well-placed call or two can quickly confirm a candidate's abilities or raise questions to consider.

In addition, many committees interview prospective candidates to be sure they understand the responsibilities and expectations of the office. "It's very difficult for a person to come onto a board and then learn of responsibilities and expectations that they didn't know about," notes Glatt.

In effect, the interview is the starting point for new trustee orientation. Catholic Healthcare Partners gives prospects information about the system's mission and board member responsibilities, including the amount of work and time expected. Nominees provide the system with a résumé, a conflict-of-interest statement, and a statement of commitment.

Gino Pazzaglini, CEO of Good Samaritan Hospital in Pottsville, Pennsylvania, a part of Ascension Health, assesses a prospective trustee's fit with the board by asking four probing questions: What are your personal values and do you see them as being compatible or in conflict with Catholic values? Are you comfortable serving on a board within a larger system, so your board has important powers but not ultimate authority? Can you represent the vision of this hospital and its role in improving community health? Can you constructively challenge management?

Stick to the Principles

When it comes time to recommend and approve the slate, the nominating committee and board, respectively, should resist the temptation to slip into familiar ways. At the 11th hour, someone will undoubtedly suggest a "great person" who hasn't been through the competency test and vetting process. The committee and the board need to stand firm. Keep the individual in the pipeline, but don't subvert competency-driven selection principles.

Assess Members Eligible for Reelection

Reappointment should never be automatic. Three possible three-year terms is not a nine-year guarantee.

The nominating committee should assess a member whose term is expiring against the board competencies. Did the trustee meet expectations for attendance and active participation? Did any issues of board conduct arise, such as breaches of confidentiality? Does a new job present a conflict of interest?

The committee also should determine whether the member contributes a competency that's still relevant to the system's or hospital's needs. One board recruited a member with strong construction management experience as it began a building program. Six years and two terms later, the project was completed and the trustee was minimally involved with the board. The committee informed him he wouldn't be reappointed because of the need to add other critical competencies to the board. The board honored him, and he left with pride. Bidding adieu to board members early won't be common, but the process of routinely reassessing performance and competencies at reappointment time reinforces the board's culture of accountability.

Reinforce Competencies through Self-Assessment

Some boards ask members to rate their own participation. At Holy Redeemer Health System in Huntingdon Valley, Pennsylvania, for instance, board members assess their own performance against written expectations. Areas needing improvement then receive the most attention. CEO Michael B. Laign says the tool reinforces performance standards.

On some boards, members complete assessments of other trustees' performance. Results are shared with the nominating committee or board chair and may be evaluated during reappointment consideration.

The knowledge-based organization of the future will rely more than ever on highly competent staff who continuously learn and expand their skills and wisdom. The governing board has the ultimate accountability and can set no less a standard for itself than it expects of management. Competency-driven selection and a commitment to board member education make the board a model for the entire organization.

Making the Whole Greater Than the Sum of the Parts

*Board Diversity Can Strengthen
Your Organization*

By Laurie Larson

In the 1999 U.S. Census, 16 percent of hospital employees reported themselves as African-American, 6 percent as Hispanic, 3 percent as Asian or Native American, and the rest as white. Hospital leadership, however—CEOs, COOs, and senior vice presidents—is still 92 percent white, according to the latest figures from the Chicago-based American College of Healthcare Executives (ACHE). In a nation with an increasingly diverse population and workforce, hospitals that expect to truly serve and represent their communities need to change those numbers—and health care boards need to lead the way.

"If we don't [work on diversity], we will lose people in the field," says Rupert Evans, president of the American Hospital Association's Institute for Diversity in Health Management (IFD). "There will be more community protest about representation, and disparities will continue."

Toward that goal, IFD began a partnership in 1994 with the ACHE and the National Association of Health Services Executives,

---

Laurie Larson is *Trustee*'s staff writer.

adding the Association of Hispanic Healthcare Executives in 1995 and the Catholic Health Association last year. Starting with a summer enrichment program for college students interested in health management careers, IFD has since added a career development track to help midlevel managers advance to executive positions, as well as a change and diversity management educational arm to help health care organizations build diversity programs. As an example of the institute's perceived value, HCA recently provided all its member hospitals with IFD institutional memberships.

"[Health care diversity] starts with governance," Evans says. "Because of rapid demographic [community] changes, if [health care organizations] are going to serve those communities, they need to bring diverse individuals to the table. It's a value change in the organization and it has to start at the top."

"Most organizations are driven by cost, but diversity transcends cost issues," says diversity expert William Guillory, president and CEO of Innovations International, Salt Lake City. "Other pressures are pushing diversity—dissatisfaction is one." The classic scenario, he says, involves an experienced employee who loses a promotion to someone he or she trained. Race, age, gender, corporate culture, or all of the above are often the reason. Cultural competence is driving diversity too, Guillory says, as physicians and other caregivers find themselves unable to speak the language or understand the culture of their patients.

"The number of people in these situations is increasing dramatically as U.S. culture itself is becoming more diverse," Guillory says. A great influx of immigrants nationwide, including a wide range of Asian and Eastern European arrivals, have sometimes "instantly" required health care systems in such far-flung areas as Great Bend, Kansas, or Reading, Pennsylvania, to become more culturally sensitive. "No one can represent another person's cultural experience," Guillory says. But hospital boards should represent their local culture as much as possible, experts agree.

"I do believe that hospitals will become increasingly concerned with diversity in their boards," says Patricia Moten Marshall, president of SynerChange Chicago, a health care management consulting firm. "There is a greater awareness of the business case for diversity, an appreciation that if you are committed to diversity, to representing your community, then you can't ignore the board of directors in reaching out on this issue."

What Are We Here For?

Trustees should begin by remembering the organization's core mission and examining how diversity figures in, Evans recommends. For example, if a core value is to increase market share in a Spanish-speaking community, more Spanish-speaking staff should be brought into the institution.

"The business case for diversity needs to be tailored for each hospital," Evans adds. "You can't skip steps. You need to ask, 'What do we look like right now? What are our values? Do we have diversity and inclusion in the organization? Do we value it?' You have to build a case first. And it doesn't happen overnight; it's a journey."

Marshall thinks diversity education comes first—and many trustees may bring insight from changes in their own corporate culture. Trustees should also clearly understand the difference between a "token gesture" of bringing a minority trustee onto the board because "it will look good" and really seeking candidates who can contribute. "If you're going into it as a token gesture, it will not be successful," she warns. To avoid this pitfall, trustees should establish a diversity goal for themselves, just as they would any other strategic planning objective, deciding over three years, for example, how to expand community representation.

Catholic Health Initiatives (CHI) has taken exactly such a methodical approach. Based in Denver, CHI is a five-year-old system comprising 64 acute care and 45 long-term care facilities across 20 states, with a system board of 14 plus the CEO. Half the trustees are from health system congregations and half are nonreligious, or lay, trustees. Nine are men, 6 are women, 13 are white, one is African-American, and one is Native American. Below this board are 40 boards organized by geographic area and called market-based organizations, or MBOs. CHI has four national senior leaders who are members of minorities, including their system chief operating officer, Kevin Lofton, who is African-American. Two years ago, CHI did a survey among all its MBOs to assess their composition, using the most diverse boards as models for the others.

"The net result was we've got a long way to go," Lofton says. "We need more nonreligious women [i.e., nonsisters], more Hispanic, and more African-American board members. But you cannot have one standard for diversity either. It depends on the community . . . you can't talk about diversity in a vanilla manner." Now the system is planning to resurvey its MBOs again to see how far they've come.

"We are committed to diversity both nationally and locally, both on the board and for executive leadership," says Sister Esther Anderson, chair of CHI's sponsorship and governance committee. She says CHI has created a board profile for new trustees, looking at what ethnic and professional backgrounds the system lacks.

Anderson says age, race, religious belief, location, occupation and professional expertise are all part of the profile. The same checklist applies at the MBO level, keeping in mind race and interfaith differences nationwide. "I really believe that to follow our mission, it doesn't take just one type of person. You need the richness of experience that [diversity] brings," she adds.

Expanding the Search

To achieve diversity, Marshall further suggests that boards may need to reexamine candidate requirements. "If you look at the selection and nomination criteria—it may be a challenge to keep [your] current criteria and [still attract diverse board members]," Marshall says. "We tend to look at senior officers in for-profit corporate America for board [members]. There is more potential for diversity in not-for-profit organizations and among professionals that own their own businesses, as well as among physicians and nurses. [You must] get away from thinking that [trustees] have to have certain incomes or be part of Fortune 500 companies." Marshall says boards often set out to "try to find an African-American or Hispanic CEO, and when they can't find one, they say, 'We tried, it didn't work,' and give up."

"The mistake a lot of not-for-profit boards make is that they put too much emphasis on notoriety among ethnic trustee candidates," says James Lowry, trustee emeritus of Chicago's Northwestern Memorial Hospital's (NMH) system board and head of worldwide diversity practices for Boston Consulting Group. "There are a lot of hardworking people out there who don't get noticed." He therefore suggests looking beyond the obvious titles and places to find trustees.

For example, if a minority professional is a manager in an important firm, even if not at the top of the executive ladder, chances are he or she has had to work at least as hard or harder to achieve goals—and might make an excellent trustee. "Look for powerful women and people of color one level or two below the top and go there to recruit," Lowry suggests. "Look just beyond the spotlight—the criteria will still apply. It's leadership's job to break out beyond the obvious candidates."

CHI looks to formal civic organizations, such as a city's urban league or minority leadership organizations, to help identify diverse trustee candidates. "It's just like any other goal," Lofton says. "If you make it a high priority, if you set your mind to something, it will get done." Lofton adds that CHI soon plans to announce a fellowship program targeted at minorities who want to move into health care leadership positions.

Comparatively, diversity figures more prominently at the local, or MBO, level, Anderson says, and local Healthy Community projects have yielded some good board members in this way. "You can't find a model of the most effective board—you create it as you go," she says. "It's not only the right thing to do; it's the smart thing to do."

"Boards should ask themselves why they want to diversify," Guillory suggests. "They need to define the key stakeholders in the community, as well as their own purpose." Each trustee should list three people who might be possible candidates to diversify the board, thinking broadly, because "boards tend to perpetuate the composition that already exists," Guillory says. A working committee for diversity should take those names, and at the same time also contacting local and national minority civic and religious leaders, to get more suggestions and "reach further with their criteria. . . . You start to learn how to describe what you want and therefore define your process," Guillory says.

Next, the working committee should get the informal background and résumés, if possible, of potential trustees. All community leaders who've been consulted should submit the names of three candidates and rank their choices. Among these options, the working committee should then determine its first choice. If that candidate declines,

Guillory suggests that the candidate be asked for a replacement suggestion. The working committee may then either check out that suggestion or interview the second choice from its original candidate list. In any case, each recommendation can be used to yield others, thereby expanding trustee choices—what Guillory calls "the multiplier effect."

Diversity Is as Diversity Does

Marshall says that often boards assume once they bring on new trustees, their job is done. "Some boards get into trouble at this point because they haven't prepared themselves for diversity," she says. "They bring trustees onto a board that hasn't or won't change the way it's been working, and therefore the new trustee quits or never speaks up."

If a board really wants the insights someone different may bring, minority candidates must be active and the board must make it possible for them to participate. This boils down to adequate orientation—that is, providing enough education so that new trustees aren't just expected to catch up as they sit through meetings, as well as a frank board self-evaluation to see if current trustees are really ready to listen to different perspectives.

"Boards need to ask, 'How do we talk to each other?'" Marshall says. Her implication is that dry reports and rubber-stamping are no way to run a diverse board—or any board. "It goes back to the structure of the board: Is it open? And does it do strategic work versus staff work?"

Trustees need to take a hard look at their corporate culture to see if it is truly inclusive, Guillory says.

"Diversity tries to break down homogeneity, to have people talk to each other. There are informal conversations that [minority or otherwise excluded employees] just don't hear about." This "cultural exclusion," or internal networking, Guillory says, can be seen as soon as a new employee walks into a job. "You see what the leadership looks like, and . . . who has the inside track," he says. Most jobs are filled before they are ever posted because of who is in or out of the loop. "You can't legislate the way people think—you have to change the belief system first. Cultural inclusion is a dramatic process," he says.

Diversity Resources

Books

- *The Business of Diversity,* by William Guillory, 2000, Innovations Publishing.

- *Building a House for Diversity,* by R. Roosevelt Thomas Jr., 1999, R. Thomas & Associates Inc.

- *Breaking Through: The Making of Minority Executives in Corporate America,* by David A. Thomas and John J. Gabarro, 1999, Harvard Business School Press.

- *Diversity Leadership,* by Janice L. Dreachslin, from the American College of Healthcare Executives, 1996, Health Administration Press.

- *Caring for Patients from Different Cultures: Case Studies from American Hospitals* (2d edition), by Geri-Ann Galanti, 1997, University of Pennsylvania Press.

- *Cultural Competency in Health Care: A Guide for Trainers* (2d edition) by Rohini Anand, 1999, NMCI Publications (National MultiCultural Institute).

- *Pocket Guide to Cultural Assessment,* by Elaine Marie Geissler, 1998, Mosby (a Times/Mirror company).

- *Multicultural Marketing: Selling to a Diverse America,* by Marlene Rossman, 1996, AMACOM.

- "The Lack of Diversity at the Top," by David O. Weber, (magazine article) in *Health Forum Journal,* Sept/Oct 2000.

Web Sites

- Institute for Diversity in Health Management: www.institutefordiversity.org

- American College of Healthcare Executives: www.ache.org

- Diversity Connection organization, a job posting/listing/ mentoring site: www.diversityconnection.org

- A daily diversity newsletter, including a career center and links to other diversity organizations: diversityinc.com

- Cultural competency: http://cecp.air.org/cultural/resources.htm

- Overview of multicultural best practices: www.diversityrx.org/BEST/index.html

- Rationale for cultural competence in primary health care: http:/gucdc.georgetown.edu/nccc/nccc6.html

Once trustee nominees agree to serve on the board, they should be asked what they expect of the board in return and what they want from the experience. Guillory recalls asking that question himself as a new trustee. He made it clear that he wanted to be given the chance to speak and be heard. Nominees therefore need to be strong individuals who will take a stand, particularly if they are the first member of a minority to serve on the board, he says. "Ask yourself who the most powerful person of your [nominee] options is," Guillory says. "Will he or she stand up and demand respect? Whom the board chooses reflects how serious it is about diversity and how open a discussion it really wants to have."

NMH'S Lowry admits that serving on a big corporate board like Northwestern's can be "intimidating" and requires candidates who "are problem solvers and who can pick up the phone," meaning that they are well connected to other people of influence. What might unite well-known and lesser-known trustee candidates, however, is the ability to solve problems, something he believes does not require wealth or corporate power.

A Comprehensive Approach

His system has long been committed to diversity, Lowry says, as best evidenced by its nine-year-old active office of diversity. NMH participates in a variety of national and local internship programs, including, but not limited to, IFD's Summer Enrichment program for minority college students interested in health care administration, as well as a postgraduate fellowship program designed to groom future health care leaders. One former fellow is now an NMH vice president and two others are directors.

NMH has a 13-member parent or strategic board, a 14-member hospital board, and a 60-member foundation board. There are 3 women and one African-American on the system board, one woman and one African-American on the hospital board, and 13 women, 2 African-Americans, and one Hispanic on the foundation board.

For the past year, Sonya Boone, M.D., has directed the NMH diversity office. Diversity recruitment is an active concern, and Dr. Boone's office takes several avenues to find candidates, from job fairs at the black and Hispanic MBA associations to medical and nursing journals with a "diverse flavor," as she describes it, tracking their mailing lists. NMH also has a recruitment program for under-represented physicians, and Boone conducts diversity awareness training at employee orientation.

"Northwestern's mission is to provide the best patient experience and attract, recruit, and retain the best people," Dr. Boone emphasizes. "It is important for an organization to have someone who can devote full time to diversity efforts because it is a business imperative." She takes pride that NMH has specifically incorporated diversity into its mission and its strategic plan.

"Studies show that minority patients prefer minority doctors, a similar cultural background. And when a health care system has a reputation for not welcoming minority physicians, it reverberates in the community . . . a minority recruitment leader will know better where to look for candidates . . . and minority leaders show by example that [the culture is] changing, validating the perception that change is on the horizon."

Dr. Boone is in constant touch with the system's CEO about her office's work, discussing how to bring diverse corporate leaders' points of view to the board. "Having a commitment to diversity at the highest level of the organization keeps it ever-present as new executives are recruited," Dr. Boone says.

Evans talks about "pushback," or resistance to change, coming from leadership or staff who want to protect the status quo. This happens when diversity is presented too abruptly, and those opposed may think some diversity quota will cost them their job—and this most often means physicians.

"Cultural change can run up against stubbornness . . . and boards need to take a stand against it," Guillory says. Board chairs need to sit down with staff leaders and explain clearly the board's diversity goals, he suggests. Those leaders in turn can meet one-on-one with resistant staff and calm their fears.

To start off on the right foot, Dr. Boone advises "something so simple as a welcoming reception," which her department does for all new minority interns and fellows. She invites all hospital leaders as well as all minority faculty, and it creates "an immediate networking opportunity—a more inviting culture."

In examining her own career, Dr. Boone knows firsthand that opportunities must be seized—and made. "Medicine is a field where knowledge can be king," she says. During medical school, she prepared exhaustively so that she could answer tough questions on student rounds, and she says that as an African-American woman, there was no question she had to work harder than her nonminority classmates to overcome stereotypic barriers. With a specialty in internal medicine and an emphasis in women's health, Dr. Boone says she has always had an interest in medical administration and policy and how to improve the physician-executive leadership relationship. For this reason, she came back to NMH to start its minority physician recruitment program. The office of diversity grew from that—and it's paying off for all.

"When boards are truly integrated, there is more compelling change in the hospital community," Guillory says. "Diversity airs all those things kept under lock before. . . . It's not a conscious cover-up, but once [everyone] is aware of diversity, receptivity comes in."

"Diversity creates a better understanding of core issues," Evans says. "The rate at which change occurs depends on leadership and management. The most important person [to have behind diversity] is the hospital administrator. If he or she is behind it, it will be an incredible program."

"It's part of being a leader in the health care industry to address diversity," Dr. Boone says. "Diversity is definitely part of being on the cutting edge. A culturally competent organization is a 21st-century organization."

Finding the Perfect Fit

*Is Your Board Chair
the Right Person
in the Right Place?*

By Karen Sandrick

Bruce Stickler learned in a hurry how it feels to be a board chair in the line of fire. In his first month as chair back in 1999, the Illinois Department of Public Health (IDPH) threatened to close the 80-plus-year-old Mount Sinai Medical Center in Chicago because of its antiquated sprinkler system. Stickler, a local attorney, mobilized into action. He met with members of IDPH, the governor's office, state legislators, and lobbyists, and worked with the hospital CEO and the governor to secure $8 million in capital financing from the state to make the needed improvements.

"It can be quite overwhelming," Stickler says understatedly, "when you don't know if you're going to be able to keep your organization open." Of course, most board chairs don't assume the gavel under such tumultuous conditions. All do, however, face extremely complex issues, and have especially in the last couple of decades.

Board consultant Michael Annison, president of The Westrend Group, Denver, acknowledges that it was hard for board chairs not to do well when health care was purely a cost-reimbursed business.

Karen Sandrick is a health care writer based in Chicago.

"If I send you a bill and everything is marked up 10 percent, and you [don't have to think twice about] paying it, the job of the board chair is pretty straightforward in terms of overseeing the organization," he says.

But expectations for boards and their chairs have changed dramatically. "Now it takes a far wider range of skills to deal with the changes in medical technology, financing, public policy, collaborative arrangements, and community services," Annison says. These days, he says, board chairmanship "is not a training-wheels job."

Stickler agrees. "Board chairs have to be much more active today in every arena, including policy. They can't leave the work to staff; they have to provide direction and leadership, and [be] involved; they must stand up and speak out for, and on behalf of, their organizations."

A Profile

Board chairs must possess a unique blend of characteristics, advises Dan Vitale, chair of Community Medical Center, Toms River, New Jersey. Chairs must be involved in their community and committed to health care; they must be able to cooperate, show compassion, support the organization's strategic plan, and work with lay and physician board members as well as senior management. "A board chair needs to be an effective communicator and consensus builder who encourages open dialogue and participation among board members, respects other people's opinions, and has an open ear for listening to their concerns," Vitale says.

Chairs must also have respect for their colleagues, a clear sense about the values that motivate their behavior and the organization, curiosity, a willingness to learn, and integrity. "They are not too tightly connected with management, keep issues open to discussion, are intellectually honest, and ask for help through personal education or outside resources when they don't have good answers," Annison says.

Very large shoes to fill, indeed. So what if a board can't find someone with the right shoe size? What if it tries to place a 9 AA into 11 EEEs? How bad can it be?

Without a knowledgeable and skillful board chair, upstart or splinter groups may vie for board control, particularly when there is a shift in strategic focus or an issue that is dividing board members. Without a steady hand on the board tiller, "boards can develop a sense of hubris and begin to think there is nothing quite like them; they can become narrow-minded, unwilling to see others' points of view, and substitute the part for the whole," Annison adds. Then, at best, disciplined two- to-three-hour board meetings turn into free-for-alls, says Carl Thieme, president of Cambridge (Massachusetts) Research Institute. At worst, a full-blown board coup erupts.

And when boards disintegrate, they can take their organizations with them. The most dramatic cases involve mismanagement, corruption, and bankruptcy. More common are lost opportunities and lack of control. Annison knows of one board and its chair that became so obsessed with management's fixation on debt income that it lost sight of the fact that the hospital was losing market share and thus missed chance after chance to prevent the organization from growing financially weaker.

Another board failed to insist on rejuvenating the medical staff and, as a result, was held hostage by one of its physicians. "The hospital was run by one hospital-based doctor who chose which contracts he would and wouldn't sign," Annison explains. "Since neither the CEO nor the board would deal with him, I told them all to go home. [I said] 'Why waste your time? Just turn over the place to the guy who's running it anyway.'"

What causes board and board chair failures? Simple, says Annison; it's poor choice in leaders—the breakdown comes because of personal foibles or failures. In other words, a board selects a flawed individual in the first place, or it chooses someone who doesn't understand what governance means and how to exercise it.

What Does the Job Entail?

The selection of a board chair comes down to finding someone who understands the job, which, Annison stresses, is not operational. Because board members typically are community leaders who have been successful in the private sector, they may believe the chair of a community organization such as a hospital is the same as that of a corporation. Although chairs of boards in the private sector tend to be extensions of the executive offices, board chairs in the voluntary sector are not. "Chairs of hospital boards need to be clear that they are not the chief executives of the organization; they are responsible for governance," Annison notes.

Chairs, therefore, must be familiar with, and willing to ensure that their boards follow, the basic rules of governance and meet expectations for fulfilling their duties. "The board chair must distinguish between the issues that matter and the fads of the moment," says Annison. The most fundamental issue for hospital boards is monitoring how their organization treats patients, which includes not only the practice of medicine but patient satisfaction. Next is service to the community, which takes many forms, including health screenings, education, and programs for the underserved.

The financial health of the organization is, of course, a core board chair focus, but it is not an end in itself. "If there's a mistake in health care, it's becoming too preoccupied with money," Annison says. He explains that a hospital's net income is nothing more than a reflection of the organization's ability to select services that meet the needs of the community, maintain a streamlined organizational structure, and foster good working relationships between staff and physicians. "If an organization is providing services that people in the community don't think matter or won't use, if it has become inordinately complex, or if its employees don't help each other, its income will go down," Annison explains.

Thieme recommends that boards prepare a job description that clearly defines the roles and responsibilities of the chair. One potentially overlooked duty is remembering the link between the hospital and its ownership, the community. Boards need to be sure their chairs are aware of the concerns of all segments of the population. "Boards need to have input through surveys and focus group about where their communities and key constituencies are coming from. We can't assume anymore that because [board chairs] are members of an ethnic group or a strata of society that they speak for those groups," he says.

Another major board chair responsibility is to decide who will be assigned to individual board committees, who will become committee chairs, and what the committees' charge will be. "Good board chairs will demand a work plan from their committees that identifies the issues they will tackle and that presents their agenda for the year," says Thieme.

Particularly important is creating boundaries between the board, its chair, and the CEO. "Who makes what decisions? What does the board reserve for itself? What does the board want to know before the CEO makes a decision? This whole area of policy development is where boards most often get into trouble," Thieme says.

Finding the Right Person

How do boards choose the right leader? The most common method is through advancement, a process that follows members of the board as they serve on committees, chair key committees, such as finance and nominations, assume the role of vice chair, and eventually rise to the chair position. "It's not an out-of-the-blue kind of thing, but an organized method of board chair selection, the theory being that if board members are exposed to enough different pieces of board operation, they eventually will be good board chairs," Thieme says.

The process of advancement through the board acquaints future chairs with both the fundamentals and subtleties of health care and hospital operation. "You [frequently] hear comments from board members [who say] that it takes two to three years to even start to understand what the health care business is all about," Thieme says.

This process also introduces board members to hospital leaders and serves as an on-the-job test. "You don't go to find a board chair who is unknown to everyone. You want someone who's been in training for a while so the board, medical staff, and administration have some idea of who this person is and how he or she responds in meetings and under stress and how this person works with colleagues," says Brian Rines, former chair of Maine General Medical Center-Augusta Campus.

At the Right Time

Board chairs with specific skills may be needed at different times in an organization's life, believes Rines, who became chair as a result of a hospital merger. "If you've just come through a merger, to some degree you need a chair who's able to say, 'We're a new institution; we have to forget the past and move on.' You need a chair who will create a new mission statement that will become the script for what the organization will become and how the board will direct that focus," he says.

When a hospital is stable, the board chair should accurately reflect the needs of the board to the CEO, balance the feelings of the board against the CEO's plans, and preserve its strengths. "Continuing stability in this field really means avoiding being whacked by the next tidal wave," Rines says.

A hospital on the brink of massive change in order to survive needs a board chair who can reassure its community that values will be preserved as the organization downsizes or restructures. It also needs a chair who can prepare the community for the inevitable— "the idea that the hospital isn't going to be doing things much more elaborate than tonsillectomies or appendectomies and setting bones and that people will have to drive six miles for more sophisticated work," Rines observes. The message is a difficult one to deliver, but, says Rines, "it's far better for the board chair and board to prepare the community than for people to wake up some morning and read in the local newspaper that the hospital is out of money and nobody is going to be there a month from Thursday."

With the Right Qualifications

In ideal circumstances, a board will have a nominating committee or a committee on governance to recommend the next chair. Many nominating committees are composed only of board members, but some include the hospital chief of staff as a voting member and the CEO in an ex officio capacity. Committees also apply a series of criteria to their selection of a chair. Regular board meeting attendance is a basic one. After all, says Joanne Meehan, former chair of Memorial Hospital in South Bend, Indiana, "someone who doesn't attend board meetings regularly is not able to get a feeling for the hospital."

Then there's the person's savvy in running meetings. "One of the challenges of a board leader is to make sure meetings are packed with substance, not simply with reports," says Mount Sinai's Stickler. "You also want lively board meetings, where people can freely express their opinions, ask questions, and explore ideas. When you bring together businesspeople, physicians, and members of the community, not everyone's perspective will be the same. And that's good;

you want diversity. But it takes a lot of energy and focus to keep the meeting active, aggressively seek the counsel of various board members, and still finish on time," he adds.

The nominating committee also considers experience and background. Meehan had chaired several not-for-profit groups in the community and served on a local bank's board before joining Memorial Hospital. As a lawyer, Stickler brought expertise on legal, audit, and financing issues.

Finally, there's the ability to meet the time commitment. "If the world is running calmly and sensibly, the board chair will have spurts of activity around the planning and budgeting cycle and community celebrations—dinners or rituals—as well as routine monthly board activities, board meetings, and subcommittee meetings. My guess is this takes up 15 to 20 percent of the board chair's time. When things are noisy, difficult, or unpleasant, it's obviously more," says Annison.

For the Right Length of Time

Although some boards allow chairs to serve as long as 25 years, others impose term limits, which vary anywhere from two years to a maximum of three three-year terms. It's probably a good idea to have board leadership change on some reasonably regular basis to provide a fresh perspective and avoid the dangers of long-term board leadership: "The board tends to become narrowly focused rather than more broadly oriented, so ideas that are different are more easily rejected, and there tends to be a habit of thought that makes it harder to hold people accountable," Annison says.

Because many boards have such short terms of office for their chairs, they tend to forgo their formal performance evaluation and opt instead for self-evaluation through interviews or focus groups that assess how well they are achieving agreed-on goals and outcomes. On the other hand, long-term board chairs can become too chummy with the CEO or start acting like the CEO, Thieme says.

The ultimate test of a board chair is how well he or she maintains balance between the board, the administration, and the medical staff. Rines likens it to having a sturdy three-legged milking stool. "If one leg is too short or too long or wobbly, the other two have a hard time holding the weight. Board chairs have as much strength and ability to support the concerns of the community as the physicians who are responsible for delivery of care and the CEO who must ensure that the medical staff can practice its craft effectively. But if the board chair exerts an overly strong influence or allows himself or herself to be bullied by the medical staff or the CEO's plan and doesn't reflect the community's needs or desires, then the stool will be unstable and the institution will suffer," Rines says.

PART TWO

The Governance Process
and Trustee Education

Successful Board Retreats: What Works and Why

By Mary K. Totten
and James E. Orlikoff

*"Regular retreats are a crucial element of infrastructure
that help boards grow, change, and become
more effective. There is, however, a big difference
between simply conducting a board retreat
and designing a successful one."*
—Dennis D. Pointer and James E. Orlikoff,
Board Work

Board and leadership retreats give trustees an opportunity to look at governance from a different perspective. Retreats can be used to update trustees on issues and trends, to engage the board in planning organizational strategy, or to conduct a focused discussion on a specific issue, such as merger, partnership, or a significant capital investment. Whatever the goal, boards need the opportunity to move beyond the constraints of the meeting agenda and participate in activities that will help them grow and develop in their role.

Mary K. Totten is president of Totten & Associates, Oak Park, Illinois.
James E. Orlikoff is president of Orlikoff & Associates, Inc., Chicago.

Conducting retreats that allow trustees to learn, tackle issues in depth, and get to know each other and organizational leaders socially is becoming particularly important as organizations need more time and commitment from their board members. In addition, some of the board's traditional face-to-face interaction is being replaced with electronic communication, which can greatly improve efficiency but lacks the personal context of live discussion and deliberation.

What characteristics make a successful retreat? Consider the following very different scenarios.

Case Studies

Mount Pleasant Hospital

The board of Mount Pleasant Hospital had recently decided to increase its size from 9 to 13 members and to use new selection criteria to attract younger members with specific expertise. The board was particularly pleased with the results of its recruitment efforts, which brought two young businessmen onto the board, as well as its first female members, two physicians. The board decided to hold a retreat to help bring the new trustees up to speed on roles and responsibilities and to help build rapport among new and existing board members and their spouses.

The board chair and hospital chief executive set a date for the retreat six weeks ahead at a golf resort about a four-hour drive from the Mount Pleasant community. The retreat was scheduled to begin with a meeting on a Thursday afternoon and end with lunch on Sunday.

The primary focus of the retreat was to be a board self-assessment that asked trustees to comment on how effectively they thought the board discharged its overall responsibilities. Each trustee was also asked to individually evaluate his or her own performance and to identify specific interests and needs. The board chair asked that all surveys be returned for tabulation at least four weeks before the retreat.

The hospital's attorney also was scheduled to provide an update on state legal and regulatory issues. Golf and tennis tournaments were scheduled for Friday and Saturday afternoons. Spouse events would include transportation to area outlet malls for shopping and an excursion to local antique stores.

Shortly after the new trustees' first board meeting, the CEO called the chair. "Only seven people are able to come to the retreat," he said. "We had 11 surveys returned; however, four were not completed because the respondents said they were too new to the board to comment on its performance, and three respondents said they had yet to participate in orientation. I called our new trustees, and three said they had scheduling conflicts that prevented them from attending. What do you think we should do?"

Big Sky Hospital

The board chair, CEO, and chair of the board's governance committee at Big Sky Hospital had gathered to plan the following year's meeting and education calendar. The system held two retreats each year—one in the fall for trustees only and a leadership retreat in the spring for the board, senior executives, and physician leaders.

The spring retreat was typically a weekend event held Friday evening through Sunday noon at a well-known resort in the state. The purpose was to update attendees on a variety of national and local health care issues and trends, with a particular emphasis on strategic issues facing Big Sky. Outside speakers and facilitators participated in the retreat, which included both plenary presentations and breakout working sessions. Golf and tennis tournaments were set for Saturday afternoon, and participants' families had events planned for them as well.

The fall board-only retreat was traditionally devoted to strategic planning or to a specific board issue requiring in-depth board discussion. The retreat was designed primarily as a facilitated session geared to produce an action plan for the board. It was held at a hotel in a nearby city and began Saturday morning with a day-long working session, followed by dinner and an evening outing for attendees and their spouses. A Sunday morning session was devoted to refinement and completion of the action plan. The retreat concluded by 11:30 A.M. on Sunday.

When the governance committee chair met with the board chair and the CEO, he said, "I recently received a brochure about a national trustee conference that also offers an option for individual boards to have an on-site, facilitated retreat in conjunction with the conference. Because our board requires that each member attend at least one outside educational program during each term of service, we could go to this conference and provide an opportunity for board members to fulfill their education requirement and have a retreat for our own board."

The board chair asked that copies of the brochure be included in the next board agenda packet for review and discussion.

Questions for Discussion

1. Does your organization conduct board and/or leadership retreats as part of its ongoing governance education and development activities? If so, how frequently did they occur over the past three years, what was their purpose, and how well attended were they?
2. Compare these examples. What aspects of Big Sky's approach make it more likely to succeed than Mount Pleasant's?
3. What should Mount Pleasant do?
4. Think about the board retreats you have attended and discuss what made the best ones work so well. What do you think is the most important ingredient in conducting a successful board retreat?

What Good Retreats Share

Although engaging, memorable, and well-attended board retreats can be conducted in a variety of different ways, successful retreats generally share some common characteristics.

Purpose: A retreat that is put together without a well-defined purpose or goal is a recipe for failure. Ask these questions:

- Is the goal of the retreat primarily to educate and inform?
- Does the board need more in-depth review or discussion about a particular function or responsibility, such as strategic planning or quality or how to assess and improve community health?
- Does the board need time to focus on setting organizational strategic priorities?
- Is retreat time best spent evaluating board performance and developing action plans for improvement?

- Is there an important issue, such as affiliation or merger, or a specific conflict that should be the focus of a retreat?
- What has been the primary focus of your two most recent board retreats? Is it time to vary the purpose or focus?

Participants: Clearly defining exactly for whom the retreat is intended can mean the difference between success and failure. Inviting physician leaders or staff members to a retreat where the board is assessing its own performance is likely to inhibit discussion and be perceived as a waste of time by nontrustee attendees. Conversely, providing on- or off-site educational opportunities to board members exclusively does little to build rapport and foster teamwork among board, executive, and physician leaders. Once you have identified a purpose or focus for a retreat, you can then determine which organizational leaders should attend.

Many organizations also invite spouses/significant others and, at times, families to their retreat. This option often makes it easier for younger board members to attend weekend retreats. Regardless of whom your organization decides to invite, it is important to clarify how these guests fit in. Spouse and family activities should be planned to coincide with the retreat schedule, and family members should be invited to social activities and meals with retreat attendees.

Location: Several factors affect the decision about where to hold a retreat. Holding a retreat at an off-site location often creates a relaxed atmosphere more conducive to learning and discussion than does the routine board meeting venue. At times, easily accessible locations can help boost retreat attendance. Alternatively, periodically taking the board to an off-site location that combines a national trustee conference with the option to hold your own board retreat may be a much appreciated "thank-you" for board members' time and talents.

The Agenda—Work and Play: The pitfalls to avoid are too much or too little work and no play. Retreats that try to address too many topics and also include a board meeting tend to seem rushed and unfocused. With time at a premium, it's important to concentrate on a few, well-chosen topics and activities that are strategically significant for the organization. Combining presentations with breakout discussions or other interactive activities is essential for keeping participants focused and engaged. It's also important to allow enough time in the agenda to fully discuss ideas and issues and to address unanticipated concerns that may arise.

Trustees who comment on the value of board retreats often say that having the time to socialize with their colleagues is as much or more important than the time spent in the formal program. Getting to know one another outside of the boardroom can help trustees improve board effectiveness and cohesiveness inside it. Retreat attendees also benefit from opportunities to informally review and discuss ideas or topics shared during the formal retreat sessions. Group meals, sporting activities, or other social events can help provide such opportunities.

Speakers and Facilitators: One of the advantages of using outside facilitators and speakers at a board retreat is the objectivity and industry knowledge and experience they provide. Outsiders can often help a board understand an issue or deliver a message that would not be perceived as objective or credible if it came from an internal source. Furthermore, if the board chair, CEO, or other staff member conducts the retreat, they cannot participate in the discussion, which casts them in a role similar to the one they play at board meetings. This makes it difficult to set a tone that differs from the typical board meeting dynamic.

Because speakers and facilitators have different strengths, watching them in action and talking with others who have used them can help ensure that you select the best person(s) for your needs. But this selection process takes time. Experts suggest securing your outside speakers and facilitators 6 to 12 months in advance of the retreat.

Results and Follow-Up: Effective retreats lead to changes in participant thinking and behavior. The outcome of many successful retreats includes an action plan to enhance awareness and understanding of strategic issues facing the organization or to improve board structure, function, or overall relationships among organizational leaders. Even if the retreat is primarily educational, it should end in participant consensus about needed changes as a result of the retreat.

Once specific changes or follow-up steps have been identified, it's critical that they be implemented soon. Many boards assign responsibility for completing an action plan and then ask a board committee to monitor its progress. Making completion of an action plan an agenda item at board meetings can help ensure that work done at the retreat does not fall through the cracks once the board resumes its regular activities.

A word of caution: One of the best ways to defeat a retreat is to allow those who failed to attend to question the rationale behind an action plan or to take issue with it. Boards that allow nonparticipants such leeway create the impression that future board retreats will be a waste of time as nothing lasting results from them. The best way to handle this type of interference is to briefly explain the rationale behind the plan and suggest that those who want input into the plan should attend the next retreat.

How to Plan and Conduct a Successful Retreat

1. Start planning your retreat early. To get the speakers, location, and desired attendance level, begin work as much as a year in advance.

2. Don't delegate planning and preparation to the CEO and staff. Board and leadership retreats should have input from trustees and other leaders as part of the planning process. The board's governance committee, for example, might take the lead in organizing a board-only retreat. An ad hoc committee of trustees, physician leaders, and staff might spearhead organizing a leadership retreat.

3. If the topic is sensitive, engage participants early. Boards or leadership groups that decide to tackle a sensitive or controversial issue at a retreat can benefit from early preparation. There are many benefits to having the retreat facilitator interview those who will be participating for their input prior to the retreat. It signals that everyone's view and participation in the retreat will be important. An anonymous summary of interview comments also can help frame the issue and provide a springboard for retreat discussions.

4. Mix presentation and interaction. A full day of presentations is a surefire way to lose participants to other activities, such as frequent calls to home or office or just slipping away for an afternoon catnap. Keeping the group engaged and attentive means making sure that "talking heads" are balanced with opportunities to interact in group discussions, work through case examples, develop action plans, or participate in other small-group activities. Giving attendees an idea or issue to talk about during social functions can help build continuity from one day to the next.

Five-Star Board Retreats

Trustees, CEOs, and governance consultants offer this retreat advice:

"I am convinced that nobody can think strategically for any length of time at a board meeting. A retreat gives the board an opportunity to look at an issue in real depth, to receive background information and then, more important, to engage in real dialogue. I think that it's crucial to have board members and physicians together at a hospital or health care organization retreat. Physicians often give me a perspective that I didn't have before. Today, with the tough decisions that boards have to make, an environment of trust is necessary. The only way to build trust is to get to know one another and work together. A retreat can foster a more trusting environment."

—Lois Green, vice chair, UMass Memorial Health Care,
Worcester, Massachusetts

"I think the most successful retreats involve attendees in a participatory way—role-playing, case studies, real-world examples, and applications. Straight lecturing is the least effective approach. Engaging participants, getting them emotionally involved in the issues, is the way to help them learn faster and remember more."

—Bob Parsons, Ph.D., trustee, Urban South Region,
Intermountain Health Care, Provo, Utah

"It's really important for board members to feel that the facilitator has his or her hands around the topics being covered at the retreat. Rather than present a canned program, the facilitator should bring a diverse perspective, timely information, and real-world examples, and then be able to connect the dots for board members—explain the significance of these issues and what it means to be a good board member."

—Rich Miller, president and CEO, Virtua Health,
Marlton, New Jersey

"The most important things for a productive, successful retreat are the following:

- CEO and board chair support, with open, candid discussion, clear objectives, and a commitment to follow up on ideas generated at the retreat

Continued →

- Partnering with the facilitator to design the retreat program, including substantive advance preparation and full disclosure of below-the-surface problems and issues
- Allowing enough time . . . some boards have major issues involving trust or relationships and yet want the facilitator to "tell them their roles" and achieve dramatic results in three hours . . . that's not realistic."

—Barry Bader, health care governance consultant,
Potomac, Maryland

"My sense is that there are five essential elements for an effective retreat:

- The purpose and importance of the retreat are very clearly stated—everyone recognizes and agrees that important, real work is to be done.
- An effective facilitator provides leadership for both the design and implementation of the retreat process. Quality planning enhances the probability of quality results.
- Analysis, briefing materials, and other information are sent to participants prior to the retreat. Board members prepare by thoroughly reading everything in advance.
- Outside resources—people and materials—are used to enrich the discourse.
- The board and management engage constructively, with openness, receptivity, respect, and candor."

—Fred Miller, president, The Chatham Group,
Chatham, Massachusetts

"'Why doesn't the board show as much interest in the quality of patient care provided at the hospital as it does in the hospital's financial performance?' This question from our medical chief of staff at a board retreat prompted quite a discussion . . . and he was right. We were so focused on the bottom line that we were forgetting why we were in the community. As a result, we formed the board quality assurance committee and have monitored the quality of patient care ever since."

—Lanny A. Kope, Ed.D., trustee, Phoenix (Arizona)
Memorial Hospital

5. It's okay to relax. We've talked about the importance of including free time during retreats to allow for socializing or group activities. Some organizations want to make every second count and worry about whether each luncheon or dinner should include a speaker who addresses an important health care issue. Many retreats benefit from having entertainment after a dinner or reception, particularly on the second night of a weekend retreat. One of our clients has a band whose members include hospital executive personnel and physicians. They perform each year at the leadership retreat and are considered a highlight of the weekend.

6. Carefully consider the length of your retreat. Most trustees and other leaders find it difficult to devote more than two consecutive days to an off-site retreat, particularly if lost time means lost income. Make it easy for people to attend. Find a convenient location, include spouses and families, as appropriate, and build in free time—it will help gain commitment and boost retreat attendance.

7. If your organization has multiple boards and subsidiaries, structure an opportunity to bring all organizational leaders together at least once a year. Leadership retreats that provide both educational presentations for all attendees and specific breakout sessions for board members or physician leaders not only help build rapport among all leaders but also help clarify relative roles and responsibilities of leaders in different parts of the organization.

8. Cultivate perspectives from other organizations and industries. Consider bringing in a speaker from an industry outside of health care to share lessons learned or solutions to problems you face in your organization. Many times the perspectives you need can be found around your boardroom table. Building in time for a board member from a local college to discuss how his or her organization handled its public image campaign or asking a board member to describe how his or her organization won a statewide award for quality and customer service can help organizational leaders gain new insights and better understand the value of a diverse board.

9. Ensure that any action plans that come out of the retreat are implemented. And make sure to link change back to the retreat. "As a result of last year's retreat, we have accomplished the following activities. This year, we want to build on last year's progress and. . . ."

10. Evaluate the retreat experience. All attendees should be asked to complete and return a retreat evaluation form before they leave

the premises. These evaluations should be reviewed by the retreat planning committee, which should also take time out to assess how it approached its own work and what might be improved. Make sure that suggestions from these evaluations are used in planning future retreats.

Conclusion

Successful board retreats should be part of an ongoing program of board education and development, including orientation, ongoing self-assessment, and other written, audio, and video materials. Retreats provide an excellent opportunity for leaders to learn about each other and issues affecting the organization in a more relaxed atmosphere than the structure and dynamics of board meetings. For many boards and leadership groups, their annual retreat has become a cornerstone of continued growth, development, and improvement.

We've Got to Stop Meeting Like This: Creating Board Agendas That Work

By Pamela R. Knecht

You are sitting in the boardroom at the appointed time, waiting for the other half of the board to show up. The meeting finally starts 20 minutes later. You spend the next hour listening to senior managers give long, detailed reports. Another half hour is wasted discussing the lack of parking. Only a few dominant board members and the CEO are talking. Most of the other trustees are trying to keep their mouths shut while yawning. You can't remember what the board was supposed to be deciding today, and a voice in your head is shouting, "I've got to get out of here!"

Does this sound like a board meeting you have attended recently? Most experts agree that two hours per month of board time is "wasted." Given that there are approximately 100,000 not-for-profit health care board members in the United States, that means millions of hours of board time are wasted every year.

Pamela R. Knecht is vice-president of Accord Limited, a health care governance, strategy, and organization development consulting firm based in Chicago. She can be reached at (312) 988-7000.

Don't Be an Irresponsible Board Chair

Too many board chairs leave the effectiveness of their meetings to chance. They believe they can show up with a brief agenda and rely on the CEO and management to do the rest. That is an irresponsible way of using a very expensive resource—that is, the board's time.

Preparation is critical for ensuring that boards are able to do their jobs well. Boards should be governing, not managing; overseeing, not doing. To achieve that, board members need to be informed, they need a fruitful forum for discussion, and they need help in elevating that discussion to the right level.

Help the Board Prepare

One of the best tools board chairs can use to help their members arrive informed is the board preparation package. Remember that the main reason for this packet is to help trustees make informed decisions about important strategic and policy issues. If you provide too many specifics in the packet, the board will follow your lead and dive into questions that are overly detailed.

Here are some specific tips for creating useful board packets:

- Include the proposed meeting agenda (see the sample agenda on page 61).
- Prepare high-level summaries of the information to be discussed; do not merely copy existing management reports.
- Use graphic, dashboard-type reports of key indicators, such as financial status and clinical quality outcomes (see "Effective Boards: Working Smarter to Meet the Challenge," in the May 2000 *Trustee*).
- Add executive-level reports from each committee.
- Provide a proposed consent agenda (see below for an explanation).
- Send the packets out at least one full week before the meeting.

When determining what to include in the board packet, it's important to balance the need to keep the packet small with the need to include required meeting information. Too much meeting time is wasted presenting materials that could have been provided earlier as background reading. On the other hand, make sure that all needed materials for each agenda discussion are included in the board meeting packet.

Create a Great Agenda

An excellent board packet alone will not guarantee a productive meeting. You must take the time to prepare a focused agenda. Such an agenda will:

- Help members prepare
- Send a message about the time to be devoted to each topic
- Provide a guide for running the meeting and staying on time
- Indicate the appropriate level of discussion on each issue
- Ensure that the discussion is focused

The chair should write a one-page agenda for a two-to-three-hour meeting (see sample). Each agenda item should include:

- The name of the meeting's presenter/facilitator
- An estimate of the time required for each discussion (Add a buffer to each estimate as discussions rarely start and end exactly on time.)
- The action being requested (e.g., informational; consent; decision; input)
- The location of the relevant background materials in the board packet

Because board members should be focused on strategic and policy-level issues, make sure that the majority of the meeting is reserved for those discussions. One way to save time for important discussions is to use a consent agenda covering the routine actions that require board approval (e.g., approving committee recommendations). Any board member can request that an item be moved off the consent agenda and opened for discussion. The items that stay on the consent agenda are voted on together as a block, without any further discussion.

Once you have drafted the entire meeting agenda, go back through it and imagine having each discussion. If you do not honestly think you can fit all the potential discussions into the time you have available, delete some items.

Be a Facilitator

Once the board packets have been distributed, the board chair's next responsibility is to run a productive meeting. The most effective chairs are facilitators, not generals who control everything tightly. A facilitator introduces the topics, keeps the meeting on track, encourages appropriate participation by each member, manages conflicts, refocuses the group on the issues at hand, and ensures that the discussions are strategic. Here are some specific suggestions for facilitating a good meeting:

- Begin and end on time.
- Start with a few quick, easy items to get the board rolling (e.g., introduce new members and guests; approve the agenda for this meeting).

<table>
<tr><td colspan="5" align="center">Sample Board Agenda
Central Health System
Board of Directors Meeting
March 19, 2001</td></tr>
<tr><td>Time</td><td>Agenda Item</td><td>Presenter</td><td>Objective</td><td>Background Materials</td></tr>
<tr><td>5:00 PM</td><td>Welcome and Introductions</td><td>Board Chair</td><td>Information</td><td>None</td></tr>
<tr><td>5:05 PM</td><td>Approval of Agenda</td><td>Board Chair</td><td>Consent</td><td>Tab A</td></tr>
<tr><td>5:10 PM</td><td>Consent Agenda</td><td>Board Chair</td><td>Consent</td><td>Tab B</td></tr>
<tr><td>5:15 PM</td><td>Executive/Key Indicator Report</td><td>CEO</td><td>Oversight</td><td>Tab C</td></tr>
<tr><td>5:30 PM</td><td>Strategic Plan Input Session</td><td>Chair, Strategic Planning Committee</td><td>Input</td><td>Tab D</td></tr>
<tr><td>6:30 PM</td><td>Break</td><td></td><td></td><td></td></tr>
<tr><td>6:40 PM</td><td>Acquisition of Physician Practice</td><td>Chair, Physician Committee</td><td>Decision</td><td>Tab E</td></tr>
<tr><td>7:20 PM</td><td>Meeting Evaluation</td><td>Board Chair</td><td>Input</td><td>Tab F</td></tr>
<tr><td>7:30 PM</td><td>Adjournment</td><td>Board Chair</td><td>Consent</td><td>None</td></tr>
</table>

- Discuss questions about the key indicator report.
- Move to the substantive issues while the group is still fresh.
- Allow time for committee chairs to highlight significant items in their reports or to ask for the board's approval of an item; remember, a board should trust the work of its committees, not rehash their discussions.

Discard *Robert's Rules of Order*

Historically, boards have used *Robert's Rules of Order* to manage their deliberations and decision making. It is the author's opinion that *Robert's Rules* are no longer an appropriate tool for running board meetings.

Although the *Rules* may still be needed when a very large group is convened (e.g., a town hall meeting) to keep order, they often cause a board to become rigid and formal. The *Rules* inhibit openness and the free flow of conversation that is needed to ensure that important topics are thoroughly discussed. Well-facilitated discussions and decision-making processes are much more important than the stiff deliberations forced by *Robert's Rules of Order*.

Learn from Successes and Mistakes

In light of the board's responsibility to ensure its own effectiveness, many boards are now including time at the end of their meetings for a quick evaluation. The chair facilitates a brief discussion in which the members state what they thought went well and what they would like done differently at the next meeting. This information is included in the meeting minutes, and the chair uses the comments to help structure the next meeting.

Conclusion

Board meetings are most effective when the board is clear about its role as an oversight body; when it has received the appropriate level of preparation material in a timely fashion; when its meetings are well managed; and when its discussions are strategic, honest, and focused. Well-crafted preparation packages and agendas help boards do their work efficiently and effectively.

Board chairs who see their jobs as facilitators are the most successful because they get and keep their colleagues engaged in interesting, strategic-level discussions. If board meetings are run well, trustees are more likely to stay (literally and figuratively) and be productive, energetic contributors.

How to Run
Effective Board Meetings

By James E. Orlikoff
and Mary K. Totten

And while the Great Ones repair to their dinner,
The Secretary stays, growing thinner and thinner.
Racking his brains to record and report
What he thinks they will think that they ought to have thought.
—London Institute of Directors' 1971 *Standard Manual*

A truly unique aspect of governance is that a board exists only when
it is actually meeting. So the most valuable commodity a board has
is the time its members spend together between raps of the gavel.
The art of governance largely involves maximizing the use of this
precious time, and the effectiveness of a board is predominately
determined by how effective and efficient its meetings are. Conducting board meetings that are as focused and productive as possible and continuously evaluating and improving them is a hallmark
of effective governance.

Long, rambling, inconclusive and inefficient meetings are a chronic
complaint of many board leaders and members. Meetings dominated

James E. Orlikoff is president of Orlikoff & Associates, Inc., Chicago.
Mary K. Totten is president of Totten & Associates, Oak Park, Illinois.

by one or two people, those focused on incidental issues, or those that get sidetracked from important agenda items are also common barriers to meaningful gatherings. Effective board meetings are the result of a clear purpose, a focused agenda, summarized governance information, and an explicit decision-making process.

The Board as a Decision-Making Body

Many boards concentrate on the content of their meetings, but very few focus on the process. A key characteristic of an effective board is that it has a clear process for making decisions. Further, the board chair clearly communicates this process to each member and makes sure that all trustees understand it. Board meetings are often rendered ineffective when different members have different ideas about the decision-making process, or different decision-making processes are inconsistently applied to different situations.

Some boards use a consensus model of decision making, where a decision is "made" without a vote as long as no member strongly disagrees. Some boards have a unanimous model of decision making, where dissenting votes are implicitly discouraged and the vast majority of votes is unanimous. Some boards have a culture where a simple majority vote will carry any issue, whereas other boards require a "supermajority" (i.e., a percentage of board votes greater than 51 percent to carry the decision) on important issues. Some boards have a culture where the issues presented for vote have been "pre-decided" by the executive committee, the board chair, or the CEO, and the board votes are simply pro forma approvals. Different situations may call for different methods, and effective boards prospectively determine when specific decision-making methods will be most appropriate.

Effective boards have a clear, agreed-on process that they routinely use to both frame and make decisions. Their meetings are facilitated by the consistent use of a defined process that addresses such issues as these:

- How much discussion is encouraged prior to a vote? Are all members encouraged to speak, or are established positions articulated by designated individuals?
- Which issues, if any, require a supermajority vote of the board?

- Does the board have a policy that, except in emergencies or rare situations, it will not vote on issues at the same meeting where they are first presented or discussed? This policy permits trustees to consider an issue between board meetings, request more information, and then make a more informed decision.

Questions for Discussion

Boards can make a decision by consensus, a unanimous vote, a supermajority vote, and a simple majority vote.

1. Which decision-making process does your board use? Why?
2. If your board uses some other process for making decisions, how would you describe it?
3. If your board uses different decision-making processes at different times, is it clearly understood which process is used in which situations and why? (For example, a board may use simple majority votes on routine issues but require supermajority votes on specified issues of importance.)
4. Is the decision-making process used by your board the result of conscious discussion and deliberation, or is it used because "it has always been done that way"?
5. Does your board routinely make decisions on issues at the same meeting where the issue is first presented?

Agenda Control

A key component of effective board meetings is an effective agenda. Efficient boards control their agendas, yet many boards are prisoners of static agendas. Many still place the most mundane, trivial issues first on their agendas and take the majority of their time discussing them. The issues of greatest significance are then placed at the end of the agenda, when there is time pressure to end the meeting or trustees are tired and eager for it to end.

This can give rise to the "Law of Triviality," that is, "The amount of time a board spends on an issue tends to be in inverse proportion to the importance of, and dollar amount involved in, that issue."

To avoid falling prey to this law, an effective meeting agenda focuses first on issues that have been prospectively identified as

Tips for Effective Meetings

Try one or more of the following tips to help make your board meetings more productive and dynamic.

1. Make sure your board understands the decision-making processes it uses and how and when to apply them. Consider reviewing this information as part of a board meeting educational session and building it into your trustee orientation program.
2. Help board members prepare in advance. Set and circulate an annual schedule of meetings and board education sessions and send out board meeting agenda materials at least a week in advance.
3. Require trustees to come prepared for meetings and evaluate their performance as part of your trustee evaluation and development process.
4. Use a consent agenda to address items such as approval of board committee minutes or reports, which require board action but do not require significant discussion by the full board.
5. Organize your agenda to allow participants significant time for discussion of strategic issues.
6. Use e-mail to distribute agenda materials in advance of board or committee meetings. Some organizations use their Web site or a designated board-only subsite to post information as well.
7. Follow an action-oriented agenda for your board meetings. Set a time limit for the meeting itself and time limits for each agenda item. Circulate the schedule in advance of the meeting.
8. Ensure strong leadership. Include information about how to run efficient, effective meetings into your board and committee chair leadership development process. A knowledgeable and skilled chair who keeps the meeting on track, ensures productive participation from all members, and handles conflict appropriately (see "Resolving Conflict," page 72) is critical to meeting effectiveness.
9. Build meeting etiquette and participation skills into trustee orientation.
10. Take time out to evaluate the effectiveness of each board meeting. Continual feedback is essential to continuous improvement.

most urgently needing the board's attention. The board identifies these critical agenda issues through the strategic plan and the organization's annual goals and objectives, as well as its own annual goals and objectives. Focusing on these issues enables a board to develop a collective sense of what is important and a shared understanding of purpose and priorities. These purposes and priorities are then reflected and emphasized in board meeting agendas throughout the year.

A very useful agenda control technique is a *consent agenda*. Agenda planners (usually the executive or governance committee, but occasionally the board chair with the CEO) divide the board agenda issues into two parts. The first part contains those items that must be acted on by the board because of legal, regulatory, or other requirements but are not significant enough to warrant discussion by the full board. Issues such as receipt and approval of reports and minutes, along with related materials, are combined into a single section, or consent agenda. Trustees review this section prior to the meeting, and if no one has any questions or concerns, the entire block of issues is accepted or approved with one board vote and no discussion. This frees up a tremendous amount of time that would otherwise be squandered on minor issues.

Important issues that require thoughtful discussion, deliberation, and action by the board constitute the second part of the agenda. Items are addressed one by one, with the board spending the time that has been freed up by the consent agenda to address these more critical issues.

In addition to the use of consent agendas, other techniques to leverage better board meetings through the agenda include:

- Placing the most important agenda items first to provide the most time for board discussion
- Clear agenda distinctions between action items, discussion items in preparation for future board decisions, and information and board education items
- Distributing a timed agenda for each board meeting to all board members in advance
- Setting a realistic agenda not packed with too many items
- Adhering to the established agenda, with the board chair keeping a tight reign on digressions, members' side discussions, and issues

that have already been addressed or that will be addressed later in the agenda

- Sticking to beginning and ending times; in this way, meetings become more efficient, and trustees are not likely to feel their valuable time is being wasted

Exercise: Assess Your Board's Agenda

1. At your next board meeting cross out the date of the agenda so that it is unreadable. Have the board secretary bring an agenda from a board meeting from two years ago and cross out that date. Now, mix up the two agendas and have the board compare them. Can the board identify the agenda for today's meeting? If the answer is no, that implies the board is addressing the same issues today that it did two years ago—it is a prisoner of its own agenda.

2. Effective board agendas change as the strategy of the organization changes and as the issues change. A "living agenda" also means that the board meetings change as well. Does your board have a living agenda or a fixed one?

3. Has your board ever fallen prey to the Law of Triviality? If so, how often and why? If not, why not?

Board Meeting Evaluation

A very useful technique to continually improve meetings is to conduct a brief evaluation at every meeting's conclusion. After each meeting adjourns, trustees take no more than five minutes to complete an evaluation that assesses that meeting's effectiveness and efficiency. The board chair, with the help of the CEO or governance committee, analyzes the results and uses them to monitor and improve all processes relating to the conduct of effective meetings. Further, the aggregate results of each meeting evaluation should be presented to the full board at its next meeting, along with any plans for improvement.

Asking each trustee to list anonymously what worked well as well as what did not and why can help a board constantly fine-tune and improve its meetings. In doing so, the effectiveness and efficiency of the board meetings will continuously evolve, and the cohesiveness of the board and the quality of governance will grow.

Personal Advice on Improving Board Meetings

"We had very traditional board meetings until our new board chair engaged members in a collaborative effort to make our meetings more interesting and dynamic. Every month we build into our meetings a half hour or so of board education. Because we felt the full board needed a better understanding of financial and quality issues, we have disbanded our board finance and quality committees for the time being and use meetings of the full board to discuss these issues. We also use a consent agenda, and everyone understands they have to do their homework and come to meetings prepared. Our board meetings are more exciting, and I look forward to them. The quality of questions that board members now ask also shows that they are more knowledgeable and involved."

—Sr. Catherine Manning, president and CEO,
Saint Vincent Health System, Erie, Pennsylvania

"The single most important ingredient for a great board meeting is having a chair who's a really good meeting manager and facilitator. Running an effective, efficient meeting is an acquired skill. To do the 'acquiring,' here are some of the best books around that board chairs can read":

- *Meetings That Work,* by Richard Chang
- *First-Aid for Meetings,* by Charles Hawkins
- *The Strategy of Meetings,* by George Kieffer
- *How to Run Successful Meetings in Half the Time,* by Milo Frank
- *How to Make Meetings Work,* by Michael Doyle

—Dennis D. Pointer, Ph.D., principal,
Dennis D. Pointer & Associates, and John J. Hanlon,
professor of Health Services Research and Policy,
San Diego State University, La Jolla, California

"The most important thing we have done to improve our board meetings is to switch the agenda around to lead with education and discussion on a topic that our board members want to know more about. We now put the committee reports and consent agenda items in the second half of our two-hour meetings. This new order of agenda topics sends a message of priority to our board members— that we want to invest time and energy in helping them keep abreast of industry issues and trends."

—Michele Serbenski, assistant to the president,
Board Relations and Communications,
Bronson Healthcare Group, Kalamazoo, Michigan

Sample Board Meeting Evaluation Questions

Consider the following:

- Did the meeting agenda relate to, or support, the mission and vision of the organization?
- Did the agenda focus on the organization's strategic priorities?
- Did the meeting have specific objectives and were these objectives accomplished?
- Did the agenda book contain information that facilitated informed decision making?
- Did every board member have an opportunity to express his or her views?
- Did every member participate?
- Was more time spent on future issues than on past issues and organizational monitoring?
- Did the board micromanage?
- Did every board member come to the meeting prepared—having read and considered the agenda information?
- Did the meeting start and end on time?
- Did you think that the meeting was challenging and productive?
- Did the chair run the meeting efficiently and objectively?
- Did the board use its meeting time well?
- Did everyone learn something from this meeting?
- Did everyone leave the meeting energized and excited?
- How could the meeting have been better?

Questions for Discussion

1. Of the preceding sample questions, which do you think would be most valuable for assessing and improving your board meetings? Why?
2. Which questions do you believe would be least valuable for your board? Why?
3. What other board meeting evaluation questions would you suggest for your board?

Who Should Attend Board Meetings?

People who are not board members often attend health care organization board meetings. These individuals may include senior executives, perhaps medical staff members, and invited guests.

Frequently, nonboard members participate freely in the meetings and can even dominate them. To an outside observer or a new trustee, it may not be at all clear who is a board member and who is not.

As a general rule, if a board is meeting, those attending should be primarily, if not exclusively, board members. Other than the CEO, management staff should be present only during their reports to the board and a follow-up question period, and should then excuse

---

Resolving Conflict at Board Meetings

One of the most difficult aspects of board meetings to manage is the eruption and resolution of conflict between trustees or others present at the meeting. Conflict is a frequent presence in health care boardrooms today and can be expected to increase as a result of the significant changes in health care that make governing a hospital or system very stressful. A consistent and rational approach to conflict resolution will help any board conduct more effective meetings.

Conflict resolution techniques that can be applied by board chairs, CEOs, or trustees to minimize board and committee meeting disruption include the following:

- Define the problem as objectively as possible and get participants to agree to the definition of the problem before suggesting or even allowing the suggestion of solutions.
- Use active listening to restate each person's perspective and concerns regarding the problem or conflict in order to both understand the problem and to demonstrate that the perspectives of all those involved are understood accurately.
- Confine the debate and discussion of the problem to principles and issues, not personalities.
- Facilitate a brainstorming session among those who are involved to generate a comprehensive list of possible solutions.
- Once a list of possible solutions has been generated, take a break from the issue or conflict (perhaps even tabling it until the next board meeting) to allow all board members and meeting participants to consider the problem, generate additional solutions, and identify the most effective solution.

It is very important to remember that how a board or chair addresses a conflict or problem will be remembered long after the actual conflict is resolved.

themselves. The more nonboard members present during a meeting, the less effective that meeting is likely to be. Having nonmembers routinely attend board meetings inhibits free discussion and deliberation, and prevents the board from developing into a cohesive unit.

Questions for Discussion

1. How many nonboard members routinely attend your meetings? Why?
2. Do you think that meetings would be more productive without the presence of nonboard members throughout the meeting? If so, why? If not, why not?

Conclusion

Every board meeting is an opportunity to build trustees' knowledge and understanding and to advance the board's effectiveness. Establishing ground rules about trustee preparation, participation, and decision making; developing agendas that allocate the majority of meeting time to discussion of strategic issues; ensuring that meeting chairs are skilled in how to run an effective meeting; and taking time out to evaluate the content and process of each meeting are some of the ways that boards can make the best use of the precious time they spend together.

Dis-Oriented?

*Are Your New Board Members
Prepared or Perplexed?*

By Janet Kalbhen

First days are never easy, whether you're the new kid in school or a new trustee at your first board meeting. Obviously, new board members can't absorb by osmosis how to be a trustee, what their hospital or system is all about, and what the critical health care issues are. So the best way to make starting out less stressful for trustees-in-training and give them the tools to make smart decisions right away is to bolster them with the basics before they come to the table.

These days, with operating margins that are slim to none and access to capital curtailed, the role of trustees is even more essential than it once was. Yet many hospitals and systems still lack a formal, organized orientation program to prep new board recruits. "Traditionally, we've taken them to the end of the dock, kicked them in the derrière, and then said, 'Start swimming,'" says Dennis Pointer, a La Jolla, California–based governance consultant. By not acclimating new members, boards squander newcomers' enthusiasm and commitment and lose the benefit of that new blood, adds Pointer,

---

Janet Kalbhen is a writer and Web site developer based in the Chicago area.

who's also a professor of health administration at San Diego State University.

Those hospitals and systems that don't ascribe to the sink-or-swim method typically begin with an initial orientation meeting or series of meetings, which work best when they aren't part of a board or committee meeting. Setting aside separate time for orientation fosters an atmosphere that makes it easier for new kids on the block to ask questions and soak up need-to-know information without exhibiting their ignorance to their more seasoned peers or bogging down a regular board meeting.

While new trustees need to start somewhere, they can't afford to take too long to get up to speed. Trustees "are legally responsible from day one on the board," warns Lois Green, vice chair of UMass Memorial Health Care in Worcester, Massachusetts. Orientation must include sufficient information to help them make critical choices, such as "at their first meeting, when they have to vote on whether they should or shouldn't renew a managed care contract," Green says.

The Big Picture

What should be in every new trustee's toolbox? Polling a panel of experts, including trustees, academics, and consultants, garnered a laundry list of answers. Use the following slate of macrotopics as an outline, or draw from the subject menu to either create an orientation program from scratch or refine an existing one tailored to your own hospital's or system's needs. Keep in mind that every trustee's knowledge base is different, so play to the strengths of each member and adjust to his or her orientation accordingly.

Experts recommend that new trustees learn:

- Background of the current national health care environment
- The effect of managed care on the health care field
- Definitions of key health care terms
- Components of the health care payer mix, including Medicare and Medicaid
- Future trends, such as complementary and alternative medicine and genomics

- How health care is delivered in the age of integrated delivery systems
- Information technology trends (including the Internet) and what new medical equipment is on the horizon
- How to serve today's more demanding health care consumer

Frequently Asked Questions

Ideally, the orientation session and the written materials that supplement it should answer most key questions for new trustees. Chicago-based consultant and *Trustee* contributor James Orlikoff suggests what questions new board members should ask, and get answered, in their orientation:

1. What is our hospital's or system's payer mix (i.e., what percent of our payments come from Medicare, Medicaid, commercial indemnity insurance, discounted fee-for-service, capitated contracts, and charity care)?
2. What percent of our revenues come from inpatient acute care, outpatient surgery, outpatient primary care, hospice, home care, nursing home care, and so on?
3. What is our organization's margin on operations? What is our margin on various lines of business (the business categories listed above)?
4. What is the current demand-capacity ratio in our market?
5. What is our organization's relationship with physicians? Consider the ratio of primary care physicians to specialists and how many physicians are linked economically to the organization through employment, contracts, hospital-physician organizations, or other mechanisms.
6. What are our organization's strengths and weaknesses? What are our strategic options?
7. What is the current managed care picture for our market? How is this likely to change in the next three years?
8. Who are our competitors? What do we know about them (i.e., What is their payer mix? their business mix? their margin on operations? their demand-capacity ratios? their strengths and weaknesses?)?
9. What is our strategic plan?

Getting to Know All about You

Although there are some excellent orientation manuals and resources available, what they lack—and where you'll need to fill in the blanks—are specifics about your hospital or system. One such publication, the *Governing Board Orientation Manual* published by the Washington State Hospital Association, recognizes this shortcoming and offers the following outline for creating a board manual with pertinent details about your hospital or system.

1. General Hospital or System Information
   - Hospital history
   - Vision statement
   - Mission statement
   - Strategic plan summary
   - Annual budget summary
   - Hospital annual report
   - Articles of incorporation
   - Enabling legislation
   - Bylaws
   - Service area
   - Organizational chart
   - Physical layout (include trustee personal tour)

2. Governing Board
   - Job descriptions for governing board, chairperson, and trustees
   - List of members
   - Committees
   - Annual board goals
   - Board policies
   - Board calendar
   - Liability indemnification policy
   - Conflict-of-interest statement

3. Chief Executive Officer
   - Job description
   - Contract
   - CEO evaluation

4. Medical Staff
   - Medical staff bylaws
   - Committee structure
   - Types of appointments and privileges

5. Quality Management Plan

6. Corporate Compliance Plan

7. Affiliations and Agreements

Presentation Is Everything

How much is too much? What's the best format to present the essentials? Again, opinions differ, but here are a few tips:

Don't bury your beginners with a blizzard of paper. "When I came on the board, I got a five-inch binder full of materials," recalls Robert Parsons, a trustee for the Urban South Region of Intermountain Health Care in Provo, Utah. "It's under my stairs. I glanced at it but never read it."

A succinct but fact-filled reference manual can become your new (and returning) trustees' bible, but it shouldn't take the place of in-person orientation. As useless as a thick binder is a presenter droning on verbatim from it at orientation sessions. Instead, put together an animated oral presentation, preferably using slides or other visual media, that hits the highlights of the written materials while including charts, graphs, and flowcharts as well as benchmarking information and other useful statistics that can be understood at a glance.

For hospitals and systems whose boards are Internet savvy, consider putting up an internal Web site offering the orientation manual and audiovisual materials from the oral presentation. Keep adding new links to pertinent Web sites, journal articles, and other useful resources. Make it even more valuable by creating an electronic index and search function to locate specifics much faster than thumbing through a dog-eared print copy.

The Buddy System

One suggestion from those in the trenches is to pair new trustees with a mentor on the board. There's no magic formula for how long that hand-holding should go on. In some cases, the twosome will stay together for only a few meetings and in others up to a year. But most agree that such a pairing is very important to a new trustee's development.

"Every new trustee needs a mentor," Green says. Mentors should attend orientation with their initiates, sit with them at board meetings, ask if the information presented was clear, and answer any questions about that meeting, she recommends.

Charity Starts Here

Every October, rookie trustees from Sisters of Charity of Leavenworth Health System congregate in Kansas for two and a half days of intensive training. Their mission is to "learn about the system and affirm their roles as board members," says Annamarie Katosh, who coordinates the program. The annual retreat is geared toward trustees who have joined the boards of one of the nine hospitals in the Leavenworth, Kansas–based system within the last 12 months.

System president Bill Murray typically kicks off the meeting by outlining overall vision, goals, and strategies. The legal counsel covers conflict of interest and confidentiality. New trustees also spend time with the vice president of planning. Crucial to this orientation is the definition of what it means to be a Catholic hospital, Katosh says. This explanation then dovetails into discussions about social and corporate ethics. Attendees also can sit in on sessions that deal with such specifics as how to raise money for their local hospital. This type of in-depth program gives the greenhorns a further opportunity to network and learn from each other.

"We try to give trustees an overview of who we are and depend on hospital boards to present info [about] their local markets," says Katosh.

Trustees leave with a succinct system orientation governance manual. They can easily look up information about the system's history; mission and vision; corporate and governance structure; systemwide programs, such as its managed care consortium and group purchasing setup; and financial data.

Trustees also get to take home their conference "bible," which reiterates everything learned in their crash course. The huge binder from the system's latest program this past fall includes:

- An overview of the nation's health care future
- A strategic plan for the ministry from 2002–2004
- Market profiles of each hospital in the system
- A snapshot of the system's finances
- A primer on how to be a new trustee
- Elements of effective board leadership
- Challenges of the Catholic health ministry
- Breakout sessions with case studies

—J.K.

Those Who Can, Teach

"The CEO is the board's chief educator, says Potomac, Maryland–based governance consultant Barry Bader. Errol Biggs, a professor in health administration at the University of Colorado-Denver, agrees. "Orientation needs to be conducted by the hospital or system CEO." The only exception to that rule relates to trustee responsibilities, Biggs maintains. Because the board is chosen to serve as an impartial outside influence and also oversees the CEO, having the CEO explain a trustee's job to a trustee may be awkward. That information should come from the board chair because the new trustee "perceives the CEO as the paid insider," Biggs says.

To solve this dilemma, Green advocates the team-teaching approach. The board chair should talk about the board's roles and responsibilities and how the board functions. The CEO or board chair should outline the hospital's or system's strategic direction. The CFO should present financial statements and benchmarks. The chief medical officer should address quality of care, and the head of the medical staff should explain how the medical staff works and its relationship to the board. And the managed care department head should go into detail about capitated contracts and relationships with HMOs and insurers.

Boards with bigger training budgets may choose to hire outside experts to help them prepare orientation materials or even present all or part of the orientation session. Why reinvent the wheel, the thinking goes, when you can pay a specialist who's helped numerous other boards educate their new members. For do-it-yourselfers, there are a variety of resources, including books, Web sites, kits, and manuals to help you shape your own orientation packet and program.

Go Local or Systematic

Some of the techniques used to get a hospital board member up to speed also apply to system board member orientation. It's the focus and emphasis that differ, Bader says. Hospital boards are more concerned with quality of care, hospital operations, and the relationship between the hospital and its key stakeholders—physicians, employees, the community at large, and patients. System boards examine issues in a broader way and focus on strategic planning affecting all their entities.

A good example of the difference is how the two board levels view capital, Bader explains. "A system board needs to determine the amount of capital that is available on a systemwide basis. The hospital board decides how best to apply its allocated capital to meet local health care needs."

Educating a New Chairperson

Because the new chair of a hospital or system board is almost always plucked from among the rank-and-file trustees, the selection process is more critical than the orientation that occurs later. If the new board chair does not have the innate leadership skills needed to run the show, no amount of instruction can overcome that deficit. "You've done 90 percent of the work if you select the right board chair," says Errol Biggs, a professor in health administration at the University of Colorado-Denver and a governance consultant for hospitals and medical groups.

Assuming the right man or woman was chosen for the job, he or she can further prepare for the position, Biggs recommends, by continually reviewing industry journals and by attending advanced governance conferences annually. The person running the board also should have an intimate knowledge of the intricacies of the hospital's or system's financial status.

In addition, Biggs came up with the following crucial questions the incoming board chair should ask the CEO:

- Are there any major confrontations or events that you see surfacing in the next six months?
- In your opinion, what are the two priorities that I and the board can help you address?
- Are we going to merge with or acquire other health care entities?
- What's the status of the board, including term limits, board members leaving who need to be replaced, and potential board members in the pipeline?

The chairperson "has to think of the board as a living, breathing organism," says current CareGroup system (Boston) trustee and former Mount Auburn Hospital (Cambridge, Massachusetts) board chair F. Warren McFarlan. "The chair always needs to be thinking about where the next generation of leadership is coming from."

—J.K.

F. Warren McFarlan, professor of business administration at Harvard Business School, a trustee of CareGroup system in Boston, and former chair of Mount Auburn Hospital, Cambridge, Massachusetts, before it affiliated with that system, recommends that anyone who serves on a system board earn his or her stripes on a hospital board first. For example, system board members need political smarts and an understanding of how their institutions interact with state and local governments more than hospital trustees do. Health care systems tend to have more economic reach and clout at the state level than do solo hospitals, which gives them more chance of influencing legislation—but not without trustees who are willing and able to lobby lawmakers effectively.

Orientation Is Ongoing

An initial meeting or two should be the beginning, not the end, of orientation. The national health care landscape and local markets are constantly shifting, which in turn affects the failure or success of hospitals and health systems everywhere. So when boards sit down to either craft an orientation program for rookie trustees or to tweak an already existing curriculum, they should keep in mind that orientation works best as a process, not as a one-shot event.

Follow-through is the key. Utah trustee Robert Parsons bemoans the fact that his system hasn't always done a great job of following up with its newer board members. Although he chairs the strategic planning committee for the Urban South Region of Intermountain Health Care, which conducts orientation for new trustees, Parsons acknowledges that there is room for improvement in their process. After that initial meeting, "I don't think I've ever gone back, sat down with new trustees, and asked them how they were doing or what questions they have."

Having realized this, Parsons, who takes board education very seriously, now plans to be more conscientious about the follow-through aspect of orientation. After all, undergoing a thorough and effective orientation is more than half the battle of being a responsible trustee on any board.

The Governance Audit: Assessing and Improving the Board

By James E. Orlikoff
and Mary K. Totten

The post-Enron/AHERF backlash against ineffective, negligent, or fraudulent governance has led to new legislation and regulations designed to hold corporate boards to much greater standards of accountability, performance, and functional transparency. The Public Company Accounting Reform and Investor Protection Act of 2002 (also called the Sarbanes-Oxley Act) and the new Corporate Governance Standards of the New York Stock Exchange both impose standards and requirements on public boards to protect investors.

Although these laws and regulations will have almost no direct impact on boards of not-for-profit health care organizations, they will likely form the foundation of expectations and standards for them and establish the framework for future legislation and case law. Clearly, board scrutiny and the drive to enhance governance performance and accountability are gaining momentum.

Thus, boards of health care organizations would be wise to "get ahead of the curve" and to rigorously examine and improve all their

James E. Orlikoff is president of Orlikoff & Associates, Inc., Chicago. Mary K. Totten is president of Totten & Associates, Oak Park, Illinois.

activities. An effective way to do this is to conduct a comprehensive governance audit.

This audit should be a detailed and integrated review of the board's structure, processes, and function, with particular attention paid to those areas of highest liability exposure or risk of performance failure (see "Effective Governance After Enron and AHERF," *Trustee* Workbook 3, July/August 2002). A governance audit is much more focused and demanding than a traditional board self-evaluation, as it requires an unflinching willingness to ask difficult questions, examine challenging and highly charged strategic situations, and to "look under the rocks" to uncover and address problems. Further, a governance audit involves a detailed legal review of the board to determine if there are any areas of function, structure, or process that are inconsistent with legal or regulatory standards.

How a Governance Audit Can Help Your Board

Many boards may resist conducting a governance audit under the theory that it is better to "let sleeping dogs lie" or to not look for problems if everything seems to be working well. Yet the benefits of conducting such an audit far outweigh the excuses not to do one. According to Monte Dube, head of the health law practice for the law firm McDermott, Will & Emery in Chicago, the many valuable benefits for a board to conduct a governance audit include:

- Minimizing the risk of exposure to litigation and legal liability
- Minimizing the risk of financial or strategic damage to the organization
- Reducing the risk of regulatory sanctions
- Minimizing the risk of adverse publicity for the organization, thus avoiding embarrassment for trustees
- Proactively enhancing effective mission and corporate stewardship
- Helping the board to adopt best practices (as opposed to simply complying with minimum legal and regulatory requirements), thereby preventing the imposition of onerous regulatory requirements

When to Do a Governance Audit: Case Studies

A governance audit is beneficial for any board at any time. However, there are particular situations or circumstances when it may be immediately useful. According to Jeannie Frey, also of McDermott, Will & Emery, and Dube, there are several such situations, highlighted in bold type below.

Evaluating a Prospective Merger/Affiliation Partner. An audit of the governance structure, processes, and practices of one or both of the prospective affiliating parties can provide insight into potential clashes of governance culture, processes, and assumptions, as well as any problem areas that might affect the synergies desired by both parties.

Case Example: Hospital A and Hospital B have decided to create a two-hospital system to provide more cost-effective service to their community. The board of Hospital A has 30 members, many of whom have served for 15 or more years. The board has had the same chair for the past 10 years, and although he presides over every board meeting, the chief executive determines the meeting agendas and supporting materials, which are often delivered to board members a day or two before the meeting. The board meets monthly and has seven committees, each meeting at least monthly. Board meetings begin with dinner and often last late into the evening, with committee reports taking up most of the time. Little discussion occurs around agenda items, and deliberation and dissenting views are discouraged. Frequently, the board simply rubber-stamps management's recommendations in order to get through an agenda packed with reports and required votes.

Hospital B has an 11-member board. The chair, a well-known local business leader who has chaired many corporate and community boards, believes in strategic leadership. He works closely with the hospital CEO to develop each meeting agenda and to provide focused agenda materials that help brief the trustees about key issues and provide multiple courses of action for board discussion. The board meets monthly for two hours. Board decisions are made early in the meeting using a consent agenda; the majority of meeting time is spent deliberating one or two key strategic issues facing the hospital. Every trustee is expected to attend each meeting, prepared and ready to participate in discussion. Healthy debate and expression of diverse opinions and perspectives are encouraged.

The hospitals are considering the formation of one parent board, with half of the membership coming from each of the current hospital boards.

Questions for Discussion

1. How would you characterize the leadership style and governance culture of each hospital board? Which governance style and culture do you think would be most likely to generate liability or embarrassment? Why?
2. Which style and culture are likely to guide the new organization most effectively into the future? Why?
3. How could an understanding of how each organization is governed help the leaders of both organizations determine how best to move forward?

Distressed Health Care Provider. When a facility or system has fallen on hard times and faces possible insolvency, it should take a good look at the adequacy of its governance structure and processes for dealing with the difficult times ahead. Even strong boards will be challenged to balance the organization's responsibility for its mission and the need to ensure continued provision of care for the community with financial and business realities. A thorough review of board structure and function can help answer the following important questions.

Questions for Discussion

1. Does the board have a firm understanding of its fiduciary duties to its creditors—and what that means to the organization's mission?
2. Are the board's audit committee, internal and external audit functions, and financial operations up to the scrutiny of potentially hostile outsiders?
3. Has the board evaluated what kinds of decisions may need to be made by the outside directors, and is there a process in place for

those directors to obtain appropriate support from corporation staff and external advisors?

4. Should the board communicate the hospital's story to key stake-holders?

Public Hospitals. As government-sponsored institutions, public hospitals are subject to several additional levels of oversight compared with their private counterparts. Elected officials, the general public, and the press have greater access to information about public hospital operations and may hold such hospitals to higher standards than they do private facilities.

That's why a public hospital board must be acutely aware of its governance-related requirements, including conflict-of-interest standards and open meeting laws—whether mandated by statute, governing ordinance, or public expectation. In addition, a public hospital board should ensure that solid reporting mechanisms exist to alert it to potential operating problems, especially in finance and compliance.

Questions for Discussion

1. Has our board ever audited its structure and function to ensure that it complies with statutory and other governance requirements?
2. What reporting processes and mechanisms does our board have in place to ensure effective operational oversight?
3. To what extent have our board members been made aware during recruitment, orientation, ongoing board education, or other methods of the specific duties and responsibilities of serving on a public hospital board?

New Board Member Recruitment. It is no secret that good directors/ trustees are hard to find. Yet health care organizations have a critical need for a savvy, hard-working, and diverse board. A governance audit can be an invaluable recruiting tool, allowing prospective directors to get an accurate sense of board operations and culture. To the extent a governance audit reveals or results in the use of "best practices" in such important areas as audit committees, D&O insurance, indemnification, and use of independent directors, the governance audit report can be an effective marketing tool for wooing qualified, desirable board candidates. Further, it makes board membership more attractive to the potential trustee by suggesting that potential liability exposure or embarrassment has been minimized.

Questions for Discussion

1. To what extent do prospective board members understand our board structure and how it conducts its activities?
2. What questions do prospective board candidates ask about serving on our board? How do we address them?
3. To what extent is our board aware of governance best practices and how, if at all, do we incorporate them into our structure and function?
4. How might the results of a governance audit help improve our recruiting process?

Executive Searches. For organizations needing to fill key executive positions, such as the chief executive, chief financial officer, or chief operating officer, a governance audit can help recruiters better understand the organization's governance culture and practices, and thus identify candidates who either complement them or who bring needed skills to shore up weaknesses. A governance audit can also help prospective executives understand the organization they may join.

Case Example: A hospital has had three CEOs in five years, and the board is in the process of recruiting a new one. The most qualified candidates have requested independently that the board explain the reasons for the high CEO turnover rate, and several wish to examine the board's policies and practices. They have made it clear that they will not consider accepting the position unless these questions are answered.

Questions for Discussion

1. Are these requests for information appropriate?
2. How should the board respond to them?
3. Has our board experienced conflicts with previous executives that stemmed from differences in leadership styles or approach?

Could these have been minimized or avoided by providing them with a better understanding of how the board governs?

Donors and Grant Makers. In light of the recent governance and financial scandals and investigations in both the public and non-profit sectors, such as Enron, WorldCom, AHERF, United Way, Baptist Foundation, Allina Health, and Bishop Estate, donors and grant makers may be very interested in obtaining assurance that the organization they are funding is well managed and governed. Especially for any institution that has recently suffered "public relations nightmares," such as conflicts of interest, federal compliance investigations, or highly publicized incidents of poor care, a governance audit and implementation of practice standards can be used to win back key donors and grant makers and provide assurance that past problems will not recur.

Questions for Discussion

1. Have we lost grants or donations because of donor concern over the integrity of our organization's leadership and governance? What have we done to address this?
2. If our organization were to approach a potential donor or foundation, how would we assure them of our board's integrity?
3. Do we have mechanisms in place to ensure continuous board improvement?
4. It was recently reported that, except for health care organizations, philanthropy rose in 2001. Why do we think this happened? How might our board address this situation?

Patient Care Quality and Safety. Quality of care and patient safety top the list of concerns about our nation's health care. Therefore, board oversight of these areas has never been more important.

In the corporate world, investors and legislators are demanding greater financial transparency and accountability in the boardroom. The equivalent of financial transparency in the health care sector is quality. Health care boards are responsible for ensuring that all aspects of their organization's quality and patient safety are exemplary and, further, that all actions of the board and other leaders are in the best interests of patients and stakeholders.

Case Example: A hospital has the highest-level trauma unit designation possible in its state, one that requires certain specialist surgeons to be on-site 24 hours a day. Several months ago, two surgeons notified the hospital that they would no longer take trauma calls or be on-site during the early morning hours. This leaves the hospital's trauma unit with no on-site surgical coverage for several 12-hour periods each week. Yet the board wants to keep its current trauma unit designation, even though this coverage gap clearly disqualifies it.

Case Example: According to several medical staff leaders who have spoken to the hospital's board chair and CEO privately, one of the physicians on staff has serious quality problems. The medical staff refuses to take any formal action against this physician. An external review concludes that the physician is indeed consistently providing substandard care. Still, the medical staff will not recommend that any action be taken against the physician; on the other hand, they will not refer their patients to him or allow their family members to be treated by him. Several medical staff leaders have privately advised their friends on the board not to use this physician's services. Unfortunately, this problem physician is the only specialist at the hospital in his field and is a major contributor to the hospital's bottom line.

Questions for Discussion

1. What do these two cases have in common?
2. Who bears the ultimate responsibility to act in both situations?
3. To be true to the hospital's mission as well as to the best interests of patients and public safety, what should the board do in each situation?
4. If each board does not "do the right thing," what are the potential consequences for patient outcomes? For the board's liability exposure? For regulatory sanctions and community embarrassment?

Effective Boards Have Effective Social Systems

A recent review of governance and leadership practices in both thriving and failing organizations suggests that boards at both types of organizations do not always follow the conventional wisdom of good governance—that is, a lean structure, age and term limits for board members, few insiders on the board, the right mix of skills and talent, regular meeting attendance, and the like. (See "What Makes Great Boards Great," *Harvard Business Review,* September 2002). What does seem to distinguish high-performing boards is that they are effective social systems. In short, effective boards do the following:

- Operate with a high degree of trust and open, honest communication among members
- Encourage healthy debate and dissent
- Allow members to play a variety of roles and encourage them to develop and debate various courses of action before making decisions
- Ensure individual accountability
- Regularly evaluate both individual member and full-board performance

Thus, boards would do well to ensure that attention to governance structure supports and strengthens effective and robust governance communication.

Questions for Discussion

1. How many of these social characteristics of effective boards does your board consistently demonstrate?
2. Which ones does your board fail to demonstrate consistently? Why?
3. Does your board encourage respectful dissent?
4. Does your board have a culture that leads to the vast majority of votes being unanimous? If yes, why? Is this a problem? If not, why not?

Getting Started

If one or more of the scenarios or case studies described here sound familiar to you or depict a situation you could see developing for your board in the future, performing a governance audit should be one of your board's near-term goals. Conducting an audit and acting on its results can enhance trustees' confidence in the board's integrity and guide governance improvement.

Listed below are sample diagnostic questions developed by health care governance and leadership consultant Dennis D. Pointer for beginning a thorough governance audit:

1. Has our board formulated a set of specific trustee expectations?
2. At least every other year, does our board engage in a formal assessment of its performance and contributions and use the results to improve governance?
3. Has our board specified the competencies and capacities that all members must possess?
4. Does our board annually formulate a set of specific, quantifiable financial objectives for our organization?
5. At least quarterly, employing specific, quantitative indicators and standards, does our board assess how well the organization is meeting its quality objectives?
6. Are management "insiders" and medical staff members less than 40 percent of board membership?
7. Does our board have an audit committee and does it meet at least quarterly?
8. Does board policy prohibit our organization's audit firm from performing consulting work for our organization?
9. On average, is less than 40 percent of board meeting time spent listening passively to briefings and reports from management, the medical staff, or the board's own committees?
10. Does our board employ a formal system, with explicit criteria, for assessing the qualifications of potential members?
11. Does our board have a written work plan that details annual priorities?
12. Does our board review its fiduciary duties of loyalty and care before it discusses, deliberates, and votes on major issues, such as mergers, acquisitions, and disposition/transfer of significant assets?
13. If we are part of a system, does our parent board review the annual audits of its subsidiary organizations?
14. Does our board have a formal conflict-of-interest policy that requires directors to disclose any and all potential material conflicts of interest annually and refrain from discussing, deliberating, and voting on any issue in which they have a material conflict of interest?

15. Does our board have a formal and explicit plan for developing the capacity/competence of the board as a whole and the knowledge/skills of individual directors?

In addition to Pointer's recommended list of governance audit questions, consider applying the following New York Stock Exchange Corporate Governance Standards:

1. Does our board have an audit committee composed entirely of outside directors?
2. Does the sole responsibility for hiring and firing the independent external auditor rest with the audit committee or another committee (such as the finance committee) composed entirely of outside, objective board members?
3. Does our board and certain board committees meet in occasional executive session to discuss issues other than executive compensation?
4. Does our board have a policy that prohibits any outside board member from doing business with the organization?

Although these lists of questions are not meant to be exhaustive, they provide insight into the breadth and level of specificity a comprehensive audit should undertake.

Conclusion

Insurers, employers, regulators, and the courts have begun holding boards accountable to higher standards of behavior and performance and punishing those organizations with ineffective governance. A governance audit can help a board prepare for this new reality. When conducting an audit, the most important questions to ask are the ones that will generate the most discomfort. However, not asking such questions can be far more damaging to the board, the organization, patients, and the community.

For more information about conducting a governance audit, go to the American Governance & Leadership Group's Web site at www.americangovernance.com. You may also call AG&L Group at (909) 336-1586, or Monte Dube, McDermott, Will & Emery, at (312) 984-7549.

What Every Board Should Know

By Laurie Larson

Today's trustees no longer merely channel the knowledge of others—they must also be well versed in that knowledge themselves. This has become an increasingly daunting and complex task.

"Health care is changing so much. The days when board membership was a feather in your community cap are gone," says Charlie Ewell, chair of the Governance Institute in La Jolla, California. "Now, it's hard work. There are outside pressures from insurers and government; you have to bear down and take your responsibility more seriously." More stringent government regs and a tangled web of payer arrangements, mergers, acquisitions, MD partnerships, and other challenges all demand an increasingly sophisticated body of knowledge. What do trustees need to know, and how do they go about learning it?

Who Governs

Before these questions are answered, the students themselves must be evaluated. Who should be doing the learning?

Laurie Larson is *Trustee*'s staff writer.

"There has to be a high degree of alignment between why people are serving as board members and what they are being asked to do as a board . . . choosing the right people in the first place," says Richard Bogue, senior director of governance programs with the AHA's Division of Trustee and Community Leadership. Trustees should also be articulate, thoughtful, and reputable, and the board should represent the community, he says.

"Boards have to be broad thinkers," says consultant John Leech, trustee of Cleveland's Health Hill Hospital for Children. "They have to know what's going on in health care, and it's hard for lay people to know this. But they [lay people] also bring a community perspective . . . and may question things because they aren't so immersed [in hospital administration]. They need to be quick studies, people willing to be courageous enough to say, 'Let's rethink things.'"

"An effective organization requires an effective board," says Chicago consultant James E. Orlikoff. "No one can do this alone. The CEO needs the board as a strategic partner to be prepared to make quick strategic decisions." The nightmare scenario unfolds, he says, when a critically important strategic issue comes up and the board puts on the brakes if members don't understand the issue. The CEO winds up doing remedial education when immediate action is what's called for.

"The main advice I would give is that boards need to get education on the [board's regular] agenda and commit to it," says Leech, who consults with the Governance Institute and is president of Riverledge Health Consultants in Cleveland.

In-depth understanding is crucial for managing risk. Boards need to understand and know about physician relationships, technology, compliance and medical errors, measuring quality, the impact of the federal Balanced Budget Act, strategic planning, tackling negative community feeling toward hospitals. . . . The list goes on.

Trustees must also know their market, linking state and regional developments, such as Medicaid financing, to national trends, says Orlikoff. Otherwise, you will repeat mistakes. Realizing this, most hospitals seem willing to provide and pay for board education. "Governance education is much more accepted than it used to be," he adds. "Everybody recognizes the critical importance of having an educated board." He stresses the need to balance education on specific topics with larger trends.

Principles of Adult Learning

- Learning is most likely to occur when the material presented is clearly related to students' needs and problems.
- Learning comes from one's experience. Learning is most likely to occur when participants experience the results of a new behavior.
- Learning is unique and individual. Each student has personal ways of learning and refines these as a result of becoming exposed to others' methods.
- Every participant's experience prior to entering the learning setting is the most valuable resource this individual has to share.
- Learning is a process based on cooperation and sharing among individuals.

Significant Characteristics of Adult Learners

- Involvement in learning is more or less voluntary.
- Learning is often a secondary activity to participants' primary roles.
- Adult learners have a rich accumulation of experience.
- Readiness to learn is affected by how students see the subject's fitting in with their other roles.
- Time orientation tends to be more toward immediate usefulness and application.

Implications for Teachers of Adults

The instructor should create a setting that facilitates learning, including:

- An appropriate physical environment—good lighting, ventilation, room temperature, and seating
- A psychological climate of acceptance, respect, and collaboration
- A definite and consistent instructional style in course organization, presentation methods, and materials

Continued →

Four Keys to Effective Teaching

1. Treat students as adults—peer to peer, not authority to subordinate:

   - Recognize competing demands.
   - Use time well.
   - Make assignments significant, not busy work.
   - Have high expectations, but do not play power games.
   - Show respect; do not put students on the spot or embarrass them.

2. Develop an effective teaching style:

   - Know your subject well.
   - Be prepared; do not "wing" it.
   - Organize for clear transmission of information.
   - Try to minimize or eliminate distracting presentation habits.
   - Build on your natural style.

3. Demonstrate sincere interest:

   - Be approachable.
   - Recognize and respect individual differences and concerns.
   - Be enthusiastic about the subject and about teaching it.
   - Be available.

4. Involve participants in educational planning and execution where possible:

   - Consider scheduling preferences.
   - Use students' experience.
   - Provide alternatives and choices where appropriate.

Adapted and reprinted with permission from *Assets and Options: A Rural Grantsmanship Education Program,* edited by Mary Walker, program director.

And education should be continuous. "Governance education should be early and often," Orlikoff says. "CEOs may assume the board knows more than it does." Executives can't rely on the orientation or seminar a trustee attended years ago. "Health care is perhaps the most arcane, complex field in this country today."

"We used to spend our time on historical issues: how we did things relative to our budget or the results of adding new staff or equipment," Leech says. "Now the demand of board [education] is the future—and the mission statement is the guidepost. There is no place to look for answers right now, just lots of experiments out there."

"I think we're heading into a new generation of trusteeship with shrinking resources and pressures," says Jane Oehm, past chair of the AHA's Committee on Governance and trustee of Denver's Exempla Healthcare. "Working with the rest of the community to share the responsibility of providing care becomes urgent." This demands an understanding of community benefit, a sometimes nebulous topic for boards to wrap their collective heads around.

"'Healthy communities' is a buzzword," Leech says. "For not-for-profit community hospitals, there is the tension of existing to serve the public but not having the financial ability to do so." The same issue of maintaining their individual community responsibilities exists for not-for-profit hospitals and systems that merge with larger not-for-profits. Hospitals must examine the risks and rewards of individual mission versus merging with a larger not-for-profit, he says, by looking down the road at their long-term community benefit mission and goals.

Mission: An Ongoing Lesson

An understanding of mission should imbue all board education. "The mission of the organization may not change, but the vision and goals will," says Barry Bader, a governance consultant in Potomac, Maryland. "These must be revisited all the time to make sure you are hitting it right. Education for the year should be based on those goals."

Mission becomes more complicated and important as individual boards merge into larger systems. Leech receives many consulting requests from system boards asking for help in carrying out their mission effectively. "System boards are asking, 'Do we need all these [individual entity] boards, and, if so, what should each be responsible for?' You can keep all your boards for a while right after a merger, but eventually you have to form a system identity."

Bader says boards need to understand how their responsibilities and level of risk change as the organization evolves from a local hospital to a regional system. "It's systems thinking versus a representational governance philosophy. The evolution to a system means every subsidiary board should be making a unique contribution that does not duplicate other boards' work."

Leadership retreats are often a good educational tool to coordinate these goals. And education in and of itself can unify diverse boards, as Robert Parsons, education initiative leader for the AHA's Committee on Governance, can attest.

Parsons is a trustee of Utah Valley Regional Medical Center, Provo, which recently integrated with two other regional hospitals. "We go through perfunctory business first and then spend the rest of the meeting on an issue that affects us all, such as Y2K or our strategic plan," he says. "We are moving beyond individual hospitals to integrated systems thinking."

Education on a Grand Scale

What Parsons is learning, the Henry Ford Health System in Detroit has down to a science. "Our system is complex. We have 17 boards—but it's actually easier for a large system to educate [its boards]. There are more resources and broader talent," says Anita Watson, corporate vice president of governance. The system educates and coordinates policy through multiple channels. Every two weeks, Henry Ford's chief executive sends out a 10-page newsletter to all trustees, medical leaders, and executive staff. It gives the calendar of trustee meetings for the next four months, system information, and clippings of important journal and AHA articles. "Trustees love it," Watson says. "It really works for busy people."

An annual educational caucus is held in Detroit—a half-day, systemwide retreat that helps trustees, management, and senior executives get to know each other while providing education in breakout groups. Throughout the year, the system chooses quarterly policy reviews on specific topics prepared by the system's planning and marketing group. A handout that includes a survey of the topic, a speaker's outline, two questions to explore on the topic, and related readings, is mailed to all trustees in advance. All 17 boards then turn in the results of their discussion to the head office, and the summary results are mailed out. "Everything is multipronged," Watson says.

Finally, a systemwide orientation for all 30 to 40 new board members is held every spring, followed by local board orientation. This explains Henry Ford's integrated delivery system and its mission, managed care, competitor information, reimbursement, and revenue streams, and includes a glossary of terms and acronyms. "These procedures give the systemwide message to all," Watson says. "They work well and simplify the individual boards' responsibilities."

Starting off right with a solid orientation is too often overlooked, says the Governance Institute's Ewell. "We don't explain very well what people are supposed to do [as board members]. We should give better job descriptions up front."

"All education should be action oriented," Orlikoff says. "And make sure prospective trustees understand what you expect them to do beyond attending meetings, and explain specifically the number of hours you expect them to devote to education."

In addition to setting the right education example to trustees within the system, boards realize they need to demonstrate their hospital's commitment to self-improvement to both managed care companies and the Joint Commission (JCAHO). For the past eight years, JCAHO has required that all health care leaders know how to go through a self-evaluation.

"There is no set model, but we would look to see if [hospital executives] have a method and process for looking at performance improvement, such as patient satisfaction surveys and self-analysis," says Susie McBeth, associate director in JCAHO's standards department. "Boards should set this stage since they set mission, vision, and values. We look to see if the board made this a priority and if they were educated on performance improvement processes."

Leech assists hospitals with their JCAHO requirement by helping them design self-evaluations. Hospitals rate themselves in 11 areas, including quality of care, relation to the community, and staff-board relations. He meets with trustees to go over their aggregate responses, seeing where they match and vary.

"It gives a feeling of where they stand vis-à-vis each other and how they are changing," Leech says. "We share what other boards have learned so they can compare themselves." From the self-evaluation, trustees pick three to four topics to work on, which provides them an educational road map for the next six months. Then they must decide when they will learn.

Finding the Time to Learn

"Time is the biggest challenge for board members," Ewell says. For this reason, education is increasingly being built into regular board meetings—15 or 20 minutes for talk or a presentation. Accordingly, he sees more hospitals and health systems setting aside line items in their budget for board education and development, including retreats and conferences. To stay on top of this, Bader says, every one to two years the board should adapt its work plan to a correlated education plan.

"There is more and more to do in less time," says Mary Walker, executive director of the Texas Healthcare Trustees in Austin. "That's why we want to figure out more ways to take information to trustees." Walker's group has been around since 1961 and has a long tradition of providing educational opportunities and vital information to members. It holds two educational forums a year, one in the spring on a broad range of issues and one in the summer on a more focused topic. Starting this summer, an orientation for public hospital trustees will delve into governance issues specific to public hospitals. The group also offers a state governance manual, updated after every legislative session; a manual providing guidelines for meeting charity care and community benefit requirements; and a newsletter on state marketplace trends. Members join Texas Healthcare Trustees as full boards, so the whole group learns together.

Where an organization like this doesn't exist, Jane Oehm recommends the state hospital association's annual meeting as a good place to inexpensively gain education and interact with other trustees—a primary benefit trustees applauded in a recent AHA regional trustee symposium, co-organized by Oehm.

"Our evaluations showed that people found great value in talking to other trustees," she says. "They found that their problems were not unique and they could get practical solutions. That can happen with any trustee gathering." It seems to work especially well for rural boards, which often don't have the staff or money to cover travel expenses and absences.

What Trustees Want to Know

The AHA's Committee on Governance recently sponsored a fax-back survey asking trustees for the two most critical issues on their boards' agendas. The top four responses in rank order were:

1. Physician alliances/arrangements
2. Long-term strategic planning challenges (foreseeing future needs and directions)
3. Systems integration and network development
4. Strengthening community relationships

Orientation

A related survey explored the essential elements of effective new board member orientation. They included board member roles and responsibilities; mission, vision, and values; community context; organizational strategy and operations; and the health care environment.

Ongoing Board Education

The committee also identified its top five priorities for ongoing board education:

1. How can boards provide leadership by fostering partnerships aimed at creating effective healthy communities?
2. What is the board's role in restructuring itself and its hospital or health system through mergers, acquisitions, downsizing, medical staff relations, risk assessment, and providing services across the entire health care continuum?
3. How can boards best stay on top of understanding changes in the health care environment, such as Medicare reimbursement, coverage and access, and advocacy opportunities?
4. What are the effective roles for trustees with regard to ethics and compliance?
5. How can board members lead the organization to better focus priorities on high-quality patient and community-centered care?

Reprinted from the 1998 Annual Report of the AHA's Division of Trustee and Community Leadership.

Oehm suggests that all trustees in a particular geographic region gather for such information-sharing or have representatives from the state association come and meet with them. Those who attend can than present a report to educate their colleagues. Exempla's board also encourages its local trustees to subscribe to at least one educational publication relative to their work on the board that they can share with others.

Travel and time impediments make cyberspace one of the most likely next waves of trustee education, Watson and Walker agree. Walker points to the Healthcare Trustees of New York State who are bringing governance information into hospitals via the Internet. "No one can know everything all the time in a changing world," she says. "You can't ignore what's going on in health care. The changes will continue—we're not going back. You cannot be an effective trustee unless you try to keep up. Yesterday's knowledge does not solve today's questions." (For a compendium of educational resources, including books, videos, Web sites and organizations, go to *Trustee*'s Web site at www.trusteemag.com).

With such time and space constraints in mind, as well as a strong dedication to the cutting edge of education, Legacy Health System in Portland, Oregon, alternates its regular board meetings with every-other-month educational meetings. Educational meetings are held either at the corporate office or as on-site tours. For the past five years, these breakfast gatherings have given management and the board the chance to spend a solid 90 minutes on a topic, without any other business on the agenda.

"This in turn frees up business meetings to be conducted quickly, since the education meetings always allow time for roundtable discussions of whatever topics are on the trustees' minds," says John King, the AHA's immediate past chair and adviser to the Legacy board.

In addition, the board always takes a two-day spring retreat to begin strategic planning for the year, including joint board and CEO decisions on what educational topics will be covered. Recent sessions have covered compliance requirements, Y2K, and understanding how to facilitate understanding between physicians, hospitals, and managed care.

All about Docs

"Physician relationships are a complex area, particularly in times of economic stress," King says. "Boards need to be alert to the root causes of this stress. It's a challenge to the health care delivery system to understand the interface between doctors and hospitals." He recommends bringing in an outside "physician statesperson" to shed unbiased light on the issue.

Building and maintaining strong management and physician relationships is currently the number one issue at the Governance Institute. "Physicians and hospitals are joined at the hip. Everything that one does affects the other," Ewell says. Says Parson, "Trustees can provide a tempering role here. We represent community balance." Mergers have intensified these quality-of-care versus bottom-line issues, he says, and working out a successful physician–health system relationship is crucial to organizational health. Both sides have to make a conscious effort to meet and talk so that doctors can better understand the hospital's mission and administrators can understand how it is carried out on a daily basis.

To address this understanding, PMH Health Resources in Phoenix holds regular clinical overviews at board meetings, bringing in physicians to discuss patient–clinical activities. The interaction is excellent, says Reginald M. Ballantyne III, past AHA chair and president of PMH.

At PMH, the approach is interactive—management provides activities to educate boards and, in turn, listens to what board members bring to the table. "I'll submit that the more useful component is learning from the trustees, as representatives of the community," Ballantyne says. "We bring in others, but perhaps the best learning lab is this organization." A portion of every board meeting focuses on a specific topic around which management "is in a solid listening mode." At every meeting of all five of its boards, a PMH colleague speaks on a topic. For example, several managed care presidents sit on PMH boards and can speak to payment issues.

"The approach itself [to education] knocks down barriers," Ballantyne says. "Using our own people to educate on these areas enhances teamwork. We look to trustees to help us understand difficulties. We ask about their own businesses—what did they learn, how did they keep their cool in a difficult time. We use the benefits of learning from those in other businesses who have been down these roads before."

To Certify or Not to Certify

Analyzing these skills, many experts debate the merits of a formal certification process for trustees. The Governance Institute will soon begin offering board certification and education. Six conferences will be offered with certification at various levels depending on how many conferences trustees attend. Ewell thinks it should help with scrutiny from the Joint Commission, state attorneys general, and federal agencies.

"All other areas of health care have it," Orlikoff says. "As we see boards becoming more professional, certification will be a coming issue." Bader agrees. "Certification reflects the increasing demand for boards to be highly professional and well qualified for their work. It's a serious responsibility for a high-risk, competitive, complex yet values-based enterprise." But Bader cautions that certification has to truly advance the field, providing value that would not be there without it. "It should not turn into a moneymaking degree mill as in other fields."

Oehm is equally cautionary. "It would be good to certify trustees, but it must be set up carefully, with several educational bodies working together. You can't mandate certification."

King and Ballantyne take the opposite view. "We have peer review and recertification [to evaluate trustee performance], which seems to work," Ballantyne says. "I prefer that to another bureaucratic process that might present barriers."

"I don't see [certification] for this group," King says. "There is more to being a board member than being informed. Leadership and experience are as important as the content of education, and it's hard to certify leadership."

"Trustees should attempt to go to meetings for 'soft' certification, but nothing hard line," Parsons says. "If you've been asked to be a trustee, you have a responsibility to learn." And on that point at least, all agree.

"You need to look for board members who enjoy learning," Bogue says. "It's the only real reward today, because this is hard work." Bader says that education needs to be integrated into every board and committee meeting, retreats, and participation in outside boards as an investment. "Education is not an add-on to the work of the board. It is the work of the board to be a continuous learning organization."

PART THREE

Board-CEO Relations

Your CEO:
Are You Short-Staffed
or Shortsighted?

By Laurie Larson

Are you ready for yet another health care crisis? Truth or rumor—we're running out of hospital CEOs. You decide. "We are observing an impending leadership shortage at the CEO level," says Christopher Press, partner with Morgan Healthcare Consulting in Atlanta. "The argument is that there's not enough talent to promote and that people are burned out and leaving health care, but I'm a little bit of a contrarian—why is there a shortage?"

Larry Tyler, president of Tyler & Company, an Atlanta-based health care executive search firm, doesn't see a crisis, but he does see the CEO's job changing dramatically.

"This used to be an easy business, but now it's extremely complicated. There's a bigger pool—a larger percentage of people applying [to be CEO]—but the percentage of people who can do the job is smaller." That in and of itself constitutes a crisis to some experts.

"Yes, there's a crisis—it's [happening] now, and it will get worse," counters Carson Dye, partner with executive search firm Witt Kieffer in Toledo, Ohio. "Ten years ago we could present a list of eight to

---

Laurie Larson is *Trustee*'s staff writer.

ten candidates [to a client] versus two or three today. It's [now] taking us a month longer to fill CEO positions." The reason, he
believes, is a profound change over the past decade in a field that
maintained the status quo for 25 years, until the "empire building"
of the 1990s. Mergers and acquisitions, reimbursement riddles, and
managed care have reduced the raw numbers of qualified candidates, Dye says, as executives have either left the field from stress or
burnout or lacked the complex expertise needed for the new system. Others think that same stress has left the best men and women
still standing.

"In my opinion, there is no leadership crisis for the most part,"
says Arnie Kuypers, president of The Kuypers Company, a health
care executive search firm in Plano, Texas. Not as many CEOs are
leaving the field now as they did three or four years ago.

"I think most CEOs have adjusted—those who wanted out were
culled out," Kuypers says. "The bench strength is out there, but you
have to know what you are looking for." Health system CEOs are
actually managing revenue dollars more intelligently than CEOs in
other industries, he believes. But it remains a question of quality, not
quantity.

"It's the ability to find the right people who are capable,"
Kuypers says. CEOs today need broader skill sets, including an in-
depth knowledge of compliance, managed care, strategy, quality
mandates, and strategies of system and relationship building.

Broaden Your Search

Press thinks such a broad palette of skills should open the field to a
wider and less traditional range of candidates.

"Leadership is [being] too narrowly defined," he says. "In many
industries, a person will rotate through several key positions in the
organization, having learned the business from all sides. Health care
doesn't do that." A typical path for a CEO begins as a department
head, followed by becoming a vice president of operations, then
chief operating officer, and then CEO, he observes.

"A CEO's job is not operations; it's strategy, policy, relationships,
and finance," Press says. "When a business is as complex as health
care, wouldn't you want everyone to know each other's area of

business?" Through their performance appraisals, boards should motivate CEOs to encourage a wide range of applicants for all jobs within the hospital, he thinks. "People are a competitive asset," Press says. "You always want [employees] to know where their work comes from and where it goes, the impact of their work on others."

At Witt Kieffer, Dye sees more CEOs coming out of finance and patient care—there are currently 135 physician CEOs in the United States, he estimates, with more to come. "We will see more physicians ascend to these positions—lots of doctors are getting MBAs and MHAs [master's in health administration]—it's one of the fastest growing graduate program areas in the country."

The American College of Healthcare Executives, Chicago, has seen an "enormous growth" in physician members, and Dye thinks it's a good trend because physicians "know how to get things done at 3 A.M."

Financial and clinical experts make good candidates, Press agrees, but someone with a marketing or human resources background, for example, could also lead through innovation or by understanding employees.

The Making of a Health System CEO

Ron Hogan is one such success story. A trustee at St. Joseph's Health System in Atlanta since 1990, he became board chair in 1992 and CEO in 1995. He came to St. Joseph's after serving 27 years with Georgia-Pacific Corp., the last three as president and chief operating officer. His transition from one of the world's leading manufacturers of paper and building products to health care was unexpected but logical.

Health care costs were skyrocketing at Georgia-Pacific, and Hogan wanted to know why, so he sought an opportunity to become a health care trustee. He became chair as St. Joseph's was preparing for a potential merger. Suspecting their jobs might be sacrificed, the CEO and the chief operating and financial officer all found new positions. But the merger didn't happen, and Hogan was asked to step in as interim CEO while the board sought a replacement.

Catholic Health East, which owns St. Joseph's, then took a good look at its "temporary" leader, recently in charge of 60,000 employees at Georgia-Pacific and with five years of board experience—and asked Hogan to stay. His broad management background and a hands-on knowledge of volatility won him the job, he thinks.

"I have dealt with change throughout my career. The forest products industry has gone from a competitive to a regulatory industry, with government involvement in environmental issues versus reimbursement issues [and regulations] in health care," Hogan says.

The Search

Regardless of where candidates come from, however, the responsibility for finding the right one rests where it always has: with the board.

As a starting point, Dye thinks it's important that everyone who will be directly affected by the new CEO be consulted before the search begins. "Get consensus among board members up front," Dye says. "Make sure everyone agrees what the CEO should be."

Next, he thinks the defining question that boards should ask any candidate is, "Have you done this before?" and that question should be honed to immediate needs.

"Boards should ask themselves, 'Exactly what do we need done?' Within the first 12 to 15 months of a CEO's tenure, specific objectives should be set [and] achieved," Dye says. He gives the example of settling a dispute between surgeons who may leave and open their own ambulatory surgery center if the hospital can't negotiate with them. "Find the candidates who have faced your specific problems and solved them. The second test is chemistry and fit."

What that means to Dye, Kuypers, and other executive search experts is that CEOs are, and should be, still coming up through hospital operations.

"I've been asked to find candidates outside health care, but they don't get hired," Kuypers says. "You need that knowledge base. There's a credibility that managing assets gives you."

Count (and Keep) Your Blessings

But the best choice of all, they agree, is not having to find a new CEO in the first place. In other words, if you like the CEO you have, do whatever you can to keep him or her.

Dye predicts that over the next five years, more CEOs will retire than in the past 15. Boards need to ask themselves the blunt question: "How easily could our CEO leave, and what would we have to pay his successor if he left?"

"You have to pay competitively to really have the advantage," Kuypers says. "If you don't want to lose people, stay on top of compensation surveys and find out how much [executives] are being paid."

"You will always pay more for a new person . . . much more," Dye says. Pay raises and supplemental executive retirement plans (SERPs), which provide more pay at retirement if CEOs commit to a longer contract, make more sense, as does considering an internal candidate, who might be happy with less money than a new person for the opportunity to move up.

Whether or not your CEO tells you his or her future plans, Dye thinks that some simple demographics may be worth considering.

"If you have a CEO who's about 50 years old and has been there for five or six years, he is a prime person to leave," partly because of where he is in his career and partly because he may have children who have left for college, freeing him up to make changes, Dye says. A 40-something CEO of comparable tenure may be scooped up by a competitor as well, he says—the CEO is young and his or her children are ready for high school, another good transition time.

When a CEO wants to talk about retirement plans or giving the CFO or COO more responsibility, that may also be a signal of impending change, and boards need to pay attention, Dye advises.

Trustees should also keep an eye out for CEO burnout, as complex responsibilities and environmental pressures take their toll. "If your CEO is burned out, look at [giving the CEO] a sabbatical of six months to a year to recharge his or her batteries. Continuity of management is a key characteristic of successful organizations," Kuypers says.

To head off burnout at the pass, he recommends finding CEOs at the "right" stage of their career—a "grow-your-own-CEO" philosophy. The right candidate should come in ready to commit to the organization with an incentive to stay through compensation and SERPs.

A Marketing Perspective

A nontraditional leader of his organization for 13 years, Phil Newbold, CEO of Memorial Health System in South Bend, Indiana, has a bachelor's degree in mathematics, an MBA, and an MHA. Between the two advanced degrees, he thinks an MBA is the most valuable one today.

"There are so many financial pressures on CEOs now," Newbold says. "You need a broader and deeper background . . . not so 'hospitalcentric' as an MHA. Now we have more retail, partnerships, outsourcing—more intersections with non–health care principles."

Newbold's health care marketing background first led to a strategic planning position at Children's Hospital in Columbus, Ohio, then to the position of vice president of planning and marketing at Baptist Medical Center in Oklahoma City. From there, he became Memorial's CEO.

Newbold describes Memorial as "an organization on the move," noted for its tithing policy (10 percent of the hospital's annual bottom line after taxes is used for community partnerships) and "community plunges." (The October 1997 article "Up Close and Personal" can be accessed from *Trustee* archives at www.trusteemag.com.)

Newbold believes his greatest strengths are his customer orientation and his ability to differentiate Memorial's quality and services from other systems through "basic marketing principles." Customer service often means making sure that staff, particularly physicians, are getting what they need. In fact, he calls physician relationships "the key to getting ahead in health care."

Succession Is Job One

You also get ahead by planning ahead—that is, succession. Newbold thinks CEOs and boards should talk about their professional development goals as part of their annual evaluation. Kuypers believes succession planning "clearly should be written into the annual objectives for the CEO or it won't get done." Tyler agrees. "CEO selection is the most important thing a board does," he believes.

"Boards need to talk about succession once a year or so," Dye says. "They should ask the CEO: 'Are you going to go? Are you happy?' It really [takes] courage to put it on the table."

Potential internal successors should be trained over several years to gain the breadth and depth of experience they will need—and that candidate list should be short. Having too many potential successors doesn't give anyone the "opportunity to rise above," Kuypers says. "Key accountability can't be split up [among too many people]; it must be given to the heir apparent you have chosen." Choosing an internal candidate sends a great loyalty message to the organization as well, he adds.

Tyler recommends that heir apparents be watched with the following questions in mind: Do they accomplish their current job well? Have they accomplished the objectives they've set for themselves? How are they accomplishing them—is staff happy and do physicians have confidence in them? At each career milestone, these three questions should be asked again.

What Tomorrow's Leaders Need

Tyler thinks CEO flexibility and adaptability cannot be overemphasized in today's market. "It's virtually impossible to control anything anymore," he says. For this reason, CEOs need far better communication skills then before. They have to be better listeners and more careful writers because of instantaneous communication (e-mail). And they have to produce.

"There is a hardworking results orientation [in health care] now. You used to be able to take your time, but now you have to get things accomplished and have something to show immediately," Tyler says. "If you don't work on your short-term [financial goals], there will be no long term." And being quick on their feet may come more easily to executives from a less conservative field.

"I think one of the best things I brought to the job as CEO was not having any baggage from old payment systems and how things used to be done," former trustee Hogan says. "I was uninformed enough to ask questions others had been afraid to ask. Sometimes I'd get different answers than [had been given to CEOs] before as to why we do or don't do something." Putting people first has served him well, too. "How you treat and manage people is the most important [CEO] trait—your staff has to have faith in you."

"Until 15 years ago, hospitals were looking for managers. Now we want leaders," Tyler says. "The world is changing so fast; it's not enough to just go through the motions—you've got to be making something happen. We need someone who has a vision, an idea, and can execute it. CEO leaders will be measured by what they accomplish, not by their number of full-time employees." In addition, true leaders have an intangible quality, according to Newbold.

"Most leadership skills can be taught," Newbold says, "but you cannot change your personality. You're [either] a people person or you're not. Leaders of the future need a passion; they have to be energetic about something. They need a zest for innovation and creativity and a [belief that] it's not [too] expensive to take chances. It doesn't cost a thing to treat patients well and to develop trust."

Synergy in Motion:
The Board Chair
and CEO Relationship

*A High-Performance Organization
Needs a Winning Team*

By Elizabeth D. Becker-Reems

When you think about critical issues in health care, personal relationships usually aren't the first thing to spring to mind. But it is the "soft stuff" of relationships that can make the difference between a good health care organization and a great one. And the CEO–board chair relationship is one of the most significant.

Consider the situation at Mission St. Joseph's Health System (which was formed when Memorial Mission Hospital and St. Joseph's Hospital merged in 1998) in Asheville, North Carolina. Over the years, President and CEO Robert F. Burgin has seen the impact his relationship with various board chairs has had on board decisions and the organization's performance. Burgin recalls an instance early in his career when his chairman was president of a local technical college. As a new CEO, Burgin was eager to assert his authority and demonstrate his leadership ability. He saw his relationship with his chairman as necessary—but not critical, keeping him informed of critical decisions rather than directly involved in them.

Elizabeth D. Becker-Reems is the organization development consultant and Robert F. Burgin is president and CEO, Mission St. Joseph's Health System, Asheville, North Carolina. They can be reached at (828) 213-4867.

"Although we don't have a significant seasonal swing in our patient volumes," Burgin says, "we did experience a major decline in Medicare reimbursement in the fall of 1984 as a result of the [initiation of] DRGs. We had just hired a large number of new graduates from the technical college, and money was tight. Management decided to lay off some of these new graduates.

"I didn't realize the implications of this move on more than the bottom line," Burgin continues. "I saw it as strictly a financial decision. Well, it was much more than that—and I received and asked for little input from our seasoned board chair or from other trustees. I didn't fully consider the impact on future graduates, who would be hesitant to come work for us. We didn't anticipate the staffing pressure that would occur in the heavy-volume months of January, February, and March because of a decision I made in November. Instead of reducing cost, we incurred overtime and recruitment incentive expenses that could have been avoided if I had made a greater investment in my relationship with my chair and allowed myself to seek his advice and experience."

Get Started on the Right Foot

Not every board chair and CEO have the benefit of a long relationship before they start to work together. In 1986, the chair-elect at Memorial Mission withdrew at the last minute because of business pressures. A relatively new trustee, Garza Baldwin, head of the board's finance committee, was thrust into the position of chair. Baldwin worked in a small town about 30 miles from Asheville. He was not involved in the city's social life, and he and Burgin had had only limited contact before that time. Neither knew how their relationship would work, but both knew it was important.

At the same time, Burgin and his management team had determined that the hospital's emergency physicians' contract should be canceled because of performance problems. But Burgin wondered if he would have his board chair's support for this decision.

Fortunately, Baldwin turned out to be a strong chair, prepared to commit time and energy to his role and to his relationship with the CEO. He wanted to learn more about the intricacies of hospital operations and the medical staff's role in decision making. He also wanted to learn Burgin's strengths, weaknesses, and personality. The two moved from a superficial relationship to one in which both felt comfortable giving and receiving advice and counsel. Baldwin and Burgin worked with the chief of staff to address potential medical staff fallout over the ED decision, and Burgin learned the value of receiving guidance from his chair.

Former Memorial Mission chair Bill Boswell says, "As your turn to become board chair approaches, you get a sense of whether you will be able to relate well with the CEO, and somehow that sense [influences] the rest of the relationship. If you believe your relationship will only be neutral, it is difficult to generate the commitment and energy to make it truly effective. It doesn't take long to form an impression, and it can be a blessing or a barrier to your relationship." Boswell believes that taking early ownership of the development, growth, and maintenance of the relationship is the key. "Its effectiveness will have a long-term impact on the organization and on the CEO's future," he says.

Work from the Outside In

It's easier to start building the structural elements of a CEO-chair relationship before trying to develop a personal one. Burgin shares this story:

> I was somewhat hesitant in my initial meetings with the new chair, Bill Boswell, not fully sharing my thoughts and ideas. I respected him and believed he respected me, but we were relative strangers. Boswell was a strong manager and comfortable taking decisive leadership action. I knew that in a short time he would be evaluating my performance and would not hesitate to speak his mind. I had to ensure that his orientation and exposure to the hospital and to me was comprehensive. We started to structure more frequent communication and build a deeper understanding of our roles. In just a few months, I was as comfortable working with him as I had been with others whom I had known much longer.

The four basic strategies for working from the outside in require both parties to clarify roles, structure time together, share information, and build a shared perspective.

Clarify Roles

Regardless of past experience or the orientation you receive as trustee or board chair, an in-depth exploration and agreement on roles is critical from the start. When the nurses go on strike, for example, whom should the newspaper call? When the ED doctors require a new contract, with whom do they negotiate? When the CEO is out of town, who makes critical decisions? Current Mission St. Joseph board chair Charles D. Owen III explains how that clarity helped him once when he first became chair:

> A community member contacted me about a potential racial discrimination problem at the hospital. This person wanted to discuss the situation with me and share details so that I could more fully understand what had happened. I felt a conflict because I represent the community but am also an advocate for the hospital. Fortunately, Bob [Burgin] and I had already spent time clarifying our roles, and I knew that I had to place this problem in his domain. That initial discussion kept me from making a mistake and from encroaching on what is more appropriately handled by the CEO and vice president for human resources.

To initiate a role clarification conversation, start by asking the CEO for a job description for the two of you. It will serve as a springboard for that in-depth discussion. Job descriptions give a good, but sparse, description of the chair's responsibilities; they do, however, serve as a catalyst and starting point for your discussion, and they can be changed. Part of clarifying the chair's role while enhancing the relationship-building process includes grooming future board leaders; coaching, mentoring, and evaluating the CEO; managing board composition; and managing policy, not operations.

The role clarification process sets the stage for how the chair and CEO will work together. The discussion should be enriched with the history, experience, and perspectives that both bring to their role of the organization's leaders.

Owen describes a trip that he and Burgin took right before Owen became chair. "We went to a meeting for board chairs and CEOs. The meeting was excellent, and the networking was very beneficial to both Bob and me. But the benefits that stay with me were the out-of-meeting conversations that Bob and I had about our thoughts and perspectives on operations, policy, and how we would work as a team.

"The forced togetherness of the trip—sitting side-by-side on the plane, meeting early for breakfast, and sitting together in the evening to talk over the events of the day and to discuss how we would work together—was the beginning of a deep and trusting relationship."

Owen remembers that conversations about the conference moved into pertinent issues at Mission St. Joseph's. "Both Bob and I talked about our perspectives and learned where we agreed and where we differed. We weren't under the stress of needing an instant decision but were able to explore our differences and share the experiences that brought us to the beliefs we hold."

Structure Time Together

Both the CEO and the chair have a full life and responsibilities. Most likely, they both work from seven in the morning until seven in the evening and then have family and community responsibilities

---

Relationship Assessment

How can you tell if you have a high-performance relationship with your CEO? Ask yourself how many of the following statements apply to both of you.

1. We have taken time to get to know one another on a personal level.
2. We check on the relationship and occasionally ask each other how we are doing.
3. We take time to discuss difficult issues and are open about our thoughts and feelings.
4. We have attended educational programs together away from the hospital.
5. We accept each other's idiosyncrasies.
6. We are clear about our roles and responsibilities.
7. I routinely hear from the CEO several times a week and always in advance of a difficult or potentially explosive hospital issue.
8. We let each other know when we have done something that was "out of line."
9. We respect each other, including our differences, and our perspectives.
10. We forge ahead to resolve problems, even when the solutions are uncomfortable to implement.

---

after that. Neither has time to spare unless there are urgent issues to address. They could decide to spend time together only right before the monthly board meeting, making sure they plan the agenda and anticipate the group dynamics. But that is not the way to build a strong relationship.

How much time is the right amount? Early in the relationship it would be helpful to travel together to a meeting like the one that Owen and Burgin took. This forced time together helps ease barriers that exist just because neither person knows the other well. As an ongoing practice, it helps to meet a minimum of one to two hours every week. Take advantage of available time before or after a committee meeting for a quick update or input. This gives both the chair and the CEO time to discuss issues facing the hospital, time to build a shared perspective on those issues, and time to develop strategies for addressing them. In addition, the two may find time to trade personal stories that will build a friendship, such as how they spent the weekend and a sports event they watched, or to update one another on personal matters, such as the great performance on the volleyball court by a son or daughter.

If you don't think you can invest all this time in your relationship, what can happen? For one thing, the CEO may start handling issues and developing strategies that you see as your responsibility or on which you can't agree. Burgin recalls past board chairs who were extremely busy in their full-time jobs and/or lived out of town. He took a much greater role in the organization because these chairs weren't available or involved.

If, as chair, you're not in touch or involved, you may discover that you are questioning your CEO's loyalty when you hear gossip in the community or are called by a physician who is bringing you information "for your own good." If you begin asking yourself, "What is my CEO up to?" you are experiencing the first signs of distrust, and it is important to begin spending more time together.

Share Information

One of the cornerstones of a high-performance relationship is sharing information. It could be as simple as letting the CEO know something that you overheard at a cocktail party or as complex as trying to describe why half the board will likely oppose the CEO's recommendation for an organizational strategy or direction. The more open and honest you are as chairman, the more likely the CEO will follow suit. It's also important to openly acknowledge your regret about an action you took or a mistake you made. This gives the CEO permission to admit mistakes and insecurities also.

Build a Shared Perspective

The board chair and the CEO need to develop a shared perspective about what constitutes a serious situation at the hospital. For instance, not having enough beds to accommodate inpatients can seem to be a boon—business is great; we are full! However, there may be long-term negative effects. For example, disgruntled physicians who can't admit their patients to the hospital may admit them elsewhere. Nursing staff who are burned out from the unrelenting stress of caring for more patients than they can reasonably handle may start to leave. These potential repercussions would not be apparent to someone outside health care. Building a shared understanding of the implications of situations, organizational systems, and trends provides a framework for future discussions and decisions.

Working on the Inside

If you have addressed role clarity, set aside time to communicate, shared information, and developed a shared perspective on what matters, you are ready to work on sustaining and deepening your relationship. You can feel your spirit or soul expand when you are involved in this deepening relationship. Those elements that reflect a deeper relationship include compassion, mutual growth, integrity, and courage.

Compassion

Compassion is a heightened sensitivity and understanding of what other persons are experiencing, true empathy for their situation, and caring. In a purely surface relationship, compassion may never be called upon or offered. It is one of the benefits of a strong relationship, and when it occurs, opens the door to deeper levels of communication and understanding.

Within the organization, the CEO has few, if any, people in whom he or she can truly confide. Most everyone has a vested interest in the outcome of a decision or situation. For example, at one time Burgin was agonizing over what to do about a key staff member whom he admired and respected but who was unable to effectively function with peers and medical staff. Burgin needed a nonjudgmental ear, someone who could really listen and appreciate the importance of the decision that he was considering and the agony he was suffering. The board chair was available and really listened. He asked a few helpful questions that clarified the issue for Burgin. And that was all he had to do—just be there and listen.

Mutual Growth

As the dialogue between the chair and CEO deepens, both have enhanced opportunities to learn. The degree of information, background, and experience that they share increases, as does their openness to new ideas and new perspectives.

For example, the local newspaper gave Mission St. Joseph's advance warning about a letter to the editor that was to appear. The letter was derogatory and signed by someone Burgin knew. His first reaction was to call the paper, explain the erroneous assumptions, and give facts and figures to prove the errors. But having been in a similar situation before, the board chair suggested a different approach. He recommended arranging a face-to-face meeting with the letter writer, holding back any rebuttal and just opening up to the writer's concerns.

The chair explained why he thought this approach might work better and shared his prior experience. Burgin followed the advice and gained new insight from both the chair and the letter writer.

Integrity

One element of integrity is to be able to depend on congruence between someone's words and actions. If the CEO says he will be at certain place at a certain time, he is there. If the chair says, "I will support you on this," he does not back down. No one easily forgives a breach of trust. For instance, if the CEO discovers that the board chair has openly derided him in the community, the two will never develop a deep relationship. If the chair discovers that the CEO is trying to manipulate the chair's opinion, trust will never deepen.

Over time, when both the chair and CEO recognize that they can depend on each other, the level of the relationship deepens.

Courage

Both the chair and the CEO need to feel comfortable giving each other constructive criticism. This means taking a chance that you are telling the other person something he or she may not enjoy hearing. But giving constructive feedback does not put a good relationship at risk; it deepens it.

CEO Burgin recalls the time when a small but influential group of physicians was determined to end his tenure with the organization. This was during the first year of the joint operating agreement between Mission Hospital and St. Joseph's. Once a full merger was completed, it would effectively eliminate the competition between the two hospitals and abolish the opportunities physicians had to play off one hospital against the other. Burgin's inclination was to dig in his heels and explain why he was not at fault for reducing their opportunities to play one hospital against another. The chair and chair-elect met individually with Burgin and suggested a different approach. He listened, took a deep breath, and agreed to follow their advice. Burgin met with the physicians and accepted responsibility for any perceived problems that had occurred as a result of the joint operating agreement. He apologized for any of his behaviors that had made them feel he was ignoring their input, and he pledged to be more inclusive in all decisions about clinical operations. It took courage for the chair and chair-elect to be honest and persistent and for the CEO to listen to their criticism and change his behavior as a result.

Barriers to High-Performance Relationships

Three frequent, but not insurmountable, barriers to building a high-performance relationship are a prior poor relationship, sabotage, and time.

Prior Poor Relationship

If you had difficulties, hard words, or an outright bad relationship with the CEO before you became chair, you have some work to do to move the relationship to a new level. Although it's true that the CEO would not willingly allow the selection of a chair with whom he or she had previously had a bad relationship, circumstances may propel someone who does not have the CEO's full endorsement into that position. Slow and planned evolution to the chairmanship is not always possible.

One of the best techniques to resolve a prior poor relationship is to bring problems into the open and talk about them. Not talking about past problems allows them to fester and erode any progress you might otherwise make in building a relationship. But don't rehash problems to prove who was right. The best tactic is to acknowledge that problems occurred, that you regret they may have caused hard feelings, and that you would like to put them behind you. This tactic can close the door on the past and give both the chair and CEO a transition to a new relationship.

Sabotage

A trustee, physician, someone in the community, or an employee may seek to undermine the existing CEO or chair. Although this person may have a legitimate complaint, it doesn't help to go behind the other's back to resolve the problem. This can undermine the leadership and governance process. If both the chair and the CEO expect and require face-to-face problem solving, it is hard for anyone to succeed in underhanded behavior.

Former Mission St. Joseph's chair Jack Stevens remembers the power struggles that occurred during the merger between Memorial Mission and St. Joseph's. "During the period under the operating agreement and prior to the merger, I and other board members became aware of challenges to Bob Burgin's continued leadership from certain medical staff members and the St. Joseph's leadership. I could see the effort to undermine Bob and to change our perception of him as a highly competent leader. There were occasions when I and a select group had to meet with individuals and groups to hear their perspectives about the future of the organization and Burgin's continued role."

Stevens remembers that these discussions were uncomfortable, and that they were held without Burgin. "I made sure to keep Bob informed of what was happening, with whom we were meeting, and what the tenor and outcome of the discussions were. I don't believe he ever felt that I was working behind his back. He was fully aware of the power struggle that was going on during that period."

Time

If the chair and CEO cannot spend time together, they will not be able to effectively build a relationship. When a CEO and board chair first meet to establish how they will communicate and how much time they need to spend together, it may be an eye-opener for both—but it is absolutely essential.

There is no question that not all CEOs and board chairs will have the type of relationship that creates performance at the level of championship teams. However, by investing time, clarifying roles, and exhibiting compassion, integrity, and courage, an improved relationship is possible. This relationship is critical—not just to the CEO and the chair but to the entire organization and community.

Side by Side: Communication Is Key to a Successful CEO– Board Chair Partnership

By Jan Greene

When Margaret Sabin became CEO of Marin General Hospital in Greenbrae, California, she knew she'd have her hands full. An ugly legal dispute over control of the hospital had been resolved shortly before she started there in early 2000, so she understood she'd be working in a fishbowl. When she decided the hospital should take a $9 million write-down (i.e., an adjustment to past financial statements) to institute a more conservative accounting stance on accounts receivable, she knew she might be inviting criticism. Most worrisome was that it might look as if she were publicly denouncing the board's financial oversight during the previous three years.

So she turned to businesswoman Etta Allen, who chairs the hospital board. "When I called her, I told her, 'Etta, I have terribly mixed feelings about this,'" Sabin recalls. "My gut tells me it's better for us to be as conservative as we can be, but I don't want to make it look like I'm reversing decisions of the last three years."

After having worked together for a year, Sabin and Allen forged a good working relationship, finding that they both like honesty, open communication, and brevity. Presented with Sabin's dilemma,

---

Jan Greene is a writer based in Alameda, California.

Allen was supportive. "Etta said, 'You know, Margaret, it's a new day and it's a new way of looking at this, and we, the board, can support this.'"

Of course, that support didn't come overnight. In fact, the write-down issue was hashed out over five of the board's finance committee meetings and three meetings of the full board. "I give [Etta] credit for the board coming to the conclusion that it was the right thing to do, that it was just a different way of doing things with new leadership," Sabin says. And Allen gives the chief executive kudos, explaining that the board was able to resolve the issue in large part because of Sabin's "openness."

Sabin knows that getting that potentially explosive issue approved by the full board was a step-by-step process. And the first step was to nurture her relationship with Allen. "As health care gets more challenging . . . it really is critical that the CEO and board chair have the ability to connect," Sabin says.

Governance consultants and other successful CEO–board chair pairs agree. Because a chief executive and board leader may work closely together for just a couple of years, it's critical that the two establish good communication patterns early. "We decided right away we needed to meet every month," says Tom Strauss, CEO of Summa Health System in Akron, Ohio. "And we have discussions on an as-needed basis about what's happening." Those early conversations should also establish a partnership.

Openness and Honesty Are the Best Policies

"The best relationships I've seen are mutually supportive . . . where [the CEO and board chair] have a very open line of communication," says Mary Totten, president of Totten & Associates, Oak Park, Illinois. "The chief executive will use the board chair as a sounding board, looking for chances to think together and plan together."

Exactly how hospital leaders communicate can differ, however, depending on their management styles and personalities.

For instance, Sabin and Allen have face-to-face meetings when a particular issue needs their attention. But much of their work together is conducted during brief phone calls. "It doesn't have to consume a ton of time," says Sabin. "After five minutes Etta will say, 'OK, there we are. Have a nice day.' And I'll ask, 'How did we get that done so quickly?'"

Allen says she appreciates that Sabin is secure enough to share both good and bad news with her. "We both have this openness about us, so it's easy to pick up the phone and chat," she says. "We both express our opinions openly without any concern about [the potential to offend] each other."

Thaine Michie, board chair of Poudre Valley Health System in Fort Collins, Colorado, shares a similarly open relationship with the hospital's CEO, Rulon Stacey. "Rulon and I have a pact: there are no secrets between us," Michie says. "Rulon needs honest feedback

---

What the Board Chair
Should Be Asking the CEO

1. How does our organization define quality, and what indicators should the board receive to monitor whether we're achieving our objectives?
2. Do we promote a "blameless culture" throughout the organization when it comes to reporting medical errors and near misses?
3. What are the organization's objectives for return on investment for our invested funds, and how can the board track them?
4. How satisfied are physicians with our strategic direction? What part do they play in helping us set that direction?
5. How do our corporate compliance policies and procedures function? What system do we have in place to ensure consistent and seamless compliance throughout the organization?
6. How sound is our organizational culture? What indicators should we use to measure our success in building a strong, cooperative, collaborative culture at every level?
7. What methods should we use to measure and report progress in achieving our strategic objectives and vision?
8. How does our audit committee function? What changes, if any, should be made in this area in light of the recent Enron developments?
9. How do we define a "healthy community," and what is our role in creating one? What indicators should we use to define success in this area?

Source: Larry W. Walker, The Walker Company, Lake Oswego, Oregon

because he might be doing something that upsets someone. He has to have someone he knows will tell him what's going on."

Stacey says he's careful to keep both Michie and the whole board aware of issues as they come up. He sends e-mails and faxes to board members 5 to 10 times a month "so they're not caught off guard," he explains.

Successful pairs report that they keep one another informed about everything they believe may be pertinent to the hospital's future. Smart CEOs use the board chair as an advisor with a valuable outside perspective and a community connection.

"I've seen the strongest and most effective CEOs willingly seek help from the board in general and view the board chair as the one person they can talk to and confide in," says Ed Kazemek, governance consultant and CEO of Accord Limited in Chicago. "That may be harder to do with members of your senior executive team. With the board chair, [CEOs] don't have to worry about information leaking out."

Some chief executives and board chairs see their partnership as more than a business arrangement. "We just nurtured it like any other relationship," says Ann Brennan, chair of the Summa Health System board of directors. She works with president and CEO Tom Strauss. "I will always count on him as a friend. And I will always be available to be a counselor or a sounding board."

Strauss and Brennan have a standing monthly meeting with each other before the system board meeting and talk more extensively on an as-needed basis. It helps that they like each other. "We enjoy each other's company," Strauss says. He even stayed with Brennan and her husband in their Florida home when the two attended a governance educational conference. "That was very positive. I got to know her husband. He and I golfed together. I can't do that with Ann because she doesn't golf," he adds with a laugh.

Actually, doing business in a relaxed setting such as the ninth tee isn't a bad idea for CEOs and their board chairs, advises Errol Biggs, director of the Center for Health Administration, University of Colorado, Denver, and coauthor of *Practical Governance* (ACHE Management Series, 2001). "If the two happen to play golf, that works out very well," he says. "Or if they're having dinner together, it makes it easy to cover the key issues."

Communication is clearly one key to success. Another is knowing where the CEO's job ends and the board's responsibility begins.

The Partners' Profiles

Marin General Hospital, Greenbrae, California

One of 27 hospitals affiliated with Sacramento-based Sutter Health System; 235 beds

Margaret Sabin, CEO since July 2000; former CEO of two hospitals in Colorado

> Favorite thing about her partner: "She's got the ability to take a [board member] who has a head of steam about something and suddenly have him come around."

Etta Allen, board chair for five years, active in the community and owner of a heating and sheet metal company

> Favorite thing about her partner: "She's very inclusive of everyone in the organization. It's a pleasure to walk through the hallways with Margaret because she knows just about everyone by first name."

Summa Health System, Akron, Ohio

An integrated health care system, including two hospitals and a health plan

Tom Strauss, CEO since January 2000; took over from a CEO who held the position for 25 years

> Favorite thing about his partner: "We both have strong personalities. But she does a great job of holding back her comments until the board can consider an issue."

Ann Brennan, board chair since January 2000; longtime board member; active in the community

> Favorite thing about her partner: "He's an extremely likable person, and his values are the same as mine. He is truly dedicated to Summa Health System achieving world-class status."

Continued →

Poudre Valley Health System, Fort Collins, Colorado
A 235-bed hospital in a growing area; affiliations with many rural hospitals in nearby states

Rulon Stacey, president and CEO since 1997; the system's fifth CEO in four years

> Favorite thing about his partner: "He gives me a lot of autonomy."

Thaine Michie, board chair since 2000; retired electric utility executive

> Favorite thing about his partner: "We're both pretty open and honest people. I don't know anything he doesn't know, and he doesn't know anything I don't know."

St. Mary's/Duluth Clinic Health System, Duluth, Minnesota
A three-hospital Catholic system and a multispecialty clinic that merged in 1997

Peter Person, M.D., CEO since the 1997 merger; ran the clinic before the merger and took on the top job afterward

> Favorite thing about his partner: "I'm lucky to have someone who understands health care so well."

Sister Kathleen Hofer, board chair; St. Mary's CEO for 16 years before the merger

> Favorite thing about her partner: "There has been a complete openness with sharing information."

—J.G.

Know Your Job

"One of the things that has made this [relationship] unique and workable is that we know our roles very well," says Marin board chair Allen. "The board carries out a policymaking role . . . but the day-to-day management of the hospital is certainly in Margaret's realm."

Board leaders say they often use common sense to decide how to draw the line between operational and strategic issues. "We talk about how we could improve our market share," says Summa's Ann Brennan. "Not the nuts and bolts of 'Are we going to cut four nurses here or do something with the laundry?'"

At St. Mary's Duluth (Minnesota) Clinic Health System, board chair Sister Kathleen Hofer says board members don't have too

---

Role Adjustment

If anyone really understands the difference between being a chief executive and being a board chair, it's Sister Kathleen Hofer. She's been in both roles as a result of a 1997 merger between St. Mary's Medical Center, Duluth, Minnesota, and the large, multi-specialty Duluth Clinic. She went from a 16-year career as CEO of St. Mary's to serving as "active" board chair of the merged entity, which meant working nearly full-time to help the physician who ran the clinic take over as system chief executive.

The situation could have been very difficult for everyone. "You've got the potential for real fireworks," says Ed Kazemek, CEO of ACCORD, Ltd., Chicago, who works with the health system. "They both had to go through significant changes."

Sister Kathleen acknowledges the transition took a lot of effort. "I worked really hard at it," she says in retrospect. She used her strong belief in communication to work things out with the new CEO, Peter Person, M.D. "Initially, we worked together a lot as we were getting this new organization off the ground," she says. Now they meet for a couple of hours every Thursday morning.

As board chair, Sister Kathleen had to shift her focus from running the day-to-day operations of the hospital and "think a little more globally," she says. "I'm having to look at the much broader picture and at how decisions may have an impact on things over the long term."

Continued →

much trouble sticking with big-picture issues, in part because there's so much to know. "The best possible situation is to have the board as highly informed as it can possibly be," she says. "Some say they'll just get involved in operations. That's possible, but we can tell the difference. Besides, the lay people feel they're never as informed as they want to be. It's just too complex."

When board members start to wander into the CEO's domain, the results can be disastrous. "The worst position a CEO can get into is having a board get into micromanaging," says Sabin. "It can take a good CEO and neuter his or her ability [to run the hospital]. When that happens the CEO really needs to go, because it's hard to bring that relationship back."

For his part, Dr. Person says he's benefited from Sister Kathleen's experience running the hospital. "We really have, over the last five years, developed a high degree of trust. We also know how each other thinks, which allows us to have open communication and prevents what I see so often, which is a lack of communication, which leads to distrust, which leads to dysfunction."

He's careful to be as open with information as possible to maintain trust. "If there's an area she's really interested in from an operational perspective, we talk as deeply as we need to rather than trying to compartmentalize ourselves in our roles," he says. "The more often you do that, the more confidence grows in decision making and trust about it, and the stronger ally I have in the board chair when we run into difficult issues."

At the same time, they have to be clear with the staff about who's running the operation. "If the culture in the past was for people to stop by her office, she has to refer them to me," Person says.

The pair has developed a joint vision for the hospital, which keeps physicians and employees from trying to use one against the other. "Because we were very committed to this common vision, there were no possibilities of an end run," Person says.

Kazemek has watched Dr. Person's and Sister Kathleen's relationship grow over five years. "From my vantage point, they have a really healthy board chair–CEO relationship. They are both very respectful of one another's opinions."

—J.G.

To avoid such a fate, organizations should strongly consider having roles and responsibilities in writing. Summa Health System, for instance, already has a job description for the chief executive. Now it has a governance committee of the board working on job descriptions for the board chair and trustees to help future members step into their roles more easily. The board also conducts a yearly self-assessment. "We're trying to move this whole self-governance to a more efficient process," says CEO Strauss.

Putting it all down in writing can help draw "that fine line between strategic leadership and operational leadership," notes Lake Oswego, Oregon, governance consultant Larry Walker, president of The Walker Company. "Often these things are taken for granted in smaller organizations. It's often handled in a very informal way. But a formal, written set of roles and responsibilities" would help prevent either the board or the CEO from encroaching on the other's responsibilities, he recommends.

The CEO can take the lead in defining those roles by providing the board with appropriate educational information. Such information should include top-level summaries of major issues, such as finance, compliance, and strategic alliances. But it's important to strike the right balance—by providing too much detail, management runs the risk of either drawing trustees too far into operational issues or overwhelming them with information they simply won't have time to digest.

Walker says board members who have a lot of business expertise may ask operations-related questions, particularly if they're not being fed a regular diet of good strategic information. He defines that as "What does the board need to know to meet the challenges of the next few months?"

But information alone is not enough. Trustees must also be able to trust the information they're given, notes Van Johnson, CEO of the Sutter Health System in northern California, of which Marin General is an affiliate. When board members stray into micromanagement, "it's usually the result of discomfort with the CEO or with individuals who are providing the information," says Johnson, whose organization includes 27 hospitals, each with its own board, plus a number of system-level boards. "In some cases I get more concerned about the board becoming complacent and not asking the questions it needs to ask."

Errol Biggs suggests that boards should be asking the following kinds of questions:

- How will our organization survive in the evolving marketplace?
- What kinds of alliances or mergers should we consider?
- Are there joint ventures with physicians we should consider?
- How are we maintaining good relations with physicians, and how could we improve them?
- Do we have the right physician mix on staff?

Looking Ahead

After putting all this effort into forging a good working relationship, it can be hard on a CEO when it's time for the board chair to step down. But in most cases, consultants agree, it's important to let new blood in and reduce the chance that the chief executive and board chair will be seen as holding on to power for too long. That's fine with Poudre Valley's Michie. "It's not healthy for me to get too close to [CEO] Rulon [Stacey] and be chair for too long," he says. "Besides, after you've been chair, you're a better board member."

Occasionally, though, the rules need to be broken. For instance, the Marin General board decided to give Allen an extra three-year term as chairperson to maintain momentum on a touchy political situation that was finally improving just as her first term ended.

When the board chair changes, the CEO has to adjust to a new person and a new relationship. For instance, Margaret Sabin already knows who is in line to succeed Etta Allen and that they are likely to have more structured communication. "With that individual I will have a set meeting and an agenda, I can tell," says Sabin, "and I will have to modify myself." But that's part of her job, she acknowledges. "I don't think a CEO in this day and age can dictate how the board chair will relate to the CEO. The CEO has got to select a communication style that the board chair is most comfortable with."

Summa's Strauss reluctantly accepts that his partner, Anne Brennan, will step down at some point. "We're really just now beginning to hit the groove," he says. "The good news for us is that [former board chairs] stay involved. Our last board chair is still on the board and chairs the nominating committee. I still call upon him. I'm sure Ann will be there as well."

Count to Ten: Board and CEO Frustrations

By Edward A. Kazemek

After more than 20 years' experience consulting with hundreds of health care boards and CEOs, it never ceases to amaze me that trustees and CEOs continue to complain about the same relationship issues. Furthermore, these complaints are usually shared with me privately and rarely brought into the open, which probably explains why the same issues continue to be a problem. In the spirit of shining a light on the scenarios that most often frustrate boards and CEOs about one another, and with the hope of stimulating discussion and action, here are the top 10 frustrations that boards and CEOs have with each other.

Boards' Pet Peeves

Boards become frustrated when their CEOs do the following:

1. Present "baked cakes" (decisions that have already been made and committed to) without adequately engaging the full board in the decision-making process.

Edward A. Kazemek is chairman and CEO of Accord Limited, a Chicago-based firm specializing in health care governance, strategy, and management. He can be reached at (312) 988-7000 or at ekazemek@accord limited.com.

Most board members realize that they do not have the education and training that administrators have, but they are insulted when the CEO assumes that the board cannot help make major decisions. Board members also resent it when the CEO doesn't take the time to educate them on the issue or project being considered.

2. Don't sufficiently involve the board in the strategic planning process.

   This frustration is closely related to the first one but is often caused by a lack of clarity on how a health system or hospital should develop a strategic plan, who should be involved, and when. With today's heightened awareness of the board's fiduciary responsibilities, many boards are beginning to assert themselves more firmly in the strategic planning process, even though some CEOs perceive it as "management work."

3. Attempt to control or dominate the board (overtly or in subtle ways).

   Many CEOs, unconsciously in most cases, feel the need to keep the board under their control. Packing the board with friends and business associates or threatening the board with dire consequences if the CEO's plans are not approved are just some of the ways that boards are made to feel powerless and frustrated.

4. Keep the board in the dark on important or sensitive issues.

   Withholding information from the board or disseminating it in a highly controlled and manipulative fashion is arrogant on the part of the CEO and implies that the CEO knows best when the board needs to know something.

5. Work with just a few board members (e.g., the executive committee or chair) instead of the full board.

   Board members who are not on the "A team" end up feeling like second-class members and eventually lose interest in serving on the board.

6. Overload board packets with lengthy reports and data without attempting to make the information more user friendly.

   Most board members either don't have the time or inclination to wade through telephone book–size information packets and will show their frustration by not reading the material.

7. Use too much jargon when communicating with the board.

    Eventually, board members pick up health care industry acronyms and slang. But newer trustees end up sitting through too many meetings without fully understanding what is being discussed and hesitate to admit it for fear of looking stupid.

8. Invite too many staff members to board meetings, leaving little time for board deliberations.

    There are times when board members may want to raise issues with the CEO that may appear to criticize the executive team. Out of politeness, most trustees will not ask the staff to leave the meeting, so they end up not raising issues that are of concern to them.

9. Don't develop trusting relationships with physicians.

    Board members often feel the heat when the CEO and physicians conflict. CEOs who become defensive and draw lines in the sand with the medical staff trigger board member anxiety and feelings of helplessness.

10. Are insensitive to the fact that the trustees will continue to live and work in the community, whereas CEOs often leave the area for other positions.

    Board members have to live with the decisions they make for a long time and don't appreciate CEOs who ignore this simple fact.

CEOs' Pet Peeves

CEOs become frustrated when their boards:

1. Concern themselves inappropriately with hospital or health system operations.

    Board members roaming the halls, giving orders, discussing management issues with physicians, and questioning tactical decisions are just some examples of behavior that drives CEOs crazy.

2. Don't show up for meetings and retreats, are chronically late, and/or leave early.

    The time wasted bringing the offending board members up to speed, as well as the disrespect their behavior represents to other board members, angers many CEOs.

3. Are not candid with the CEO.

   Board members who discuss issues concerning the CEO, the senior management team, or the institution behind the CEO's back breed an atmosphere of mistrust between the CEO and the board.

4. Don't function as advisors and "partners" with the CEO but act more like "cops," keeping an eye on the CEO.

   Over time, this behavior will lock the CEO and board into an unhealthy, counterproductive relationship.

5. Dwell on minutiae instead of dealing with strategy and policy matters.

   Board members unable to elevate their perspectives (focusing on fixing the cracks in the parking lot versus long-range capital investments) disappoint CEOs who genuinely want help in thinking strategically and long term.

6. Accept gossip or criticisms of the hospital (from the community or staff) as fact without checking with the CEO.

   Board members who raise issues in an accusatory manner based on rumor or hearsay stimulate a defensive versus a problem-solving response from most CEOs.

7. Fail to set clear performance expectations with the CEO and do not give candid feedback on a regular basis.

   Not knowing where one stands in the eyes of the board creates insecurity for even the most capable CEOs. Contrary to what many board members may think, most CEOs value having clear goals and expectations agreed on and receiving timely feedback on their performance.

8. Don't attempt to learn about the health care industry, especially regarding reimbursement, quality, and physician relationship challenges.

   CEOs don't expect board members to know as much as they do, but they do expect the board to take every available opportunity to learn about the crucial issues related to governing a health care facility.

9. Don't keep sensitive information confidential.

   Board members (including physicians) who share confidential hospital information with outside parties are in violation of their fiduciary duty of loyalty and often create difficult (and legal) problems for the CEO.

10. Disrupt meetings by dominating discussions, ignoring the agenda, or not participating at all.

    Board members who behave like unruly children, causing meetings to run late, exasperate CEOs.

Fortunately, not many hospitals or health systems experience all of the frustrations described here. However, any one of these board-CEO dynamics can become a significant barrier to effective performance. Therefore, it would be worth spending some time at a board meeting or retreat and using this list of frustrations to stimulate discussion on the board-CEO process and performance. After all, in an industry as frustrating as health care, who needs self-inflicted frustrations?

Orchestrating the New Leadership: What It Takes to Be a CEO Today

By Patrick Plemmons

In a few terrible moments on the morning of September 11, our world changed forever, and one of the more striking changes came in how we viewed our leaders. Suddenly, our nation's priorities and needs changed dramatically, and we found we wanted and valued a whole different type of leader, with different skills and personal characteristics. Fortunately, President Bush, Mayor Giuliani of New York City, and many other lesser-known leaders rose to the occasion and showed us character traits we had not seen previously.

The lesson is clear—when the basic rules of the game change significantly, we require a different type of leadership. Admittedly, changes in the hospital industry have not been as sudden as those the nation experienced last September, but the field has experienced sweeping and almost continuous change over the past 10 to 15 years. And the hospital CEO's job has had to change accordingly. When a board has to recruit a new CEO, what skills and qualities should it seek? And given the tremendous complexity and difficulty

Patrick Plemmons is a vice-president in the Atlanta office of executive search firm Tyler & Co. He can be reached at (770) 396-3939 or by e-mail at pplemmons@tylerandco.com.

143

of leading a hospital today, how long can any CEO hope to be effective? Does an effective leader have a "life span" in one organization, after which he or she needs to move on?

The Good Old Days

David Hannan, the CEO of South Shore Hospital in South Weymouth, Massachusetts, remembers an easier era of hospital leadership before the mid-1980s when DRGs were first implemented: "It was easy to run a hospital. It was a cost-plus environment, and you could function in isolation and get by. You just had to be a cheerleader and adequate supply sergeant. Now things are more global and interconnected, and you must be a leader in the real sense of the word," he says.

The complexity of leading health care organizations has been increasing incrementally since DRGs, managed care, and, most recently, the Balanced Budget Amendment. Employees, especially nurses, have unionized, and physicians have become disaffected and contentious as their own profession has come under increasing scrutiny and attack.

Certainly, definitions of *leadership* are subject to interpretation. Faced with declining margins, workforce shortages, and seemingly relentless pressures from patients and payers alike, the "kinder and gentler" leader has had to toughen up.

Joe Swedish, CEO of Denver-based Centura Health System, agrees that the business of providing health care has changed and not necessarily for the better. "This business does not have the gentility it used to have," says Swedish. "And the customer today is markedly different from earlier days in hospitals."

He adds that with the current emphasis on access to capital and financial issues, a CEO must have much stronger financial skills now than in the past. "I see the job today as a combination of leadership and technical skills. Finance has been a critical part of my job at Centura. I am passionate about performance metrics, and to implement those you must understand the technical aspects of running the organization. I can't afford to be disconnected from operations and function exclusively at a strategic level," Swedish says. Since he was brought into Centura to carry out "a pure [i.e., financial] turnaround," such a strong emphasis on financial skills has been an important part of his job description. And it brings up another important point: job descriptions are not monolithic but differ according to the needs of the organization at any given time.

"Different phases of organizational life require a different CEO job description," says Swedish. "Be realistic as a board about where your organization is on the continuum and what kind of leadership you need." For many board members, this is a challenging exercise because they are relatively new to the organization and may not have a historical perspective. Still, boards must take the time to learn where the organization is today if they hope to identify a CEO who can lead it effectively tomorrow.

The Vision Thing

For South Shore's Hannan, the key element of real leadership is vision. "You must have a vision for the organization, and then you implement that vision by getting good people [to work with you], teaching them, listening to them, and learning from them." Jim Hinton, CEO of Presbyterian Healthcare Services, based in Albuquerque, New Mexico, also believes in the importance of a CEO's vision: "The job is to create a rational plan [i.e., vision] for the future of the organization and make sure that the operational chassis and indicators are in sync with that plan." Gary Strack, the former CEO and principal architect of the Orlando (Florida) Regional Healthcare System, agrees. "A CEO must see further, have greater cognitive ability, and greater emotional maturity than those he is leading," he says.

But vision alone is insufficient for good CEO leadership. To complement a clear and far-reaching vision, the CEO also needs an intimate understanding of how to provide and finance health care. Hinton puts it this way: "Your business has to be coherent and focused; most businesses fall down because of a lack of clarity. The focus must be on the organization, not the leader."

Michael Rindler, a former hospital CEO and president of The Rindler Group, a health care leadership and financial performance improvement consulting firm based in Hilton Head Island, South Carolina, agrees. He takes a decidedly dim view of what might be called the "captain-of-industry" model of the hospital CEO, prevalent since the 1970s. In this dated model, the hospital CEO is expected to be running a diversified, vertically integrated business, in which providing health care services is de-emphasized. In actuality, the CEO is preoccupied with system building, acquisition of non–health care businesses, creative financing, and corporate staffing. Rindler believes that the CEO of 2002 must "get back to basics and focus on running a better hospital." That means concentrating on high-quality medical care, improved medical staff leadership, and achieving at least a 3 percent operating margin.

Being There

Leading, inspiring, and motivating the organization's employees were vital to all of the CEOs with whom we spoke, but Sue Brody, CEO of Bayfront Medical Center, St. Petersburg, Florida, takes it a step further. Brody, the recent ACHE Young Healthcare Executive of the Year, says, "You have to personify the institution; you have to be its physical presence. You should be visible and accessible to all the groups and people in the organization so they know they can come to you for advice or reassurance, or just to be heard." Of course, in a stand-alone hospital, such as Bayfront, this accessibility is still possible. In a system, especially a large, multistate one, it's impossible for a CEO to be physically available to all staff. So the system CEO must rely on a management team and processes to unify the organization.

In order to benefit most from other people's talents, Presbyterian Healthcare's Hinton still believes in constant communication from the leader. "Far and away, the most important skill of the CEO is understanding the importance of, and carrying out, active communication," he says. Sue Brody agrees: "A large part of my job is inspirational and motivational. How you communicate to people, in all settings, is so important, maybe the most important thing." Gary Strack adds, "Seventy percent of the [CEO's] job is creating a climate that generates mutual trust and respect so people can learn, grow, and develop. You have to force a planning process and set goals and objectives. Give people a challenge so they can stretch, and give them support by training and leading. Challenge is toxic without support. Create an inclusive organization—open and non-secretive. Use the minds and energy of your people and drive fear out of the system."

Encouraging CEO Leadership Qualities

To help develop CEO and senior management leadership skills and qualities, you can do the following:

- Ensure that job descriptions explicitly detail desired leadership qualities and behaviors. These should be emphasized at least as much as technical skills and experience.
- Use leadership criteria in CEO formal and informal evaluations. By including leadership effectiveness in the formal evaluation process, you signal the importance of these skills to the organization's overall success. To be most effective, leadership skill evaluation should be continuous, not just a part of the formal review.
- To really gain the CEO's full attention, link leadership goal achievement to financial rewards. Bonuses can be a powerful motivator for leaders to further develop their skills.
- Include leadership qualities in the organization's mission and values statements and in the formal strategic planning process. Because so much of leadership depends on developing the optimal organizational culture, this action will emphasize the importance of leadership to both internal and external stakeholders in the organization.
- Give leadership substantial weight in the hiring decision whenever the organization recruits a new CEO or other senior manager. This will not only add to an overall culture of leadership but will also reinforce to existing managers the importance of leadership values.
- Include leadership topics in the board's continuing education. Trustees and the CEO can attend seminars or conferences about leadership, and experts in leadership may also be invited to speak to the board.
- Model the behavior you seek to encourage in your CEO. By the questions you ask, by the issues you hold most important, by all the contributions to governance you make, you can be a positive role model in stimulating the CEO to be the best possible leader he or she can be.

Brody also notes the importance of the CEO's energy and enthu-siasm. "Energy is so important—or maybe it's just stamina. You have to keep going and stay positive and consistent. That's what people respond to best." But in uncertain times, consistency often falls vic-tim to crisis management. The predictable leader becomes unpre-dictable. Unfortunately, those are precisely the times when it's most important for CEOs to be consistent about what they say and do.

But CEOs do not have to have all the answers. In fact, Hannan notes, humility is a helpful quality. "It's much more important to know how to ask really good questions and then know if the answers make sense," adds Brody. Ray Budrys, CEO of Craven Regional Medical Center, New Bern, North Carolina, uses this metaphor: "The CEO is an orchestra conductor. You need to know what a violin looks like and how it should sound, but you don't need to be a violin virtuoso."

Gary Strack sums it up nicely: "The higher up you go, who you are matters a lot more than what you know."

That's why teamwork is important to all the CEOs with whom we talked. Hospitals are extremely complex organizations, and the demands placed on them are so great that no one person can hope to solve every problem. The CEO cannot be seen as someone who has all the answers. Indeed, one of the most important functions of a CEO is choosing a team of outstanding senior managers and sup-porting and developing them. As Jim Hinton says, "If you are a set of solutions looking for problems to solve, you are going to be inef-fective in short order. The success of our organization is directly related to the activities of our senior team, and all of them are involved at the board level."

Sue Brody believes that people respond as much with their hearts as with their minds. "The people in this organization are mission-driven, but I don't think that's why they do things. They do things for other people in the institution."

View from the Boardroom

Larry Davis, M.D., board chairman at Bayfront Medical Center, believes that 70 percent of a hospital CEO's job description revolves around personality. He sees the CEO's role today as providing a vision for where the medical center is heading and putting together a strong, autonomous management team. Interpersonal relations with physicians are also a very important part of the job. Basically, he says, "a CEO makes decisions, works with people, and gets things done."

Lottie Kurcz is a senior vice president with FirstHealth, a managed care company in Chicago, and chair of Holy Cross Hospital in Chicago. After a difficult search process, Holy Cross hired a new CEO about six months ago. The hospital needed a CEO who could develop and implement a strategic plan—someone who could act quickly and decisively on tough issues. The board struggled with how to evaluate and measure the candidates' real operating style. It's much easier to get a handle on financial measures, or number of employees, or similar "hard" metrics. But Kurcz believes the board hired the right CEO because it did not rely primarily on interviews but conducted broad, in-depth referencing.

The importance of references cannot be overemphasized. In our experience, it is virtually the only way to thoroughly evaluate and predict leadership skills and styles. And it is vital that whoever checks references understands the context in which the candidate has operated. A skilled interviewer, with in-depth industry knowledge and contacts, can develop the best picture of a prospective CEO's personality, behaviors, and track record with people.

It's easy for a charismatic candidate who is a skillful communicator to fool interviewers. In fact, there have been several recent high-profile instances of résumé fraud by senior executives in the corporate world.

Careful reference checking is one of the best ways to uncover dishonesty among job seekers. And the best way to conduct these checks is by using the "360-degree" method, which entails talking to superiors, subordinates, and peers. Most important, it means not relying on a list of references furnished by the candidate. The board needs to develop its own list of key references based on the candidate's experience and current situation. If a reference is "off limits," there needs to be a very good reason. The board needs to look for themes across references, and when a problem surfaces in one reference, it should be tested against others. A search committee should not settle for generalities—it needs to press for specifics and be prepared with questions that are germane to the specific recruitment.

Where Are the CEOs?

There was no shortage of qualified candidates in Holy Cross's search. "I would be very surprised if there were not a lot of qualified people just waiting for a chance to run [your] hospital," says Bayfront's Davis. "They are out there; just give the young ones a chance."

Jim Hinton was 36 when he became CEO of a multihospital system, and he sees no shortage of leaders. "I see lots of capable young leaders out there," he says. "Granted, we're not seeing the same

---

Evaluating CEO Leadership

As a board or CEO evaluation committee, first decide on the specific criteria you want to evaluate, and then develop questions that will give you the information you need to reach an informed opinion. This need not be an overly formal and structured exercise. Just come up with a few questions that deal with the most important aspects of leadership. For example: Do employees feel valued? What is the organization's reputation in the community and in the health care field? Has the CEO assembled and developed a strong management team? How visible and accessible is the CEO? Questions such as these, when posed to the right people, will develop a true picture of the CEO's leadership effectiveness. So who are the right people to ask?

For starters, ask those who know best—employees. And not just senior managers but employees at every level. If the CEO is doing an outstanding job of creating a positive culture where employees feel empowered and valued, and where everyone is working toward shared goals, staff will confirm it. Don't delegate this task to someone in human resources or just send out a survey. Trustees should talk directly with a cross-section of employees to get a true picture of the CEO's leadership effectiveness.

People outside the organization can be helpful as well. Former employees will sometimes be more honest than current staff, and vendors, consultants, and other external parties can offer valuable insights too.

Continued →

career paths as before." Today, CEOs are coming from the ranks of planners, nursing, human resources, and even from boards of trustees (see the article "Your CEO: Are You Short-Staffed or Shortsighted" starting on page 109 of this book). Operations is no longer the sole training ground for hospital leaders. David Hannan advises, "Don't be afraid to look in nontraditional places; one-third of my senior team [was originally] from outside of health care. Leadership skills are not much different in this field from any other." Trustees are advised to be open-minded to both youth and change, experts agree.

Any evaluation of CEO leadership must also include the medical staff. Of all the relationships a health care CEO must cultivate, his or her relationship with the medical staff is the most important to the organization's success. Physicians are usually very frank when expressing their opinions about the CEO, and their insights can be most useful in assessing top leadership.

Industry rankings and awards can also aid leadership evaluation. For instance, *Working Mother* magazine presents an annual award to the top 100 corporations that are especially supportive of issues important to their female employees. Bayfront Medical Center in St. Petersburg, Florida, won this award in 2000 and in previous years, indicating that Bayfront's CEO places a high priority on creating a welcoming, supportive employee environment. Such actions are one of the hallmarks of effective CEO leadership.

Evaluating CEO leadership is a task that trustees should not delegate, but there are times when outside expertise can be helpful. Executive search consultants, management psychologists, or management consultants can bring an outsider's perspective and many years of experience to the evaluation process.

But in the end, trustees themselves must make the final judgments when evaluating CEO leadership.

"I think you are seeing a generation passing, and they might think that they can't be replaced. Maybe it's a case of boards not giving young people a chance," says Bayfront's Brody. During the many tough years hospitals have endured, it could be expected that boards would be more risk-averse in choosing leaders and would opt for the most experienced leaders. But Brody also points out that "it's more acceptable now to 'have a life' and to balance work and family. I'm not sure the existing [CEO] leadership buys into that yet."

The Time of Your Life

How long can a CEO be effective in the same organization? Brody thinks "there are waves of organizational life, and you have to recognize the new ones coming along and reenergize people and yourself along new lines." Michael Rindler is more specific: "Ten years is the optimum tenure. That takes you through two complete strategic planning cycles. After five years, you start facing the consequences of decisions you have made." Craven Regional's Budrys is equally precise. "Five to seven years is probably the optimum life span of a CEO in one organization. Medical staff conflicts will inevitably grow over this time and reach critical mass. If you're trying to do the right things for the organization and community, you will eventually face serious conflicts." Gary Strack sees CEO tenure as a structural issue. "The problems in leading a hospital organization are so systemic that doing the right thing for the institution, over time, [leads to] falling on your sword," he says. Hannan sees the CEO's organizational life span as being divided into five-year segments. He believes that the first five years are spent serving the community and hospital; the second five trying to realign the medical staff; and "during the next five years, you need to reinvent yourself or get out."

Even though the exact timetable may be debatable, it's clear that there is some effective life span in which a CEO can optimize leadership and performance. Just as organizations go through life cycles or waves, so too, it appears, do CEOs. There is no "one-size-fits-all" model of hospital leadership and no date carved in stone for when it makes sense to move on.

FirstHealth's Lottie Kurcz believes that the two most important responsibilities a board has are choosing a CEO and then ensuring that he or she remains the right leader as the organization changes. David Hannan agrees: "Leadership is a long-term thing, and it takes courage." Boards can show their own courage by seeking out CEOs who are true leaders and by giving young leaders a chance to take their place on the stage.

And what characterizes a true leader? The message from the CEOs represented here is clear—the "softer" skills are the ones that ensure effective leadership. Vision, focus, integrity, communication, consistency, energy, team building—these are some of the essential skills of today's CEO. The challenge for boards is to recognize and measure such inexact skills as best they can when evaluating existing and prospective CEOs. It's not easy, but it can and must be done.

Tough Love:
Ten Questions to Ask
Your CEO

By Paul B. Hofmann
and Wanda J. Jones

If your board is typical, there is an unspoken agreement between management and trustees to let management bring issues to the board for discussion. This gives CEOs control over timing and process while not requiring the board to expend a lot of energy searching out problems. In exchange, the board will pay attention to the issues of the day and generally support management's recommendations. After all, the CEO has a major role in trustee selection and orientation to achieve just this level of predictability and comfort.

The tacit understanding among trustees is that CEOs may not be telling the board all that they know or worry about, especially if they do not yet know what to do or if they believe it will unduly worry the board. In this atmosphere, the highest risk is not what is on the table but those subjects that are out of sight, unaddressed.

The following ten questions are a starting point for a new relationship between the board and management—one where the trustees

Paul B. Hofmann, Dr.P.H., is senior vice president of Aon Consulting's health care industry practice and chairman of New Century Healthcare Institute, San Francisco. Wanda J. Jones, M.P.H., is president of New Century Healthcare Institute.

can probe for areas of risk in keeping with their fiduciary responsibility to the public. The list follows a hierarchy of importance.

Level I: Manage against Increasing Risk and Declining Revenues

Question 1. What are the main areas of risk in the future, especially in regard to the different rates of change in revenues and costs, and what are our compensating strategies for each?

Corollaries. On which external organizations are we most dependent (e.g., health plans, government payers, individual physicians, or medical groups)? On what are our relationships based? How secure are they? What is our contingency plan in the event that any relationship fails? Are we equally adept at managing both revenues and costs?

Question 2. How and when will we adjust expenses to revenues (at the same time, after the fact, or in anticipation? by cuts, redesign, or reprogramming)?

Corollaries. How do we protect our quality standards? How do we promote those standards to payers? How do we demonstrate that high quality is cost effective? How do we separate the issue of quality performance from the accusation that price negotiation is all about professional and staff income and corporate profits? Do we give consistent messages to our staff or do we require them to keep quality high while starving them for resources? What do they think? Are we preserving uneconomical programs because of resistance from physicians, staff, unions, or the community? How can we position ourselves to make sound resource decisions in a timely, open way?

Question 3. What is the status of our reserve accounts, and how are we protecting them? What is our policy for use of these reserves?

Corollaries. Are we using money earned from patient care activities to invest in nonpatient care activities, such as purchase of medical practices or creation of health plans? If so, how can these investments be returned to our reserves? Do we have a policy concerning the level of reserves we should maintain relative to our risk exposure?

Level II: Capture and Hold Market Share

Question 4. Are we gaining or losing market share—that is, do major payers consider us an essential provider? Why? What is our strategy for attaining a stronger buyer-seller negotiating position?

Corollaries. Do employers and consumers know which delivery system is included in their plans? Do they know enough about us to insist that we be included? What is our reputation with health plans? Why? How can we enhance it? How do we measure market share (share of hospital admissions, share of health plan contracts/enrollees, and/or share of the regional health care dollar)?

Are we paying attention to the market share of consumer-paid health care (e.g., for complementary care therapies and plastic surgery, not just insured health care)? Do we still consider only the medical staff our market, or do we now understand how to treat health plans and buyers as our market, along with the general public?

Level III: Restructure and Redesign

Question 5. What proportion of management's work is spent on maintaining the status quo compared with building the next-generation delivery system? Does management have a 5- to 10-year vision of how health care services should be redesigned? Are projects based on delivery redesign, or are they rehousing old concepts?

Corollaries. Does management accept that one role of this organization is to be a community partner in the redesign of health care delivery? Has it added to its own skill mix? Has it engaged with community organizations? Has it brought out the leadership potential in its professional staffs and on this board? Does it demonstrate an understanding of the early trends that hint at how the health care system is being restructured from the outside?

Question 6. In the same time period that costs are being cut, is innovation being protected and preserved?

Corollaries. Is management encouraging innovation in both operations and clinical programs? Is innovation being driven by population need, or provider competition, or only by technology? What are the barriers to innovation and what is being done to reduce or remove those barriers? Is there congruence between operations and finance on the need to protect innovation? Is the organization geared to learning and changing rapidly, or is innovation slow, tentative, and painful? How can the board show its interest in continued innovation as a broad business strategy?

Level IV: Manage Key Relationships

Question 7. What are the organization's key relationships—those that can either support or hinder our development or longevity? What is the status of those relationships? How do we manage them (consider both internal and external relationships, local and nonlocal)?

Corollaries. Are we geared for cooperation with our primary external partners, or is there an atmosphere of self-protection, competition, or fear of government's role? Do our internal stakeholders understand the nature of our external relationships, especially buyers and payers? Is there a shared understanding of general health care economics as a basis for mutual planning and cooperation? Do we have plans for improving our perceived value to organizations that we consider valuable to us? Are there relationships that are too costly to sustain in their present form?

Question 8. What are the ethical foundations of our relationships and behaviors? How do we know how well we are maintaining our standards? Are there areas where we are at ethical risk? Are we open with the public about issues the public considers important to it?

Corollaries. Do we scan for the ethical breaches of others as a signal to audit our own practices? Do we have a "crisis management" policy that favors prompt disclosure and problem solving (e.g., billing abuses, mistreatment of patients, or an infectious outbreak)? How recently has an ethics audit been conducted?

Level V: Advocate for the Community

Question 9. Do we see ourselves as advocates for the health of the community? If so, how do we fulfill this role? Does the community expect us to represent its interests? To whom?

Corollaries. Are we skilled in interpreting our own experience in community health terms (prevalence of diseases of poverty, for example, or diseases produced from addictions or the environment, or diseases related to stress and depression)? Do we view advocacy as the responsibility of other organizations and not our own? Do we expect management will make time for this role? Do we assume the medical staff will advocate as it sees broad health care problems? Are there areas that affect the public in which we may be practicing benign neglect? How do we show the public that we care as much about meeting its needs as we do about our own survival or financial success?

Question 10. Do we contribute to public policy development in health care as we see the increase in public distrust and the growth of activism toward more regulation? If so, how and in what areas?

Corollaries. If we were standing outside looking in at our work, knowing what we know about how health care works, what changes in public policy would be in the public interest? Do we take on the responsibility of educating our publics so policy decisions are at least better informed? Are we open about sharing data and helping with its interpretation? Do we know how to make allies of the media and elected officials? Is the board useful to the organization in translating health care policy proposals to its home organizations and public bodies?

If, over the course of a year, the board's agenda could address these questions in some reasonable order and then visit them again, its positive influence on the course of the organization would greatly increase. All of these questions would signal to management that the board is ready to see the organization through some rough waters—that management need not be reticent to bring up worrisome, but crucial, topics.

PART FOUR

Board Work

Trustee Development: Starting with the Individual

By Mary K. Totten
and James E. Orlikoff

Because boards don't really exist apart from their meetings, efforts to improve the way the board as a whole functions make sense. Much has been written about the importance of effective board functioning as a team, even as the most important team in an organization. Beyond the trustee recruitment and selection process, most governance activities—meetings, educational conferences, retreats, evaluation, and restructuring activities—are largely directed toward, and intended to engage, the full board.

Yet like any team, if a board is to work well, its individual members must understand their roles and contribute to the success of the whole. When boards perform poorly, blame can often be traced to members who don't pull their weight, who pursue their own or constituent agendas, or who don't have the information and tools they need to govern effectively.

High-performing boards that add value to their organization's leadership have members who are committed to their organization's mission and vision and who work continuously to improve

Mary K. Totten is president of Totten & Associates, Oak Park, Illinois. James E. Orlikoff is president of Orlikoff & Associates, Inc., Chicago.

their own performance, often with a helping hand from other trustees as well as from management. On high-performing boards, individual trustee assistance is deliberate and planned. It begins during the recruitment and selection phases, is reinforced through an organized orientation, and is refined and expanded through regular performance evaluation and ongoing education and development.

Begin with Trustee Selection

As governance strives toward greater professionalism, there is a growing recognition that, not only must boards be more focused about what types of members they need, but they must also provide more and better education and support for them.

Today's demanding and competitive health care environment requires decisive, knowledgeable leadership and trustees who have skills tailored not only to a hospital's or system's particular needs but to a more sophisticated marketplace. Consequently, trustee selection and board composition are becoming more focused, systematic, and driven by an individual organization's strategic priorities.

Many health care organizations, especially those with multiple entities and boards, are developing specific trustee selection criteria that go far beyond the traditional board expectations of attendance and residence in the organization's service area (see examples in the following section).

Trustee Criteria

System Board

- Ability to understand that the needs of the whole organization or system supersede those of any of its components
- Capacity to be strategic and future oriented; able to create and sustain performance toward accomplishing mission and vision
- Expertise or knowledge in specific fields, such as strategic alliances or partnerships, systemwide information systems, or the Internet
- Experience on the board of a multiunit business or health care system
- Experience as a CEO or senior executive of a health system

Hospital or Other Provider Board

- Experience with quality assessment or improvement programs
- Clinical experience
- Health care governance experience
- Expertise or experience in community health issues

Foundation Board

- Experience governing a fund-raising organization
- Experience in fund-raising, planned giving, or other development activities
- Relationships with community groups, individuals, or corporations that could assist the organization
- Comfort with fund-raising activities or soliciting money

Finding such specific talent can be a challenge, especially in small towns or rural areas. That's why some boards are beginning to turn to professional recruiters who can help zero in on the specific governance needs and the type of talent the board is seeking. Recruiters can help open up a board's search process and identify candidates who may be particularly suited to the board's needs although coming from outside the organization's service area.

The traditional perspective that governance on behalf of a community can best be accomplished by drawing board members from that community alone is giving way to an appreciation for the particular skills and unbiased viewpoints that an "outsider" executive or trustee can bring (see "Outside/In," in the July/August 1999 *Trustee*).

They may have had experience leading an organization in a different market or geographic area that has already dealt with issues and problems similar to those facing your board.

An outsider can also bring a fresh perspective to the organization and its board, unfettered by internal politics, traditional ways of doing things, or fear of local reaction to a difficult or potentially unpopular board decision. An outsider can hold a mirror up to the board, allowing it to examine its reflection and see itself in a new light.

Questions for Discussion

1. Does your board use specific criteria to help identify new trustees? If so, what are they?
2. If your board uses selection criteria, do the criteria help to identify candidates with expertise that will help you address strategic issues facing your organization? Are the criteria tailored to your specific governance responsibilities, and do they differ among the different boards in your system?
3. Does your board include any members from outside the communities you serve? If not, under what circumstances might your board be willing to bring in an outside member?

Expanding Orientation through Mentoring

Once a candidate joins the board, a cycle of "learning, doing, and leading" should begin. Most orientations, however, fall short. They rely on a brief presentation and supporting materials focusing broadly on health care and specifically on the organization but without much sense of the board or the organizational culture. They usually raise more questions than they answer.

Rather than viewing orientation as a onetime event that largely leaves the new trustee to his or her own initiative, boards are more frequently viewing it as a process that may take up to a year to complete. Included in this long-term orientation are:

- One-on-one interviews between the trustee and key executive staff to clarify the organization's activities and services
- Opportunities to attend outside educational events about governance processes and practices as well as issues facing the organization
- Pairing the new trustee with a more seasoned board member who gives perspective on how the board works and background on major board issues and decisions—mentoring

According to the *AHA/Ernst & Young LLP 1997 Hospital and Health System Governance Survey,* only 15 percent of system board chairs reported that their new trustees were assigned mentors.

However, pairing new trustees with more seasoned peers can have several benefits: It provides an ongoing resource for new members for answering questions and checking out their perceptions; it helps them gain greater awareness and understanding of board dynamics and operations; it brings new trustees up to speed more quickly while building board member relationships; and it gives senior board members a chance to gauge new trustees' educational needs and leadership potential.

Boards have used trustee mentoring in different ways. Some set up a trustee-to-trustee connection and then let the relationship develop on its own. Others pair a new trustee with two mentors, one a board member and one a senior executive, each of whom works with a manual that clearly defines the mentoring role, suggests topics to cover and time frames for completion, while providing background information and other support materials. The senior trustee's role is to help the new trustee understand board culture—the norms and expectations of group interaction, decision-making processes, and other aspects of how the board works. The executive's role is to help new trustees better understand health care and market issues facing the organization.

Boards that have used a mentoring process report that it has been well received, especially in multitiered systems where trustees may move among boards. Those being mentored appreciate the opportunity to have information tailored to their individual needs, with an emphasis on filling in their knowledge gaps rather than reviewing system governance information they already know. Participating executives appreciate the opportunity to get to know trustees individually in a casual setting outside a board meeting or other formal context.

Experience also shows that the connection made during an initial mentoring process often remains long after orientation concludes, with newer trustees continuing to seek out their mentors for questions and guidance.

Questions for Discussion

1. Which type of orientation did you go through as a new trustee?
2. After your orientation, did you have additional questions or issues you wanted to pursue? If so, how did you address your needs? Did they get resolved?
3. Does your board's orientation process include mentoring? If not, what value might it bring to new trustees?

Trustee Performance Evaluation

Boards that want to help trustees make the most of their service develop and share their performance criteria with current and potential trustees. These criteria should clarify the level of participation and performance the board expects from its members and are framed to be specific and measurable (see "Performance Criteria" below).

Sharing criteria with prospective trustees during the recruiting process gives them a "heads up" about future commitments and can help them decide whether to accept a board position. New trustees also should review and discuss these criteria during their orientation and understand clearly how they are used in individual performance assessment, development, and reappointment.

Performance Criteria

The following criteria can be used for individual board member's performance evaluations:

- Consistently attends board and committee meetings and does not miss more than three consecutive meetings
- Seeks to continually improve individual performance
- Participates actively and thoughtfully at board and committee meetings; listens and solicits others' opinions
- Serves on at least one board committee
- Keeps the organization's strategic direction in mind when making decisions and encourages the board to focus on strategic priorities
- Attends at least one outside educational program each year
- Respects board confidentiality
- Understands the board's conflict-of-interest policy and does not violate it
- Expresses dissenting opinions or votes, but publicly supports the board's final decisions

Trustee evaluation is beginning to evolve from a cursory, private assessment usually conducted by the individual as part of a full board evaluation to a more formal, broad-based process that includes outside input. Many trustees are understandably hesitant or uncomfortable about bringing individual evaluations to light, and this probably explains why such processes are less than universal.

A 1996 study by the consulting firm Korn/Ferry International indicated that only 16 percent of *Fortune* 1,000 companies evaluate individual directors. Yet survey data also indicate that boards that evaluate individual members rate their board's effectiveness significantly higher than those that do not.

Some corporate and not-for-profit health care boards have combined self-assessment with trustee ratings conducted by a designated board committee or a team of board leaders that may include the CEO, board chair, and the chair of a trustee development committee. This assessment is based on preestablished performance expectations, and each member of the evaluation team is asked to comment on strengths and opportunities for each trustee. The group then meets to discuss and finalize the assessments.

Every member of the evaluation team is then assigned specific trustees to mentor. The mentor meets with each trustee to review the team's assessment and the individual's own self-evaluation to create a plan identifying specific growth opportunities. The mentor then follows up with trustees to ensure that they have taken advantage of the opportunities identified in their development plans. This process is repeated every one to two years.

Peer evaluation, in which each board member anonymously evaluates other members, also adds perspective and objectivity to individual trustee evaluations. Peer assessments are coordinated by a designated board leader or an outside facilitator. The facilitator summarizes comments and ratings and shares them with each member of the board. Preserving evaluator anonymity, the facilitator might also provide full assessment results to the board's nominating or governance committee to be used for board reappointment.

Questions for Discussion

1. Has your board developed trustee performance criteria? Are they used to help evaluate, further develop, and reappoint trustees?
2. Does your evaluation process allow trustees to reflect on the personal meaning, importance, and value of their trusteeship and either reaffirm their commitment or make plans to move on?
3. Does the process include perspectives on an individual's performance from other board members or leaders?

4. Do you think that evaluating individual trustees improves overall board performance? Why or why not?

When Performance Crosses the Line

No trustee evaluation process is worthwhile without a performance improvement plan. However, if performance does not
improve, the board must be willing to take corrective action. A
1997 study of corporate governance conducted by Russell Reynolds
Associates showed that investors felt strongly that boards should
be more aggressive in removing underperforming members. Few
would argue that it makes good sense to formally assess individuals and either quickly turn around poor performers or remove
them.

In their book *Board Work,* Dennis D. Pointer and James E.
Orlikoff recommend that boards establish a clearly specified subset
of criteria that signal when immediate removal of a member is
advised. Examples of such criteria might include:

- Violation of the board's conflict-of-interest or confidentiality
  policies
- Failure to attend a specified number of board meetings over time
- Verbal or physical abuse of other board members, physicians, or
  employees
- Subverting board policies or decisions

Such criteria should also include a clearly worded written policy
for trustee removal. Both the criteria and the process should be
shared with all trustees as part of their recruitment and orientation.
Such criteria not only help define inadmissible behavior but also
create an impartial and speedy way to resolve egregious problems
that have a negative impact on overall board performance.

Questions for Discussion

1. Does your board have specific criteria and a mechanism for
   removing a member midterm?
2. Are the criteria meaningful?

3. Has the process been used? How did it work? Could it be improved?

Tips for Trustee Development

These suggestions can help strengthen your organization's board by ensuring that trustees get the information and support they need.

- Assign trustee development responsibility to a board committee or leadership team and ensure that the oversight group has a work plan to address this responsibility.
- Develop trustee selection criteria specific to the strategic needs of the organization and the specific issues facing the board.
- Develop written job descriptions that include individual performance expectations.
- Make sure that all candidates receive job descriptions and understand performance expectations before they accept a seat on the board.
- Consider seeking trustees from outside your organization's service area if needed and compensating them to attract and retain the specific talent you require.
- Develop mentoring opportunities for trustees, both as part of orientation and ongoing development and performance improvement.
- Consider expanding performance evaluations to include assessments from board leaders or peers for greater input and objectivity.
- Ensure that each trustee has a development plan and that your board provides a variety of personal development opportunities for its members, including on-site and off-site education, opportunities to participate on committees or ad hoc groups, access to governance and health resources, and encouragement to take on board leadership roles.
- Consider developing a set of criteria and a clearly written policy to remove trustees and ensure that the process is implemented when the criteria are met.
- Have a full-board discussion at least once a year to evaluate how well trustees are supported and how development opportunities could be improved.

Self-Assessment Questionnaire

The following questionnaire can be used as a stand-alone survey or as part of a board evaluation process. Each trustee should independently and anonymously rate the board's performance on the following questions. Pay particular attention to any questions that produce significantly diverse responses. The ensuing discussion should produce an action plan for improving trustee development and support.

1. Trustee development is part of the ongoing work of our board and is coordinated and implemented by a designated board committee.

   □ Strongly Agree   □ Agree
   □ Somewhat Disagree   □ Disagree

2. Each board in our organization has selection criteria tailored to the issues, responsibilities, and needs of that particular board.

   □ Strongly Agree   □ Agree
   □ Somewhat Disagree   □ Disagree

3. Our board has sought new expertise from outside our organization's service area.

   □ Strongly Agree   □ Agree
   □ Somewhat Disagree   □ Disagree

4. Our board has developed trustee performance expectations that are shared with every new candidate and used as part of ongoing performance assessments and reappointment.

   □ Strongly Agree   □ Agree
   □ Somewhat Disagree   □ Disagree

5. Our board views orientation as a formal process that provides specific resources, educational opportunities, and support for new members during their first year of service.

   □ Strongly Agree   □ Agree
   □ Somewhat Disagree   □ Disagree

6. Senior board members participate as mentors, both during orientation and as part of a trustee's ongoing performance and assessment.

   ☐ Strongly Agree   ☐ Agree
   ☐ Somewhat Disagree   ☐ Disagree

7. Performance evaluation is a formal process that includes perspectives from other board members.

   ☐ Strongly Agree   ☐ Agree
   ☐ Somewhat Disagree   ☐ Disagree

8. Each board member has an individual development plan that identifies specific needs and opportunities for that trustee to gain additional knowledge and governance expertise.

   ☐ Strongly Agree   ☐ Agree
   ☐ Somewhat Disagree   ☐ Disagree

9. Our board has a written set of performance criteria and a process for removing members.

   ☐ Strongly Agree   ☐ Agree
   ☐ Somewhat Disagree   ☐ Disagree

10. Our board regularly reviews its trustee development processes and seeks input about how those processes could be improved.

    ☐ Strongly Agree   ☐ Agree
    ☐ Somewhat Disagree   ☐ Disagree

Conclusion

A board is only as strong as its weakest member. That's why high-performing boards expend effort and energy to ensure that trustees get started right—with a clear understanding of their roles and responsibilities and what performance expectations the board has of them. The boards then follow up with strong orientation and ongoing trustee development opportunities that are tailored to the specific needs identified in each trustee's development plan. Having informed, engaged trustees committed to continuous learning and performance improvement is essential to board effectiveness.

Top Ten Policies
for the Board

By Michael W. Peregrine
and James R. Schwartz

The board of directors of a not-for-profit hospital or health system should adopt and maintain a core of governance policies that address how it takes action on both a collective and individual basis. A "Top Ten" list of the most important board policies should include:

1. The **governance policy,** intended as an overarching summary of the individual trustee's core duties. Its purpose is to provide the framework within which the board and its members will execute their fiduciary duties. As such, it contains a clear statement of the corporate mission, as well as the board's and trustees' core duties of care, loyalty, and obedience to purpose.

2. A detailed **conflict-of-interest policy** that goes beyond the basic financial interests of the IRS and that extends to specific hospital/physician considerations, to nonfinancial potential conflicts, dual directorships in general, and concurrent service on an affiliate or competing board in particular.

Michael W. Peregrine, J.D., is a partner in the Chicago law offices of Gardner, Carton & Douglas. James R. Schwartz, J.D., is a partner in the Los Angeles law firm of Manatt, Phelps & Phillips, LLP.

3. A policy on **corporate opportunity** that establishes the basic prohibition against "appropriation of corporate opportunity" (i.e., where one board member takes advantage of a business deal that the corporation would have otherwise pursued). The policy should establish what to do when an appropriation issue arises and provide guidance to the board on how best to identify strategic matters as system opportunities.

4. A straightforward and strongly worded **policy on confidentiality** that emphasizes the trustee's fundamental obligation to maintain the confidentiality of board actions, as well as all other information regarding the corporation's activities until they are disclosed to the public by the corporation or are otherwise in the public domain. The penalties for breach of this duty (e.g., removal) should also be stated in the policy.

5. A policy that sets forth the board's position on **outside board service** by trustees and senior managers. Of course, concurrent board service is not a breach of any duty, per se. It can, however, raise issues related to conflict of interest, compensation, full-time board service, and mission conflicts, among others.

6. An **oversight of senior management** policy that outlines this basic board obligation. To be effective, the policy must not undermine the board's ability to delegate day-to-day operations to senior management but should clearly remind it to be sensitive to potential management-activity red flags.

7. Although most states allow trustee compensation within not-for-profit corporations, it is still not a common practice. For those not-for-profits that choose to pay their trustees, it's important that they create a specific **policy on board compensation.** Such a policy should summarize the rationale for compensation, how trustees are to be paid, limitations/ceilings on total compensation, and how compensation decisions will be approved by a disinterested body.

8. Given the importance of investment portfolio return to many not-for-profit hospitals and systems, it's very important for boards to adopt an **investment management policy.** Such a policy would delineate the basic guidelines and premises the board should use to invest the organization's funds through its investment committee and financial advisors. The policy should stipulate that investment practices be made in a manner consistent with governing

law (e.g., the Uniform Management of Institutional Funds Act) and with a clear articulation of the organization's investment needs. This policy should also include guidelines for the use/application/monitoring of restricted funds and how charitable gifts are to be solicited.

9. A policy that sets forth the organization's commitment to **maintaining the independence of the corporate audit.** Such a policy should establish board protocol for evaluating an independent audit firm as well as specify when the board would engage an audit firm (or its affiliate) to perform nonaudit services.

10. A policy that supplements the **corporate compliance plan**— that is, a board statement confirming its commitment to the plan and to providing its corporate compliance committee and compliance staff with the administrative and financial resources they need.

Through adopting corporate board policies such as those above, the governance of not-for-profit hospitals and health systems can achieve two worthwhile goals: It can clearly demonstrate to regulatory bodies the seriousness with which the organization and its board treat their obligations under the laws governing charitable organizations; and it provides a concise reference to all trustees on their core fiduciary duties.

Whose Job Is It Anyway?

Governance Restructuring Clarifies
Board Roles

By Pamela R. Knecht
and Edward A. Kazemek

"Exactly who has the authority to make this decision?" asks a trustee during a local hospital board meeting. The trustee, a prominent community leader, is new to the board. Her fellow board members, many of whom have served for years, shift uncomfortably in their seats. The new trustee rephrases her question: "Does our board or the system board have the ultimate authority to approve this $5 million expansion project?"

Some of the trustees argue, "Of course, it's our decision; we are the hospital board." Others are less sure. They remember addressing this issue at the time of the merger. However, that was three years ago, and the trustees cannot now recall exactly what the revised bylaws said about capital expenditures of this size. Because the board cannot agree on an answer, the chair says that she will contact the system chair for clarification, and the discussion is tabled until the next month's meeting.

Pamela R. Knecht is vice-president and Edward A. Kazemek is chairman and CEO of Accord Limited, a Chicago-based firm specializing in governance and organizational change. They can be reached at (312) 988-7000.

The Problem: Confusion and Inefficiency

This conversation highlights what is happening in many board-rooms today. The numerous mergers among health care providers over the last 5 to 10 years have produced many systems with multiple layers of governance, numerous boards, and many committees. In one system, the corporate organizational chart grew to 16 boards and 57 committees, and spread across five layers, involving more than 200 people.

Confusion Regarding Authority

Even relatively small health care systems have ended up with separate boards for the hospital(s), the long-term care facility, the home health organization, the foundation, and other entities. All of these boards (and their committees) are supposed to report to a system or parent board. In many cases, this reporting relationship exists only on paper.

In reality, final decision-making authority may lie with any of a number of bodies within the governance structure. Sometimes the hospital board makes all the decisions for its own institution; sometimes the system board's finance committee is the final arbiter; at other times, the board's executive committee of the system's largest hospital has the most power. As a result, many new board and committee members become justly confused about their board's role in the decision-making process.

Slow Decision Making

The ungainly governance structures we have created also make for slow and arduous decision making. Jeff Wendling, president and CEO of Northern Michigan Regional Health System, Petoskey, says that before governance restructuring, some staff and board members served on as many as 13 governing bodies within the system. It took too long for decisions to work their way up through the multiple levels of committees and boards. In addition, trustees and managers became frustrated with hearing the same report over and over. Most felt that they were devoting an inordinate amount of time to governance.

Unmanageable Board Size

Merger and acquisition activity may also spawn unmanageably large system-level boards. In order to accomplish mergers and assuage the reservations of trustees from previously independent hospitals, a certain number of seats may be reserved on the system board for the trustees of the acquired entities. We have seen system boards grow to more than 40 members as a result. Because experts in group dynamics believe the optimum size of a decision-making body is between 8 and 10, these large boards are, by definition, inefficient. Either it takes a very long time to hear the opinions of 40 people, or, as is more often the case, the majority of trustees do not speak up for fear that the board meeting will last until midnight. The board, therefore, loses the opportunity to hear all of the relevant facts and opinions before it votes.

Governance Design Principles

Here are some principles a system may want to use to evaluate the appropriateness of various structural options. The new organizational structure must:

- Help create a successful health care delivery system
- Ensure effective resource allocation throughout the system as needed
- Clarify the locus of power and authority
- Clarify roles and relationships among the various entities
- Enable governance to hold management accountable for its performance
- Provide more opportunities for physician input and governance participation
- Increase community input and involvement
- Allow more strategic thinking at the board level
- Expand the diversity of those serving in governance
- Use board members' time wisely
- Ensure that future governance leaders are knowledgeable about, and prepared to deal with, the changing health care industry
- Be legally sound, factoring in regulatory and reimbursement issues

---

Underutilized Trustees

This situation leads to one of the worst consequences of governance confusion and inefficiency—the loss of talented board members. Board members check out (mentally and/or physically) because they do not believe they are making a significant contribution; because their roles are unclear; or because, as successful, busy community or business leaders, they cannot tolerate being part of an inefficient organization.

Given today's need for active boards, we cannot afford to squander this valuable resource. Without the total involvement of trustees, it's difficult for executives to understand the needs of the communities they serve and to determine how best to meet those needs while maintaining financial stability.

So what can and should be done about this situation?

A Solution: Governance Restructuring

The answer for many systems is governance restructuring. According to The Governance Institute's 1999 *Biennial Survey of Health System Boards,* 53 percent of the 77 responding systems had conducted comprehensive governance assessments in the past two years. Of those, 63 percent had fundamentally restructured their governance model as a result.

Restructuring looks different for each organization, but it generally entails a comprehensive assessment of:

- The corporate structure (e.g., the "boxes" on the organizational chart representing each board and committee)
- Board and committee composition (i.e., the number and types of skills of members)
- Governance functioning (i.e., roles, responsibilities, and authority; meeting effectiveness, decision-making processes; orientation and education)

Although on the surface this seems like a straightforward process, governance restructuring can be fraught with difficulties.

An Organizational Change Initiative

When Sister Gretchen Kunz, president and CEO, and Bill McGee, board chair, of the St. Joseph Health System in Bryan, Texas, decided to initiate a governance restructuring effort, they were concerned that their trustees would be uncomfortable with the discussion. In fact, they thought that talking about changing board members' roles, responsibilities, and authority would create fear and uncertainty and could lead to resistance to governance restructuring. In other words, they recognized that the restructuring must be viewed in the context of an organizational change initiative.

Start with Education

To counteract this potential reaction, St. Joseph began the restructuring process with a multiday, systemwide governance retreat. Everyone who served on boards throughout the system was invited to this event, where board and committee members participated in a highly interactive educational session about national health care trends, governance best practices, and organizational change dynamics. One hundred and twenty people—trustees, physician leaders, and senior managers—participated in the retreat.

Engage Key Stakeholders

Next, St. Joseph used a participatory approach to its governance restructuring. Many of the system's key stakeholders (e.g., board members, physicians, and senior administrators) provided input into and feedback on the process. They identified obstacles to effective governance and offered suggestions for needed changes. As a result, the key stakeholders strongly supported the final recommendations to streamline the structure and to change other aspects of their functioning because they had been involved in defining the problems and creating the solutions. Their fears had been allayed through education and conversation.

Be Participative and Efficient

To succeed as it did, the St. Joseph restructuring process needed not only to be highly participatory; it had to be efficient. No one had the time or the desire to make a career out of governance restructuring.

To balance the "competing goods" of participation and efficiency, a small task force was created. This group of 10 board members, physicians, and senior administrators met a few times to analyze the information gathered during the input and feedback sessions, to review the options presented by the facilitators/consultants, and to make recommendations to the system board. In this way, St. Joseph got the best of both worlds: involvement from a large number of stakeholders and an effective, efficient decision-making process (see the figure below for a graphic depiction of this process).

Common Changes

What kinds of organizational changes occur as a result of governance restructuring?

The Corporate Structure

Although there are many different ways of organizing governance, the ultimate goal is for "form to follow function." In other words, the structure should be aligned with, and support, the system's mission and vision.

Generally, governance restructuring results in a more streamlined corporate chart. By consolidating and/or eliminating legal entities, there are fewer layers, fewer boards, and fewer standing committees.

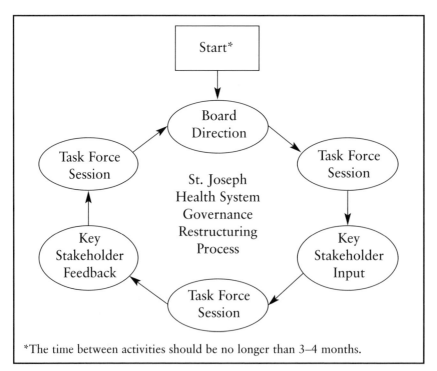

For example, the system that started with 16 boards and 57 committees was able to decrease its structure to one system board, 2 hospital boards, and 12 advisory entities.

However, decreasing the total number of boards and committees does not necessarily result in fewer individuals serving in governance. In the above example, boards of subsidiary organizations were converted to advisory boards and committees. In this way, the system retained community input, but it clarified decision-making authority among governing bodies.

Board and Committee Composition

The next stage of governance restructuring reconfigures board and committee composition. Generally, 12 to 15 trustees serve on each fiduciary board and five to nine people on each committee. Many systems have also instituted the "rule of three," in which no one individual can serve on any more than three boards or committees. To fill the seats, nonboard members are included on committees. This increases the number of community members serving the organization, creates a pool of potential future board members, and decreases the likelihood of trustee burnout.

After restructuring, many systems begin to use selection criteria as well as term limits for board and committee members. Selection criteria ensure that people with the right skills and perspectives are included. The use of term limits (e.g., three three-year terms) helps boards and committees recruit new people with energy and fresh ideas.

Governance Functioning

As a result of a comprehensive restructuring, many of the following changes may be included in the board-approved recommendations:

- Quicker and more effective decision making
- Improved communications across the system
- Mandatory orientation and education sessions
- Annual goal setting for the board
- Annual evaluation of board and committee members
- Increased focus on strategic and policy issues

Tips from the Trenches

St. Joseph Health System and other systems that have restructured their boards recommend the following as critical components of successful initiatives:

- The chair of the system board must fully agree with the need for the process and champion it. Otherwise, it will be a meaningless exercise, whose recommendations will not get implemented. Even worse, negative feelings among trustees could be dredged up, leaving the organization in worse shape than before the restructuring began.
- Because governance restructuring is a complex organizational change, it is helpful to have an experienced external consultant/ facilitator to assist with the design of the whole process, to facilitate the task force meetings, and to act as a coach to the CEO and board chair.
- A restructuring effort should include all the key stakeholders in the process (i.e., sponsors, system boards, subsidiary boards, senior administrators, and medical staff leaders). Strong, influential individuals who feel they have not been included in discussions can cause the initiative to fail by stimulating conflict and resistance to the changes among board members.
- In some cases, governance restructuring efforts have been initiated by physicians who want greater involvement in and/or access to the board. At one system, the medical staff had taken a vote of no confidence in the CEO and wanted to deal directly with the board. A highly inclusive governance restructuring process provided the forum for the physicians, board, and administrators to discuss the physicians' concerns and work out a series of structural and functional changes that have significantly improved relations and improved governance efficiency.
- When presented with governance structure options, it is difficult to know which one would serve the organization best. Creating and using a set of design principles to guide the restructuring effort can help a task force determine which of various alternatives are most appropriate for the system (see "Governance Design Principles" on page 177 for examples).

- The governance structure should be aligned with the system's purpose and strategic intent. If necessary, the boards and CEO should clarify the system's mission and vision before embarking on, or as part of, the restructuring effort.

The ultimate benefit of governance restructuring is an enhanced ability to perform the key roles and responsibilities of the board. Restructuring enables everyone connected to governance to better focus on the future, ensure high-quality clinical care and patient satisfaction, protect the financial health of the organization, ensure effective executive leadership, reflect the communities served, strengthen relationships with key stakeholders, and perpetuate effective governance. The ultimate goal for systems is to improve the health of those living in our communities. And isn't that why you agreed to serve as a trustee?

Accountability Stops Here: Educating the Board to Meet Its Responsibilities

By Shari Mycek

We've all been there—stuck bumper to bumper in a sea of fuming cars and SUVs—deadlocked on the highway, unable to turn back or accelerate forward. Inevitably, we resign ourselves to our place in line—make a phone call, turn up the radio volume, creep forward ever so slowly. When we finally reach the site of the accident, our necks crane. We can't help it. We look.

If it's only a minor fender bender, we may resume our previous pace. But if the accident is serious, if people are hurt, or, worse yet, if there appears to be a fatality, we slow down and heed the reminder.

It's that same type of moment to which Seattle-based governance expert Dennis D. Pointer says health care trustees must increasingly pay attention. In the past five years, the governance highway has witnessed two fatal crashes: first, the collapse of AHERF (Allegheny Health Education and Research Foundation in Pennsylvania) in 1998; and, most recently, the demise of Houston–based Enron, which declared bankruptcy in December 2001.

Shari Mycek is a contributing writer to *Trustee*.

Pointer raises the question, "Where were the boards?" in his presentation to trustees around the country. He works with more than 500 trustees, 70 percent of whom are on health care boards. And although he doesn't claim to have all of the answers in this new age of accountability, he does offer this insight: "Boards are as high up in organizations as one can go and still remain inside them. They bear ultimate fiduciary responsibility, authority, and accountability for their organization's affairs. As the plaque on Harry Truman's desk said: 'The buck stops here.'"

But increasingly, the governance "job" is tougher than it used to be.

"Ten years ago, health care trustees served on boards because it was a feather in their cap and a nice thing to do for the community," says Pam Knecht, vice-president of Accord Limited in Chicago, a national consulting firm specializing in governance and organizational strategy. "What's expected of trustees today is very different. The world of health care—with its mergers, acquisitions, takeovers, dispositions of assets—has become very complex, and trustees are being held accountable in ways never seen before." She also points to Enron, AHERF, and Intercoastal in West Palm Beach, Florida, where a community didn't want its hospital turned into an ambulatory care center.

"Communities are speaking out; attorneys general are stepping in, but trustees cannot and should not count on the state attorney general or the community to hold them accountable," says Knecht. "Accountability has to be self-imposed. Boards have to create and maintain a culture of holding themselves accountable."

But how?

Both Pointer and Knecht first suggest board education. The old adage that knowledge is power is perhaps nowhere more true than in the health care governance arena. But educating well-meaning, time-stretched trustees may be easier said than done.

Mary Walker, president and CEO of Texas Healthcare Trustees in Austin, speaks fondly of a trustee in her home state. Like many, this individual serves on multiple boards, is committed, and is a hard worker. But like many, he feels unsettled about his new responsibility as a not-for-profit hospital trustee. "Health care looks a little complicated," he told her. "But I'm sure I'll figure it all out. I didn't need any special training to be a bank trustee."

But "special training" is exactly what Walker and other governance experts are prescribing.

"Being on a board today is not about sitting down and having a cup of coffee," says Walker. "There are consequences to making bad decisions—of not having the right information, not asking the right questions."

"Health care governance is definitely not a competency-free zone," says Pointer. "Knowledge, skills, and experience (of the right type) are a board's most important and precious assets. Trustees need to understand the industry, the market, and their organization. What we're asking of them is really a lot."

And the job doesn't come without a hefty time commitment. The typical not-for-profit hospital or system trustee already clocks more hours in a given year than a director of a Fortune 500 corporation, so it's difficult to ask trustees to give more. The issue, therefore, is not how to get more time out of trustees but how to make the time they already spend more effective. Following are some thoughts on how to do that.

Focus, Focus, Focus

"Many of the boards I work with simply don't have a clear sense of what their obligations are and [what] type of work they need to do to

---

Board Skills

What are the core competencies that all health care trustees must possess to keep themselves and their organization accountable? Governance expert Dennis Pointer, of Pointer and Associates, Seattle, says that all trustees must understand:

- Governance obligations, functions, processes, and best practices
- The health care industry as well as their individual market and organization
- Key success factors, including strategic, financial, operational, and clinical variables
- How to read, analyze, and interpret basic financial statements

Pointer further notes that at least some board members must possess specific competencies in law; accounting and financial expertise; and clinical care.

---

fulfill those obligations," says Pointer. "They spend a great deal of time on issues that are irrelevant, inconsequential, and don't add a lot of value. If you have a 15-member board and five members think the board should be concentrating on A, B, and C; another five think the focus should be on D, E, and F; and the remaining five haven't much thought about either, that board is going to be ineffective by definition. To be effective, a board must have a collective notion of what it needs to do and how to go about doing it," Pointer says.

"One of my favorite quotes comes from the greatest philosopher around, country-western singer Willy Nelson, who says that 'if the next pot of chili tastes better than the last, it's probably due to something you left out versus something you put in,'" Pointer says. "I think that's true for governance. If the board has a laserlike focus on the things that will add value and make a difference—if it can clear everything else from its plate—it will be effective."

Defining Expectations

Knecht adds that trustees should be aware—up front—of what is expected of them. "When the nominating committee is out there trolling for potential board candidates, it is critical [that they] ask, 'Are you aware of what it is we're requesting of you?' Otherwise, we do our trustees a great disservice." She tells of one health care system that has instituted a covenant that board members must sign when they agree to serve on the board, stating how many hours they will spend in meetings, the number of educational sessions they're expected to attend, and so on.

"It takes guts to do this," she says. "In wooing potential board members, you don't want to make them feel like [governance] is a big bad job, but the truth is that it is a very serious responsibility."

In Kalamazoo, Michigan, former Borgess Health Alliance CEO Tim Stack demonstrated exactly that type of "guts." While at Borgess, Stack and his board chair sat down with the board and created a very realistic job description detailing the commitment required to serve on the board, the amount of time it would take, and the number and types of mandatory meetings. Now, as the new president and CEO of Piedmont Medical Center and Piedmont Hospital in Atlanta, Stack has asked the board there to follow suit.

"Right now, we're getting to know each other [at Piedmont]," says Stack. "But in a few months, we're going to start laying some serious expectation groundwork. Trustees have an awesome responsibility. The better prepared they are, the better off the organization is. Trustees of nonprofits do a great job, but it's a tremendous amount of time, and I think we have to be sensitive to their time—make it a little easier for them by letting them know what the expectations are ahead of time."

Stack describes the time spent with the Borgess board as "a wonderful process. It really set in place—in front of the board—the requirements. Then there's no surprise down the road when we say, 'Okay, we're going to meet 10 times a year, once a month on Tuesday mornings for three hours,' everyone knows the expectations. When the dialogue took place, some folks—for a variety of reasons—chose not to proceed because they couldn't meet the demands."

Board Development

Formal, didactic education is yet another critical way to help trustees. But rather than budget for a once-or-twice-a-year educational session, Knecht suggests that boards themselves create a complete development curriculum.

"Most often, boards hold a retreat, figure out the 'hot topic,' bring in a speaker to talk to the board, and that's it. We should approach board education and development the same way we would management education and development. Board members [usually] say that it takes two years to really learn—to be a good, functioning board member. That's a crime. We have to figure out how to orient our board members so that within two months they are feeling relatively comfortable, and by six months they're functioning."

And that begins with a comprehensive orientation.

Pointer says he has personally served on all different types of boards: nonprofit, hospital, health care system, and corporate. And despite his knowledge of governance and health care, there is a learning curve on every board.

"So many times, the idea of orientation is to grab new board members by the hand, walk them along the dock, throw them in the water, and tell them to have a nice swim," he says. "I can't tell you how many times that's happened to me. Orientation should instead be a series of well-designed activities that last the better part of the first year of a board member's tenure. I'm a huge advocate of orientation through mentoring—of pairing a new board member with a really excellent, experienced board member so that after a meeting, the new member can ask, 'Hey, what just happened in there?'"

Teaching Moments

As important as formal education are "teaching moments"—opportunities (Knecht advocates 30) built into every board meeting, where education is framed around a specific issue or challenge that trustees are facing.

If the hospital is contemplating a merger, a "teaching moment" might be to offer trustees insight into the board's roles and responsibilities for its fiduciary obligation and mission. Monthly reporting mechanisms (such as the well-known "Dash Board" approach—see "The Data Game" in the April 1997 issue of *Trustee,* available from the archives on www.trusteemag.com) are also recommended. But more important than the actual dashboard format is the assurance that every trustee knows how to interpret it.

"How can you serve as a member of the board and really govern if you can't read the basic financial statements of the institution?" asks Pointer. "How can you sit on a hospital board and not truly understand the factors that affect the quality of medical practice? The answer: you can't. So when trustees come on board, when we get the people [we want] to serve, we have to help them read, analyze, and interpret the data."

And, finally, trustees must continually engage in self-assessment.

"Feedback," says Pointer, "is the breakfast of champions." As with orientation, Pointer asserts that self-assessment needs to be a serious board activity. Boards must constantly ask themselves whether they are focusing on those issues that make a difference to the organization. Are they executing their proper roles? Meeting their obligations and responsibilities, their fiduciary duties? And they must courageously broach that "third rail" of governance—individual trustee assessment.

"Everyone knows [individual assessment] is important," says Pointer. "But no one wants to touch it. Yet it is critical in making reappointment decisions and for individual board member development."

In his presentation to trustees, Pointer repeatedly draws striking comparisons between what went wrong at Enron and what failed at AHERF (both of which he calls the "poster children of bad governance").

"Both boards formulated flawed business models, stumbled badly in executing their strategies, were blindsided by unanticipated industry and/or market forces, employed hyperaggressive accounting [practices], and engaged in highly questionable management and financial practices," he says.

The two boards also shared specific and similar behavioral characteristics. On both were highly intelligent, competent, experienced, and successful individuals, yet, according to Pointer, "most knew very little about their organization's industry, markets, business, and key strategic, financial, or operational success factors. Board meetings were highly scripted events, produced, choreographed, and performed by executives (board members spent meeting time listening passively); proposals were floated as faits accomplis; and board members who questioned or objected and expressed reservations were pushed aside or removed.

"Essentially, executives employed a 'mushroom management' strategy—keep the board in the dark and feed em' manure," Pointer adds.

One of the most effective strategies against such "mushroom management" is to raise flags and ask questions. The issue of decreased reimbursement provides a perfect example.

"Decreased reimbursement continues to be a problem," says Knecht. "As it becomes more and more difficult, hospitals have to figure out where to get revenues. Creative strategies are devised—some of which are great and fit directly with the mission of the organization and employ good ways of utilizing resources. Other strategies may be on the edge. Boards need to be educated about health care in general, and about various strategies in particular, to recognize a bad idea when they see it. And they need to call a 'stop action' if they find themselves in a position where management is suggesting something they think may be a little harebrained. Trustees need to be able to say, 'Hang on a sec,' and ask intelligent questions," Knecht says.

The same concept holds true in maintaining individual trustee accountability, and for this the board chair is key.

"The board chair has to be a person knowledgeable in governance and in health care, and also an individual who has the strength to make sure the board is, indeed, doing what it is supposed to be doing," she continues (see "Board Skills," page 186). "It's the board chair who really sets the tone for whether the board is going to serve as a social entity or whether it's going to do real work. If, for some reason, a person ends up on the board who simply shouldn't be there, the chair must be able to privately take that person aside and say, 'Hey, you haven't attended the educational meetings; you haven't even been to the last three board meetings. Shape up or ship out.'"

Show Them the Data

*What Do Trustees Need to Know
and How Do They Need to Know It?*

By Michelle Bitoun

As dubious business and accounting practices at U.S. corporations continue to dominate the news, hospital trustees aren't above the fray. The hospital industry, too, has its share of boards that have not lived up to their oversight responsibilities. (See the article "Accountability Stops Here" on page 184 of this book.) These cases are a sobering reminder of the professional and personal liabilities that hospital trustees face if they're not regularly reviewing the data and activities at their institution. In fact, many experts say these cases have underscored the need for board members to track more information than they have in the past.

"Boards need to know more than they used to—about business, the organization, competition, all those sorts of things," says L. Edward Bryant, Jr., a partner in the Chicago law offices of Gardner, Carton, Douglas, specializing in health care and governance. Bryant has served as counsel to many hospital boards and is currently board chair of the Sisters of Charity of Leavenworth (Kansas) Health System.

Michele Bitoun is an assistant professor at the Medill School of Journalism, Northwestern University, Evanston, Illinois, and a freelance writer.

Unlike the past, when "there wasn't a great deal of oversight" and board members who weren't involved in committees or leadership roles "just came [to meetings] and participated in social events," the stakes are now higher, Bryant says. "Boards have fiduciary obligations to [the hospital's] employees and medical staff to [govern] an enterprise that doesn't go bankrupt."

The same goes for unethical practices.

"I think [trustees] have concluded, based on AHERF, Allina, and other cases, that they [have] personal liability for a number of things," he says. Federal intermediate sanctions adopted in 2001, for example, assess serious penalties for deriving excess benefits from a tax-exempt entity. "This pertains to every transaction, including compensation, between the tax-exempt entity and an insider," Bryant adds.

But in order to stand firm at the helm, trustees need to be knowledgeable. Bryant refers to "The Sergeant Schultz Defense," a term coined by one of his partners and inspired by the *Hogan's Heroes* television sitcom character who feigned innocence with the frequent refrain, "I know nothing." Says Bryant, "Many hospital trustees or directors take the position, 'Nobody ever told me.' That's no longer a viable excuse . . . they're supposed to ask about these things."

What information do trustees need? James Lifton, a director with Arista Associates, a health care consulting firm in Northbrook, Illinois, emphasizes the difference between reviewing mere data—which is, no doubt, available to any hospital trustee in truckloads for the asking—and reviewing meaningful information that's presented by the administration in a clear, concise format.

"What we're really talking about is information. . . . Voluntary trustees can get a lot of data and not understand what they mean or not have time to review all of them," Lifton says. "I've seen boards get a three-ring binder or a large packet, and sometimes they don't know what to make of it, or they're unwilling or unable to take the time to go through it."

That's where a tool commonly referred to as a "scorecard" or "dashboard" comes in. The tool's indicators reflect the organization's goals and help trustees quickly gauge how well they are meeting their targets. "It's a very powerful approach that allows the board to look at information as you would on the dashboard of your car," Lifton says. More detailed information can be scrutinized in committees.

Experts have different opinions on the exact indicators to use, in part because they depend on a hospital's or health system's goals and strategies, which can change over time. Richard Umbdenstock, president and CEO of Providence Services, a nine-hospital system based in Spokane, Washington, and former head of the American Hospital Association's division of governance, says boards should be regularly reviewing indicators in several areas: finance, quality, patient and employee satisfaction, operations, and community benefit.

"I think within each [area], you have to decide what the important indicators are, and then within those [determine whether] the bells and whistles are going off on one or two of them. If they are, how are you attending to them?" says Umbdenstock. "It would be good if the board and management agreed on the critical 10, 15, or 20 indicators that span the the enterprise and [treat] them as a balanced set of indicators so that they're not just looking at finance, which is the general tendency, because it's the universal language [that most people understand]."

Lifton agrees. The dashboard or scorecard concept isn't new, particularly in the business world, but what is changing, he says, is the breadth and complexity of chosen hospital indicators evolving from basic financial measurements to criteria reflecting a variety of strategic goals, including quality, staffing, and even charity care.

"I think that most boards, in fact the majority, probably started with financial indicators because that's what they're most comfortable with. They understand operating margins. They understand [patient] days and accounts receivable. They understand equity as a percentage of total capitalization," Lifton says.

Umbdenstock says it's the CEO's job to recommend a set of indicators to the board, "but it's up to the board to then say, 'Yeah, that makes sense,' or 'I'd be interested in these, and, oh, by the way, maybe quarterly I want to know what our liability experience and lawsuit experience has been,' or 'In my business, X, Y, and Z are really important. How come they're not here?' " Some of the current significant issues to track include medication errors and overall patient safety issues, such as wrong-site surgery, he says, as well as pain management for those with chronic or terminal conditions.

For instance, Providence uses four indicators to monitor quality: medication errors; risk-adjusted mortality rates; severity-adjusted length of stay versus expected length of stay; and severity-adjusted complication rates. In the area of charity care, the system looks at dollars as a percent of nongovernment patient revenue. Umbdenstock says the format was challenging for the individual hospitals of the system to implement because:

> People have been defining these [indicators] their own ways for years. They're not used to having to change those definitions to conform to a group process. Secondly, sometimes they're not set up to collect this particular set of data, so it's either costly or culturally challenging to get people to organize their systems to produce the data. But generally, I think, what most people would have on this type of balanced scorecard is stuff that the field has started to focus on as key potential hot spots that a board ought to be aware of.

The Sisters of Charity of Leavenworth Health System, a nine-hospital system spanning four states, instituted a 30-indicator report (see pages 196–197) for its 15 board members about a year ago. The approach has streamlined meetings and reduced confusion at board meetings. In fact, the approach has cut the number of board meetings from six to four per year.

"It really allows the board to get a good sense for whether the administration is moving forward and whether, in fact, the organization is moving toward its vision for the future," says Bill Murray, president of the Sisters of Charity system. "In the past . . . as [trustees] would look at reports, they had a difficult time determining whether we were actually making progress. And . . . this report has helped them . . . to look at the total operation and understand whether or not we're doing the things we need to do."

The indicators reflect the system's four strategies: mission and culture; physician relations; health care transformation (such as new service lines); and consumer value. Within each of those four areas, the board tracks specific quarterly indicators delineated by red dots (which means the target has not been met), white dots (which means the target has been met), or green dots (which indicates that the target has been exceeded). The indicators include traditional financial markers, such as profit margin, but also cover employee vacancy rates and turnover, free care, community service, medication errors that cause patients harm, and physician and patient satisfaction.

SISTERS OF CHARITY OF LEAVENWORTH HEALTH SYSTEM

Performance Indicators

Outcomes as Compared to Internal Targets for the Fiscal Year Ended May 31, 2002

			Providence Health			Montana Region				
		SCLHS	Providence Medical Center	Saint John Hospital	St. Francis Health Center	Holy Rosary Healthcare	St. James Healthcare	St. Vincent Healthcare	Saint John's Health Center	St. Mary's Hospital & Medical Center
Mission and Culture										
Quality of Worklife										
Nurse Turnover	E	X	◆	◆	X	X	◆	■	X	◆
RN Vacancy Rates	I	X	◆	◆	X	X	X	X	X	X
Employee Turnover	E	X	◆	◆	X	■	X	X	X	◆
Employee Satisfaction	E	X	X	X	■	X	X	X	X	X
Social Accountability										
Social Accountability/Community	I	X	X	X	X	X	X	X	X	X
Benefit Expense										
Care of the Poor Expense**	I	X	X	X	X	X	X	X	X	X
Physician Relations										
Physician Satisfaction										
Physician Admissions Growth	I	X	X	X	■	■	X	■	X	■
Physician Satisfaction	I	■	◆	◆	■	X	◆	X	X	■
Health Services Transformation										
Growth										
Adjusted Admissions**	I	■	X	■	X	X	■	X	■	■
Inpatient Surgeries	I	■	X	◆	X	◆	◆	■	X	■
Outpatient Surgeries	I	X	X	◆	■	◆	X	X	■	◆
Emergency Room Visits (Admitted)	I	◆	X	X	■	■	◆	X	◆	◆
Births	I	■	X	◆	◆	X	◆	◆	X	■
Open Heart Surgeries	I	◆	X	na	◆	na	na	◆	◆	◆

Consumer Value

	Benchmark						
Quality							
Unscheduled Readmissions	E	O	O	O	O	O	O
Pain Management	E	O	O	O	O	O	O
Patient Falls	I	O	O	O	O	O	O
Medication Errors	I	O	O	O	O	O	O
Surgical Site Infection Rate— Hip Arthroplasty	E	O	O	O	O	O	O
Post CABG Mortality	E	O	na	O	na	na	O
Financial*							
EBIDA Margin**	I	◆ ■ ◆	◆ X ◆	■ X X	◆ X ◆	◆ X ◆	◆ X X
Days in Net Accounts Receivable	I	X	X	X	X	X	X
Days Cash on Hand	I	◆ ■ ◆	◆ X ◆	■ X X	◆ X ◆	◆ X ◆	◆ X X
Debt Service Coverage Ratio	I						
Operational*							
Paid Hours per Adjusted Admission	I	■ ■	■ ■	■ ■	X ■	■ ■	■ ■
Total Expense per Adjusted Admission, CMI Adjusted**	I	■ ■	■ ■	■ ■	X ■	■ ■	■ ■
Compensation Ratio	I	◆ ◆	■ X	■ ■	◆ ■	◆ ■	◆ ■
Medicare Average Length of Stay, CMI Adjusted	I	◆ ◆	■ X	■ ■	◆ ■	◆ ■	◆ ■
Customer Satisfaction							
Adult Inpatient Satisfaction**	E	■	■	■	■	■	■
Emergency Room Patient Satisfaction	E	X	X	X	X	X	X

*Inclusive of System Office (net of Eliminations) and Exempla/Saint Joseph Hospital

**Key Performance Indicators

Legend:

X Greater than 3% Favorable Variance

■ Within 3% of Internal Targets

◆ Greater than 3% Unfavorable Variance

O Not Available

E- External Benchmark or Target

I- Internal Benchmark or Target

Source: Sisters of Charity of Leavenworth Health System, Leavenworth, Kansas.

Murray and all the system's hospital CEOs created the indicators together. "Some came out of our strategic plan, some of them are actually the measures we use for performance-based [manager] compensation, and some of them are indicators we would be tracking anyway," Murray explains. The targets, plus or minus 3 percent, reflect either internal standards (systemwide goals) or external standards (such as industry norms).

Bryant says dashboard indicators have been key to improving his trustees' efficiency, setting incentive compensation, making strategic moves in local markets, setting agendas, and bringing in speakers to discuss trouble spots. Especially for a diverse board that may have difficulty reaching consensus on specific issues to study, "this helps you do it," he says.

"It's amazing how much time you save and how much it helps you focus your interest," says Bryant. "You don't have to spend 40 minutes going over 60 pages of financials. Literally, within 2 minutes, you can figure out where your problems are, then go to that part of the financial statement or the feasibility report, or whatever it is."

Homing in on what criteria to put on a dashboard does take some trial and error. "It's a couple of years before you fully feel these systems work," Bryant says. For example, his board initially used AOIM (area of interest management) to measure operating margin until trustees finally switched to EBIDA (earnings before interest, depreciation, and amortization) to factor out depreciation, over which the hospital board had no control.

"Sometimes it's those accounting nuances that you [need to] keep adjusting your dashboards to pick up," he says.

But for Bryant, the 30-indicator dashboard now used by the Sisters of Charity of Leavenworth provides just the right amount of depth because it encompasses every area in which board members need to be informed, including incentive compensation, strategic planning, and operations. "We started out with 16 and worked our way up to 30," he says.

"[The indicator report] is really a red flag report, if you will," adds Murray. "It's a rollup of a lot of other reports that [the board] might have been seeing." But it works better. Previously, he says, board members "were frustrated that as they would look at reports periodically, they had a difficult time determining whether we were actually making progress. And that's what this report has helped them to do—to be able to look at the total operation and understand whether or not we're doing the things we need to do. And we're not looking just at finance. We're really looking at volume growth and quality indicators to get a sense of whether there are any areas of concern."

The approach has also helped board members spot trends that could affect their future significantly. "There's a change taking place in cardiovascular surgery—with the introduction of beta-blockers and the use of stents, the number of open heart [surgeries] is going down . . . and . . . we saw it right across the whole system, and we're able to take that [finding] into consideration as we're projecting our long-range plans," Murray says.

Murray adds that the approach has also allowed the system to zero in on nurse vacancies and turnover rates to such an extent that it's now looking at them on a systemwide basis. "We're able to really get a sense for [which hospitals in the system] have problems," he says. No more than 30 indicators are used at one time, but they may change with shifts in the system's priorities and long-range plans.

Committing to the targets associated with these indicators, especially financial ones, such as operating margin—and holding management accountable by tying them to compensation—is critical to a hospital system's success, says Nathan Kaufman, senior vice president for health care strategy with Superior Consultant Holdings Corp., San Diego. For-profit hospitals operate this way as a matter of course, but the same should hold true for not-for-profits, he says.

"Even when tax-exempt hospitals quantify things and hold people accountable, they achieve [their target], so that's what the game's all about," he says. What often happens, however, is that management will look at a margin that isn't 5 percent and cite a nursing shortage or some other problem to justify why the goal was not achieved, he says. "What the board of trustees should be asking is, 'Okay, what are we going to do to get it to 5 percent?'" The board may not achieve the target immediately, but it should adopt a sense of urgency about working toward it, he says.

The critical performance indicators Kaufman recommends tracking, with some targets subject to modification to reflect local market conditions, include: operating margin (at least 5 percent); earnings before depreciation, interest, taxes, and amortization (at least 15 percent); personnel expense (less than 45 percent of net revenue); supply expense (less than 16 percent of net revenue); growth in net revenue per adjusted patient (at least 6 percent); growth in net revenue (at least 8 percent); inpatient surgery per 100 admissions (at least 28); bad debts as a percent of net revenue (less than 8 percent); accounts receivable (less than 65 days); growth in ER visits (at least 3 percent), as well as other key services; RN turnover; employee turnover; patient satisfaction; and quality indicators (see "Strategic Vision" in the July/August 2002 issue of *Trustee*).

Kaufman says these indicators should be reviewed by the board every month, and if the system isn't within its targets, "there has to be an action plan to get them back in place. . . . When there's a variance from the target, there needs to be some sense of urgency and some activity and action plan in place that brings it back over time into compliance." For instance, if staffing costs went up because the hospital raised nurses' salaries, one option might be to raise prices in the next round of pricing, even if it's not for another six months.

Methodist Hospital in Arcadia, California, starting tracking about a dozen performance indicators a few years ago, including inpatient and outpatient activity, patient satisfaction and quality information, cash position, and a case mix index. Holding itself to these targets has encouraged the board to improve its operating margin significantly, which started out at 1.3 percent, says CEO Dennis Lee.

"Nate's message to us [during a retreat] was that even though we're tax exempt, most hospitals need a 5 percent operating margin in order to generate sufficient cash surpluses to be able to replace our equipment, buy new equipment, invest in new technologies, and invest in our facilities," says Lee.

The 5 percent goal prompted the 18-member board to assemble a task force comprising board members, medical leaders, and administrators to identify three or four "attack points" to boost their profit margin. One of those strategies was to negotiate higher rates with managed care companies. It worked.

"Virtually all the HMOs have [agreed to] our rates," says Lee. "Sometimes they jockey for position, and they do it at the 11th hour. Sometimes [they miss] the expiration date and then come back a week later and agree to [the new rate]. There's that kind of game-playing going on. But in just about every case, we've been successful in getting higher rates." The board expects to hit a 3.3 percent operating margin this year, followed by 4 to 4.5 percent the next year, and 5 percent after that.

Methodist's scorecard is designed as a bar graph using individual months, as well as a 12-month rolling average. To the left are targets (set internally) and prior years' performance so that board members can see trends. "The variances that occur from month to month—that's really what a board needs to see," Lee says.

He says the dashboard format has been well received by the board. "My impression and the direct feedback [I receive] is that [trustees] really do understand it; they like seeing the graphs; it's meaningful information to them; and they really do have a sense for how well the hospital is doing—for example, is our volume growing? Are our inpatient admissions going up or down or remaining stable? Is our outpatient activity going up, down, or remaining stable? Are revenues above our costs?"

In the past, Lee says, he'd get all that information to trustees, then ask them for their general impression of the hospital's status. "They'd say, 'Gee, I don't know,' because it was too much detail for them. Now it's a digestible amount of information."

The targets used have been established in the budget," Lee says. "We don't routinely give industry standards on the key performance indicators, because we don't have access to that information on a real-time basis, but generally once every year or two we will engage a consultant to get us the benchmark information to show the board how we compare."

Bryant says that boards must track services that make their hospitals and systems unique, as well as typical financial indicators. And they need to be just as vigilant about tracking losing operations as they are about winners. "In hospital language, cross-subsidization was what always solved everything," says Bryant. "It didn't matter that you lost money in arthritis center operations because you made money in cardiac. Or it didn't matter that you lost money in the emergency room because you made money in oncology. But you never quite knew how much money you were making or losing on a per-service basis, so you could never make actual tactical or strategic decisions about what to do and what not to do. It's that discipline that [boards] can bring to hospitals—knowing whether an enterprise is viable or not doesn't mean looking at just the bottom line."

Diagnosing the Health of Your Organization: Early Warning Signs

By Mary K. Totten
and James E. Orlikoff

Trustees who believe it is their role to help create their organization's future understand that good stewardship first requires a solid understanding of their performance today. Tools and processes that allow boards to routinely assess and compare their hospital or health system's performance over time can identify potential problems early on that might erode the organization's overall health—sometimes more rapidly than board members could have thought possible (see "*Trustee* Workbook 1: Stewardship of the Future," January 2000 issue of *Trustee*).

Rather than being forced to confront a turnaround or other drastic crisis measures, governing boards should engage in ongoing performance monitoring, getting the information they need to keep their organizations on track. In order to be a good steward, anticipation is the name of the game. So to help boards identify the early warning signs of a business failure, we talked with John Tiscornia, principal, Wellspring Partners, Ltd., Chicago, a financial consultant with more than 30 years' experience advising health care organizations.

Mary K. Totten is president of Totten & Associates, Oak Park, Illinois. James E. Orlikoff is president of Orlikoff & Associates, Inc., Chicago.

"Prudent health care organizations routinely engage in risk management activities to help evaluate and improve the quality of the services they deliver," says Tiscornia. "Boards need to conduct risk management from a business perspective to help their organizations regularly assess and improve their overall performance. Once problems hit the bottom line, it may be too late."

He adds: "Research tells us that about 70 percent of health care organization failures are due to flawed strategies. All of us are familiar with some of the more high-profile failures, such as hospitals or health systems engaging in large-scale purchasing of physician practices or getting into the insurance business by buying a health maintenance organization. Yet the problem of flawed strategy runs deeper.

"Some hospital boards will authorize the purchase of expensive imaging equipment, such as an MRI, without asking for a specific business plan, what risks [the purchase of such equipment] might pose for the organization, and what plans management has to minimize those risks," Tiscornia says. "After the purchase, the board may never look back to assess results."

Trustees often fail to ask whether the programs or services they approved actually fulfilled their volume or financial projections and, if so, over what period of time, Tiscornia says. And unlike many of their corporate counterparts, health care boards, for whatever reason, often fail to act when performance is not on target.

"I know organizations that purchased physician practices and planned to lose money in the first year and break even after four years," Tiscornia says. "Four years later, the practices were still losing money, and no action had been taken. In an uncertain environment, boards need to be tolerant of risk-taking, yet they also must act appropriately when a project doesn't deliver."

What's on Your Board's Radar Screen?

Although most boards and their finance committees regularly review selected indicators of the organization's overall financial performance, many need to perform a more comprehensive evaluation. And though boards will frequently step back and study the big picture once their own organization is in trouble, Tiscornia says a better approach is to look for cracks in the dike—early warning signs that, if addressed, can prevent financial disaster.

Governing boards should routinely complete a diagnostic checklist that broadly assesses overall organizational performance. Tiscornia recommends that boards and executives complete and review such a checklist two to four times a year to help diagnose potential problems in market, money, people, management, medical staff, and governance.

Market

Tiscornia believes "it all starts with the market." Health care organizations, however, often focus too much on their internal indicators. They look at how many inpatients are on today's census or how many outpatients came through the door during a given period. Many don't spend enough time looking at market share trends; and when times get tough, marketing is often one of the first areas to see staff or budget cuts.

Boards need to receive monthly or, at least, quarterly revenue and expense summaries for their hospital's top five product lines in order to track profitability, Tiscornia advises.

Having ongoing processes in place to monitor how strategies are carried out can help prevent failures down the road. For example, "if an organization has a strategy to improve employee satisfaction through recruitment and retention, yet no additional dollars have been budgeted for recruiting or retention activities, the likelihood of success is slim," he says.

"It's also important to know where board members and their families receive their own health care. The answer to that question is a 'gut check' about what trustees really think of the organization's quality," he adds.

Money

Even though boards should routinely review financial indicators, some health care boards don't pay enough attention to their cash position until they have difficulty paying their bills. Tiscornia recommends developing and using daily cash flow projections and trends to help both executives and the board stay current on their performance and prevent denial.

Assessing Your Organization's Market Orientation

To assess its market orientation, the board should answer the following questions:

	Yes	No
1. Are key strategies and investments aligned?	☐	☐
2. Do you monitor your corporate strategy?	☐	☐
3. Do you and your families use this hospital when you need care?	☐	☐
4. Are your top five product lines profitable?	☐	☐
5. Is market share increasing for your top five product lines?	☐	☐
6. Are customer perception and organizational image key strengths?	☐	☐
7. Is satisfaction improving for these groups:		
• Patients	☐	☐
• Physicians	☐	☐
• Employees	☐	☐

Board Checklist for Monitoring the Organization's Financial Position

	Yes	No
1. Are your financial, quality, and other key indicators identifying the right information?	☐	☐
2. Are your operating, financial, and quality reports providing timely information in a format you can understand and use?	☐	☐
3. Are your operating and financial projections on target?	☐	☐
4. Do you have a consistent program to evaluate revenue improvements?	☐	☐
5. Do your net revenue/admissions compare favorably with those of your competitors'?	☐	☐
6. Do you review monthly and daily cash flow projections?	☐	☐
7. Is your operating cash flow sufficient to meet future investments?	☐	☐
8. Has your revenue cycle—from admission, treatment, and discharge—been evaluated and updated recently?	☐	☐
9. Are nonsalary contracts competitive with others in your market?	☐	☐

Continued →

Board Checklist on Workforce Issues

	Yes	No
1. Do you have appropriate performance indicators for the organization and each business function?	☐	☐
2. Have you developed benchmarks for each performance indicator?	☐	☐
3. Does the organization support management's educational and skill needs with appropriate resources?	☐	☐
4. Are accurate performance data available to key users?	☐	☐
5. Are protocol-driven processes in place to support the appropriate use of resources?	☐	☐
6. Are managers accountable for the deployment of resources to enhance their staff's performance?	☐	☐

Board Checklist for Monitoring Management

	Yes	No
1. Have you reviewed your organizational structure recently?	☐	☐
2. Is management accountable for organizational performance?	☐	☐
3. Does your organizational culture support your vision and mission?	☐	☐
4. Are managers trained to use performance management tools, such as mentoring and evaluations?	☐	☐
5. Does the incentive compensation formula encourage "stretching" accounting rules?	☐	☐
6. Is financial management focused on the future rather than on past performance?	☐	☐
7. Are finance executives and managers rather than members of your finance department accountable for operating variances?	☐	☐
8. As labor costs are reduced, are adequate internal and business controls maintained?	☐	☐
9. Is the hospital's infrastructure adequate to handle additional patients?	☐	☐

Continued →

Board Checklist for Monitoring Medical Staff Issues

	Yes	No
1. Does physician compensation align with your strategy and mission?	☐	☐
2. Do you have a system for monitoring the value the organization receives relative to physician compensation?	☐	☐
3. Do physicians have communication channels outside of the formal medical staff organization?	☐	☐
4. Does the hospital have an active and effective medical staff human resources plan?	☐	☐
5. Does the hospital or system offer a leadership training program for physicians?	☐	☐
6. Are periodic physician satisfaction surveys completed and reported?	☐	☐

Governance Checklist

	Yes	No
1. Are the roles of board committees and the full board clear?	☐	☐
2. Are the roles of the board and management clear?	☐	☐
3. Are decisions made appropriately and effectively?	☐	☐
4. Are decisions made in a timely manner?	☐	☐
5. Does the board have no more than 15 members?	☐	☐
6. Does the board use specific criteria for selecting new members, including personal characteristics and functional skills?	☐	☐
7. Does the board conduct a self-evaluation each year?	☐	☐
8. Does the board spend 60 percent of its time on strategic issues?	☐	☐
9. Do the board and individual trustees have good relationships with key physicians?	☐	☐

Source: John F. Tiscornia, principal, Wellspring Partners, Ltd., Chicago.

"A 'bad month' can easily become a 'bad six months' unless the board recognizes the trend, asks how soon management plans to get 'the train back on track,' and then holds everyone accountable," Tiscornia says. "Focusing on the organization's performance in this area can help avoid the need for big year-end adjustments."

People

If people are an organization's key asset, then it's important to know how the organization invests in them. The board and management need a real-time picture of employee satisfaction to help assess staff needs. The problem with satisfaction surveys is often in the lag time—frequently as long as a year—between when a survey is fielded, the results analyzed, and problems addressed. Tiscornia recommends that health care organizations conduct satisfaction studies on a rolling basis, surveying a portion of employees or physicians each quarter to provide more timely data and faster problem identification and resolution.

Management

So much of an organization's performance relates to its culture and to the tools and resources available to managers. In many hospitals, managers of clinical services have had little or no management training, Tiscornia says, and performance accountability is lacking. Boards and executives need to monitor regularly the extent to which they provide clear expectations for management's performance, as well as whether they provide appropriate training and incentives to help managers achieve desired results.

Medical Staff

Many organizations have development and succession plans for their key employees and executives, but few have such plans for their medical staff, Tiscornia says. The lack of such a plan should be a warning sign to boards of a potential problem. Board members should ask for a breakdown of medical staff by highest admitters, age, and specialty. If data show that all of the medical staff's heart surgeons are 55 years old or older, for example, it's time to begin recruiting

Tips for Using a Performance Diagnostic Checklist

Listed below are several suggestions boards can use to help them note early warning signs of performance problems in their own organization.

1. Customize the checklists shown here to enable the board and executive management to broadly evaluate the hospital's or system's overall performance.
2. Consider completing and reviewing the results of the checklists on a quarterly or biannual basis as part of a scheduled board meeting or retreat.
3. Have both trustees and executives independently complete the checklists and discuss results.
4. Clarify and discuss every negative response and follow up with corrective action where needed.
5. Make sure the board has processes in place for timely follow-up and resolution of identified performance problems.
6. Move toward implementing organizationwide, ongoing processes for gathering and tracking performance-related information.
7. Board committees should incorporate specific performance indicators or sections of the performance checklist into their work plans to promote more frequent board performance monitoring.
8. Make participation in performance monitoring part of the board's job description.
9. Include an evaluation of how well the performance monitoring process works as part of the board's self-assessment.
10. At least annually, summarize and share performance problems with the full board that were resolved through performance monitoring.

new, younger surgeons. Other medical staff issues to consider are shown in the Board Checklist for Monitoring Medical Staff Issues (p. 207).

Governance

Dysfunctional governance is a clear indication of organizational performance problems. For example, boards that don't understand the distinction between the role of the board as a whole and the role of committees or that increasingly cross the line between governance and management often see their organization's financial performance deteriorate eventually, Tiscornia says. Other board performance questions include those listed in the Governance Checklist (page 207).

Discussion Exercise

In "The Success Syndrome" (in *Leader to Leader*, Jossey-Bass: San Francisco, 1999, pp 201–212), David A. Nadler and Mark Nadler write that sustained success can foster organizational complacency, which can lead to reduced innovation, increased costs and bureaucracy, and an organizational inability to act, adapt, or learn. Nadler and Nadler suggest that leaders take the following eight steps to prevent the success syndrome from infecting their organizations:

1. Create and sustain an external focus. Leaders need to communicate constantly and reinforce by personal example that the organization must continuously focus on customers, competitors, new technology, and market forces.
2. Maintain a contrarian mindset. Even if things are going well, performance can always be improved.
3. Never underestimate your competition. Don't assume your competitor's recent win is just a flash in the pan. Understand that even a small competitor might have a better strategy, market assessment, or product than you.
4. Anticipate change through systematic, periodic environmental scans. Anticipating disruptive change can give your organization time to experiment with ways to minimize potentially negative effects.

5. Think of yourself as your own biggest competitor. Don't be afraid to innovate and be out front with a new product or service, even if it means getting out of existing business lines or taking business away from a profitable product or service.
6. Don't wait until a crisis to bring in new, experienced leaders from outside your organization or industry. Be willing to question why your organization does things the way that it does.
7. Pay close attention to the observations of frontline employees. These people are often the first ones to sense when something is going wrong.
8. Create formal processes to analyze your successes and failures so that lessons learned can be applied throughout the organization.

Conclusion

To secure their hospital's future, boards must first find firm footing in their present performance. Tools and resources that help governing boards routinely and systematically monitor their organization's performance and provide early warning signs of performance problems can give boards the information they need to make corrections today that can avert disasters tomorrow. Although hindsight can help us see the past more clearly, foresight is the foundation of true vision.

PART FIVE

Finance

Finance:
What Trustees Need
to Know

By Timothy G. Solberg

Hospitals are currently addressing some of the most significant financial challenges they've ever faced. Budgets are tighter and margins are narrower than ever before. Government regulations—from the Balanced Budget Act to Medicare and Medicaid cuts—have constrained revenues for many hospitals. Public and private payers are demanding more information and accountability. And market forces—from closures to mergers and consolidations of hundreds of hospitals—are placing new pressures on boards and senior executives to protect their bottom line while, in many cases, their revenue shrinks.

Hospitals thinking ahead—to new buildings, renovations, and capital improvements—may find it harder to obtain needed funds. Not-for-profit hospitals typically fund major building projects through municipal bonds backed by private markets. These bonds are usually secured with assistance from state and/or local government authorities that help hospitals obtain affordable capital. But financial markets now see hospitals as a riskier investment. Bond and credit ratings for hospitals are dropping (in 1999 Moody's

---

Timothy G. Solberg is an investment consultant in Chicago. He can be reached at (312) 518–5599.

Investors Service downgraded the bond and credit ratings of five times as many hospitals as it upgraded, an unprecedented ratio), which makes it harder for some hospitals to obtain needed capital.

But the picture isn't entirely gloomy. The growing economy and booming stock market have created millions of jobs and billions of dollars in new capital. Trustees have significant control and influence over how they invest the hospital's assets and can leverage good economic times to shore up their fiduciary responsibility.

The key issues for trustees are:

1. Fiduciary responsibility and requirements
2. Investment management practices and responsibilities
3. Traditional versus new investment strategies and long-term considerations for "staying ahead of the curve" to deliver and expand services

Fiduciary Responsibilities

The definition of "fiduciary"—involving a confidence or trust—is a significant responsibility for trustees. Basically, it means managing and investing the institution's assets prudently with an eye toward maximum return at minimum risk.

Hospital trustees are not brokers or fund managers; they should not be micromanaging a hospital's portfolio, but, instead, they should be providing oversight, asking sound questions (see below),

---

Questions to Ask Your CFO, Investment Advisor, or Fellow Trustees

1. How frequently should the board receive information about hospital investments and their performance and make investment decisions?
2. What proportion of the total budget is manageable for investing?
3. What do I need to know to manage both short- and long-term needs and demands?
4. What is our asset strategy and mix?
5. Does the board retain an investment counselor and/or fund manager?

and, most important, recruiting and turning to investment counselors and managers to handle the organization's assets wisely.

Given that many trustees have business and financial experience, the "risk-return" concept shouldn't be difficult to fathom. But, in reality, a trustee's fiduciary role—regardless of his or her personal comfort with risk—typically changes when managing a public trust.

Trustees traditionally behave conservatively, investing assets in low-risk bonds and cash equivalents like certificates of deposit.

These comparatively safe and highly liquid options typically generate returns comparable to the rate of inflation. A decade ago, when inflation was 9 to 10 percent and the stock market was relatively stagnant, these investments generally met the standards of fiduciary responsibility. But today, with low inflation, the booming stock market of 1995–1999, and constraints on revenue streams, the same portfolio not only produces comparatively lower returns but most likely doesn't keep up with revenue losses. If, however, the downturn in the stock market during the first half of 2000 persists, trustees will need to make corrections to their hospitals' portfolios.

Investment Management Practices— Retirement and Corporate Assets

Retirement Funds

Hospitals typically offer and manage assets of one or more of three types of retirement plans.

Traditional defined benefit (DB) plans guarantee fixed payouts to beneficiaries at retirement. These plans are established so that the amount of the employee's retirement income is preset, with employer contributions (determined by actuaries) sufficient to enable the fund to meet liabilities as they come due. According to the 1999 Hewitt Associates, LLC *Survey Findings: Hospital and Multi-Hospital System Investment Practices*, more than 70 percent of independent and system hospitals still maintain DB pension plans.

Defined contribution plans—known as 401(k) plans—are those in which beneficiaries contribute from their pay. Payouts are based on how plan funds perform. Until 1997, these plans were limited to for-profits and a limited category of not-for-profits, but now hospitals and other not-for-profits may offer them—29 percent of systems and 15 percent of hospitals did so in 1999.

Tax-sheltered annuities (TSAs) have typically constituted the mainstay of not-for-profits' retirement offerings. Employees take money from their paychecks and put those funds into a flexible annuity for retirement. Three-quarters of systems and two-thirds of hospitals offer these plans, though these numbers have decreased since the advent of 401(k) plans for not-for-profits.

It's important for trustees to know how these plans are managed. DB plans, for example, are overfunded if returns on investment exceed promised liabilities. (They are underfunded if their investments have poorer-than-expected returns.) Overfunded pension plans are, of course, preferable because hospitals can contribute less for every year of overfunding, thereby freeing resources for other priorities.

That's why, in today's market, many defined benefit plans have shifted assets into equities with generally good results. In 1999, nearly 75 percent of systems' defined benefit plans generated returns of 10 percent or more, with more than 40 percent realizing more than 15 percent returns. Virtually all pension plans responding to the Hewitt survey allowed nearly two-thirds of their total portfolio to be equity based. Among hospitals' defined benefit plans, the average 1999 return was nearly 12 percent.

Corporate Assets

There are typically five types of these assets managed by hospitals:

1. Short-term operating funds are used for immediate needs. They help pay salaries and other day-to-day bills, usually for up to 180

Retirement Fund Investments			
Type of Fund	1999 Median Return	Median Asset Size (in Millions)	Proportion of Total Assets
Independent Not-for-Profit Hospitals			
Defined benefit pension	12.0%	$30.4	45.7%
Funded depreciation	7.5%	$19.0	28.6%
Foundation/endowment	10.8%	$5.5	8.3%
Multihospital Systems			
Defined benefit pension	13.6%	$100.0	29.5%
Funded depreciation	10.0%	$130.1	38.4%
Foundation/endowment	11.0%	$16.6	4.9%

Glossary of Key Terms

Fiduciary: involves a confidence or trust and describes the legal role and responsibility of a trustee or board member for hospital, pension, or foundation assets

Actuaries: financial experts who calculate how much is needed to pay all expected or promised benefits and cover expected liabilities in a benefit plan based on employee demographics

Retirement Plans

Defined benefit plan: the traditional retirement plan with a preset, guaranteed payout made at retirement

Overfunded: a defined benefit plan that has assets exceeding promised future liabilities and can easily meet retirement payments

Defined contribution plan (401k): a retirement plan in which beneficiaries contribute specific amounts from their paychecks (often matched in part by employers) and whose payouts are not preset but are simply based on investment returns earned by plan assets (Until 1998, these were available only to for-profit institutions, but now the IRS has relaxed restrictions on not-for-profit institutions offering 401(k) programs.)

TSA (tax-sheltered annuity) 403(b): the defined contribution plan most not-for-profit institutions offer; usually offered with an insurance contract

Corporate Assets

Funded depreciation: funds typically used for plant and building expenses, new construction, renovations, and purchases of major equipment

Working capital: funds typically used by hospitals for short- to intermediate-term needs

Foundation/endowment: funds (sometimes charitable entities) typically used for long-term planning and major projects; can be considered a hospital's "rainy-day" fund (When a hospital is sold, its trustees may become board members of community foundations established from proceeds of the sale.)

Self-insurance: funds maintained for workers' compensation, malpractice insurance, and similar activities typically requiring matched liquidity

Short-term operating funds: funds providing cash-on-hand (for payroll, etc.) typically up to 180 days

days. Given their uses, it's clear why these funds maintain extremely conservative and liquid investments (short-term bonds and CDs) in case they need to tap into resources quickly. As a result, their return on investment tends to barely exceed the inflation rate.

2. Self-insurance plans usually cover workers' compensation and malpractice insurance. The assets are invested in bonds with maturities matched to the timing of liabilities (payouts), which may change over time.

3. Working capital is used for a range of short- to intermediate-term needs, such as when a project costs more than expected and additional funds are needed to cover the difference. The investments needed for these assets should be relatively low risk and therefore have low returns.

4. Funded depreciation and foundations and endowments offer trustees more leverage for higher-risk investment strategies. The former are used for longer-term initiatives like new construction and major renovations and the latter for large-scale, community-focused projects. These funds make up roughly 40 percent of hospitals' assets and offer trustees the greatest flexibility in carving out a long-term, more aggressive investment strategy.

5. Because budget constraints, closures and consolidations, and Y2K issues limited major building projects in the '90s, many hospitals will soon undertake new construction and capital improvements. Many—even those in good financial health—now have to build new facilities or retool existing ones to respond to outpatient care and market demands. Trustees need to look closely at their financial plans for ambitious capital projects.

Market Issues and Trends

As the economy expanded in the 1990s, some hospital boards realized they were missing out on double-digit returns from investment in equities and changed their strategy. In turn, many hospitals have altered their asset allocation to reflect more moderate-risk opportunities in the stock market.

Both independent hospitals and systems have steadily increased equity investments in pension plans while reducing investments in CDs and bonds. Independents now devote 61 percent of these assets

Investment Management Benchmarks

Investment management benchmarks typically are categorized by stocks and fixed income, and measure different mixes of companies and funds.

Stock Benchmarks:
- S&P 500—the 500 core companies with large market capitalization (blue chips) as measured by Standard and Poor's.
- S&P BARRA/Value or Russell 1000 Value—large-cap, "value-oriented" stocks. The most common attribute of these stocks (utilities, chemicals, and airlines) is their low price-to-earnings ratio. They are considered more defensive in "down" markets.
- S&P BARRA/Growth or Russell 1000 Growth—large-cap stocks that focus on earnings-per-share growth. Technology companies tend to fall in this segment. These stocks tend to be more aggressive in bull markets.
- Russell 2000 Growth Index—small-cap indexes tilted toward growth stocks.
- Russell 2000 Value Index—small-cap indexes tilted toward value stocks. (The small-cap growth sector includes the new Internet companies and the smaller technology stocks. In the "bull" market, investors poured resources into these stocks, betting on their future profitability as opposed to short-term returns.)
- EAFE International Index—the Europe, Australia, and Far East index of established international companies as measured by Morgan Stanley Dean Witter.

Fixed Income Benchmarks:
- Lehman Aggregate Index—5000+ bonds, including U.S. government, corporate, and mortgage-backed securities. Average maturity ranges from 9 to 11 years.
- Lehman Government/Corporate Index—covers the U.S. bond market, excluding mortgage-backed securities.
- Lehman Intermediate Government/Corporate Index—covers the above index, limited to a five- to seven-year average maturity range.
- Lehman Government or Merrill Lynch One to Three Year Treasury Index—a short-term index of U.S. government or Treasury issues.
- Treasury bills or Donaghue's Money Market Index—measures cash equivalents.

Case Study I

Dearborn County Hospital, in Lawrenceburg, Indiana, uses funded depreciation as the "hospital's pension plan," money targeted for long-term (8–10 year) programs, according to Philip Meyer, director of finance. In 1997, more than 90 percent of its investments were in low-risk certificates of deposit. Then management changed its strategy. The $8 million fund was augmented by a $6 million loan, and the hospital diversified its portfolio so that today 30 percent of investments are in a variety of equity mutual funds. Since mid-1997, that $14 million has grown to $18 million.

"We did not feel we would need to spend these moneys in the next three to five years," Meyer says. "So we had an opportunity for a more aggressive strategy." The hospital board moved some of the fund's money into moderate-risk equities, Meyer says, and is happy with the results.

"The hospital is much better off today having expanded our investment options," he says, adding that there's a larger pool to tap if resources are needed sooner than expected. Moreover, he notes, the hospital now has added flexibility to borrow and invest down the road.

"We're a more attractive credit risk now," he notes.

Case Study II

There are degrees of "conservative," even to bank executives known for their conservative approach to finance and investment management.

At Lee Hospital in Johnstown, Pennsylvania, the pension committee chair is a former bank executive and trust officer. A decade ago he saw the need to add a greater share of equity investments to the hospital's pension plan. Over a period of several years, the pension committee has gradually expanded the share of equities in its pension portfolio from 40 percent to close to 60 percent today, including a small portion in international equities. As a result, the hospital pension plan is now overfunded. That means Lee Hospital can easily meet retirement commitments and free up resources for other capital needs.

"We still have what we feel is a conservative outlook," the committee chair says. "I'm quite satisfied with the overall outcome."

Continued →

Case Study III

For many hospitals, the foundation or endowment is more than just a "rainy-day" fund. It's there for short-term needs, too.

The Galesburg (Illinois) Cottage Health Care Foundation is an example. For most of its history, it placed its funds in CDs and money market funds and had little guidance on investment strategies and options, says James L. Bjorkman, its executive director. Then it hired an outside investment counselor to advise the foundation and manage a share of its assets. The results, according to finance committee chair Lincoln Phillips, are outstanding.

Initially, the foundation shifted some of its assets to equities. Then, as it identified specific programs to support at 189-bed Galesburg Cottage Hospital, it needed more liquid funds, so the hospital converted some of those equities to a highly liquid short-term bond fund. As a result, the foundation has recently supported the hospital's educational/customer service programs and an MRI program, and contributed in excess of $1 million toward the hospital's construction of a new medical office facility.

"We decided we could be a little more aggressive on the equity side," Phillips says. "We're still pretty conservative but recognize what the market's done and that we need to have that working for us."

---

to equities (including international equities), up from about 33 percent in 1990; systems devote 58 percent to equities, up from about 42 percent in 1995.

Most dramatic, hospital trustees have used equities to beef up funded depreciation pools. Equities made up about 8 percent of these investments in 1991 and grew to 33 percent in 1999, at the same time that CDs' share has dropped from nearly 60 to 16 percent over the past decade. Short- and intermediate-term bonds make up the remainder. (Recent rate increases invoked by the Federal Reserve are designed to stop "irrational exuberance" in certain sectors of the economy, to quote Chairman Alan Greenspan and may slow the trend toward higher equity exposure).

Foundations and endowments—that typically constitute hospitals' long-term, "rainy-day" funds—have dramatically shifted asset allocation toward stocks and away from CDs. Since 1989, hospital foundations have increased equity investments from about 40 percent to 51 percent in 1999, while cutting their CD assets from 55 percent to 12 percent; systems now invest 56 percent of assets in equities, up from just under 50 percent in 1995. Some of the shift can be accounted for by appreciation of equity assets already held during the market run-up of the past several years. Much of it is due to deliberate asset allocation changes, placing heavier weight on equities.

By and large, these shifts are producing solid returns. Hospital trustees have seen returns on pension, funded depreciation, and foundation and endowment investments grow significantly from 5 percent in 1994 to double-digit returns. In 1999 alone, independents' pension fund median rate of return was 12 percent against 13.6 percent for systems; 7.5 percent for funded depreciation against 10 percent for systems; and 10.8 percent for foundations and endowments against 11 percent for systems. Considering the scope of these funds in a typical hospital's or system's assets (see table, page 218), it reveals how a more aggressive strategy in today's market can reap significant benefits.

Conclusion

Many hospitals are taking advantage of the recent growth of the stock market by shifting significant amounts of assets from CDs and bonds toward equities, generally with strong rates of return. These strategies enable them to offset losses in other revenue streams and maintain or expand existing programs. This shift sheds a great deal of light on hospitals' and trustees' strategies for future growth and expansion of services through prudent investment management practices that take into account the risk profile of the hospital given its financial condition. Again, if the bullish trends of the stock market over the past several years slow significantly, as the first half of 2000 may signal, trustees will need to carefully examine investment strategies with an eye toward longer-term objectives.

Capital Planning:
Competing
in the Marketplace

By Karen Sandrick

Cedars Sinai Health System (CSHS) in Los Angeles started formulating a capital plan for major construction projects in the late 1980s and early 1990s. Then managed care turned health care economics in California on its head. It wasn't until 1997 that the system could come to terms with the new health care financing realities and grow fiscally comfortable enough to develop a master facilities plan. Then it took two more years to gear the plan specifically to current competitive market demands, such as increased patient volumes and bed shortages, and identify future capital needs and cash balances.

The board of trustees was involved all along the way. "We took a bottom-up look at what we thought we needed and at the same time what we could achieve in financing the project, and both the finance and master planning committees of the board were represented from the very beginning," recalls John Law, chair of the master planning committee.

Trustees heard not only about projections but also their underlying assumptions—the expected population growth, especially among the elderly—best, worst, and expected case scenarios, each with a

---

Karen Sandrick is a health care writer based in Chicago.

complete set of variables, nuances of fixed and variable debt, and contingencies for completing the buildings on time and on budget.

No mean task, as CSHS trustees reviewed and signed off on a $500 million-plus building and renovation plan that will add 80,000 square feet to the health system's research facility; consolidate five magnetic resonance imaging machines, four computed tomography scanners, four radiotherapy rooms, mammography, ultrasound, and nuclear medicine in a 120,000 square-foot inpatient and outpatient imaging center; construct a 300,000 square-foot acute care tower with 125 new intensive care units and eight floors of bridges to other buildings in the main campus; create a diagnostic and treatment center for neurology, urology, and cardiology; centralize all laboratories in an 80,000 square-foot location; pipe a new pneumatic tube system throughout the hospital for transporting documents and laboratory samples; and install an automated guided-vehicle system for distributing materials.

"Trustees didn't do the grunt work in pushing the pencils on paper or the buttons on the computer, but the members of those committees were so active, they could speak to the projections, assumptions, risks, and variability as well as management could," says Ed Fortunis, senior vice president of finance.

Trustees have always trained a careful eye on capital planning as their institutions strive to compete in their marketplaces. For example, updating information technology in order to enhance administrative functions and patient care is a highly intensive capital undertaking. Increasing numbers of hospitals are responding to concerns from employers, state agencies, unions, and consumers to improve patient safety and purchasing computerized physician-order entry systems (CPOE). According to a survey of 241 hospitals by The Leapfrog Group, only 3.3 percent of hospitals have a CPOE but 30 percent will have one by 2004. One hospital well on its way to a CPOE is Brigham and Women's Hospital, Boston, which has earmarked $1.9 million to implement the system, which it expects will cut medication error rates by 55 percent and slash other serious errors by 86 percent.

Health care organizations also prepare for population growth and medical advances by upgrading facilities and clinical technology. The driving forces behind Cedars Sinai's master facilities plan is varied, but demographics are clearly part of the mix. California's population has been projected to grow by 16 million in the next two decades and by 32 million in the next four; the number of elderly will rise by 183 percent by 2022. The hospital, which was built in 1975, has had an extremely high occupancy rate for the last few years, and its critical care areas have not been able to accommodate the enormity of some of the latest medical equipment. The master facilities plan therefore "tried to estimate what the demand would be for beds overall, but probably more significant than population growth were [estimates of] advancements in medicine and science that might become available on the horizon," says Rick Jacobs, senior vice president of system development.

Hospitals also are on the lookout for ways to capture new markets. The University of Illinois Chicago (UIC) is one of a handful of facilities that have a 3.0-tesla MRI, which is 1.5-tesla more powerful than standard workhorse MRIs and about $2 million more expensive. But the machine will allow radiologists to assess patients they couldn't image before—those with cognitive disorders related to aging or disabilities because of head trauma.

Operating margins for many hospitals are so tenuous today, however, that board members must pay even greater attention to the factors that make their organization creditworthy—a strong revenue/cost position, a clear response to marketplace trends and investment downturns—as well as to the fine print in covenants. In the process, they practically need to trade places with lenders. "Trustees have to look at the hospital as a credit analyst or potential bondholder might look at it and ask questions from that perspective, not purely from the perspective of either a hospital system or a vested party," says Peter Young, a financial analyst with Healthcare Strategic Issues, Fort Myers, Florida.

Good News, Bad News

The health care credit picture coming out of 2001 is surprisingly favorable. According to Standard & Poor's, for the first time in at least three years, not-for-profit median health care ratios have stabilized in many categories and risen modestly across the board, with operating ratios and balance sheets improving because of increased revenue from third-party payer contracting as well as growing federal and even state reimbursement. Hospitals are also enjoying

Evaluating Capital Projects

A hospital wants to finance a nine-figure capital program to stay competitive in its market. What do its trustees need to know?

First, the board has to assess whether the program is the most appropriate place to direct limited capital and get a return on investment that will make the hospital more attractive going forward, says James Grobmyer, president of Grobmyer Associates, St. Petersburg, Florida. He recommends setting a specific rate of return and using a weighted cost of capital calculation to determine whether a project will add to, or detract from, the organization's value. "If you are not doing that analysis and not looking at a project in a fair amount of detail, you're playing with dynamite," he says.

Trustees should also compare the specifics of a capital plan against predetermined parameters and guidelines. Martin Klein, trustee of Mount Auburn Hospital, Cambridge, Massachusetts, and president, Institutional Strategy Associates, Inc., Belmont, Massachusetts, boils those parameters down into three foci: the program, the resources it will require, and the price tag.

Klein acknowledges "one of the chastening things you learn as a hospital trustee is that there are limits to what you can do." One way trustees can help management is by rationalizing the sequence in which capital projects occur. "People will be content to realize that some projects must be deferred as long as there is a rational plan, a sequence that makes sense, and a commitment to get them done eventually," he says.

Board members won't be combing through capital financing documents to review covenants in detail, but they should at least know the bond services' requirements and whether the new covenants are permissible in terms of those on existing bonds and the hospital's ability to cover payments. "The art is to see that you protect yourself against the things you can protect yourself against by having a process for getting the best deal you can and for making hard decisions," says Klein. Such a process ensures that the hospital's audit committee will look at covenants line by line, that the board finance committee will press for clarification of covenant language, and that the board as a whole will have a reporting system that flags potential difficulties, like sudden changes in accounts receivable days that can compromise debt service payments.

Continued →

"Trustees have to make sure they know what's going on and that they have an information system they can depend on for . . . openness and transparency between the board and the administration," says Klein.

Boards have to accept that a certain amount of loss from investment income will never be recouped in the stock market, but they should expect management to address that loss by increasing the organization's overall profitability. "If your hospital's investment has been in stocks and you've taken a hit, what's your plan of action to replace the value of those lost assets, to continue to make yourself attractive? The principal ways are by improving operations and cutting major expenses," Grobmyer says.

It's a matter of balancing the cost and revenue sides of the equation and the ups and downs of individual lines of business. The process is not unlike balancing a portfolio in the stock market. "If you're in long-term value funds, you may find that's the wrong segment of the market to be in right now, and you need to switch to short- or long-term growth," Grobmyer says. "With a portfolio of assets, it's a question of how you balance those assets so if one goes down, the other will sustain you for a while. That's the kind of analysis trustees have to request from management."

—K.S.

growth in patient volume, greater market power through consolidations and mergers, and, after divesting noncore services in 1998 and 1999, they're no longer feeling a drag on operations from underperforming assets.

Operating margins are still far more vulnerable than they were five years ago, however, Young says. Even with better reimbursements from Medicare and managed care, many hospitals are posting negative or barely positive operating margins, and they are vulnerable to niche revenue cutouts from physicians who siphon off revenue normally captured by hospitals by opening their own surgicenters or other services.

Weak operating margins block easy access to affordable capital. As Greg Scrine, analyst with the Tiber Group, Chicago, points out, "When margins slide, players cannot go to the public market and issue debt, certainly at rates that make any sense, that they can afford."

Tepid margins are also prey to fluctuations in cost, and costs have changed so fast in some areas that Young doesn't call them fluid anymore; instead, he says they're volatile, because the cost swings associated with labor, pharmaceuticals, supplies such as implants, and casualty and malpractice insurance can be so dramatic. Malpractice or liability insurance premiums can jump $700,000 and wipe out 10 percent from the bottom line of a hospital that has a margin of only a few million dollars.

Funding sources that shore up teetering margins are rocky, to say the least. Hospitals, like other investors, are suffering from dismal returns on their investments. Just a few years ago, hospitals that had a negative 3 percent operating margin, for instance, could net a positive 7 percent because of 10 percent returns on their investment portfolios. But no more.

Donations to hospitals have slowed since September 11, because small ($300 to $1,000) donors are sending their charitable contributions to terrorism victims. And because of uncertainty about the effects of estate tax reform, major donors are holding off on hospital philanthropy, says Young.

Nevertheless, there is a genuine need for replacement and replenishment of capital assets to improve efficiencies in operations; hence, a pent-up demand for capital, says James Grobmyer, president of Grobmyer Associates, St. Petersburg, Florida. In the face of lower interest rates, such tactics as short-term financing, balancing long- and short-term debt more actively, making adjustments that lock in helpful interest rates, and matching long-term debt with long-term assets have become attractive strategies. "Hospitals have an opportunity to look at their total long-term debt in various capacities and components. To miss this window of opportunity would be very foolish," Grobmyer adds.

The question is: how do executives and board members get the capital they need?

Paper Trails

Hospitals clearly can't issue paper without backing it up with enough substance to make investors comfortable. And the same factors that lead to success in local markets make hospitals attractive to capital lenders and investors.

That means recognizing and adapting to trends shaping the industry, such as the Health Insurance Portability and Accountability Act (HIPAA), the shift to outpatient care, and labor shortages, says Ernie Butler, president of I. Butler Securities, Little Rock, Arkansas. "Hospitals need to be sure they are preparing themselves from a nonfinancial standpoint to improve the quality of their information technology to be HIPAA-compliant. They have to have adequate ambulatory facilities, because outpatient care is claiming a higher percentage of revenue, and a consistent and continuous recruitment program to attract licensed nurses," Butler says.

Addressing these trends will be costly. Hospitals, on average, will spend about $9 million to prepare for HIPAA alone, concludes the Gartner Group, Washington, D.C., on the basis of 121 providers studied in 2001. Large health care organizations stand to gain nearly $15 million in yearly revenue in the process, however, by reducing the number of rejected insurance claims, and moderate-sized facilities can speed reimbursement and cut administrative costs by $4 million a year, Gartner says.

Hospitals also need to focus on asset turnover and resource use. Grobmyer's hospital clients are asking first how they can maximize returns on assets, balance assets and liabilities, and free up capital through divestitures; then how they can direct capital to core lines of business. "They are asking the right questions: where are we now and where do we need to be?" he says.

Credit markets are scrutinizing revenue stability, in particular, says Young. "After experiencing a number of shortfalls on the part of providers relative to actual versus budgeted performance, especially 'surprise' or unexpected shortfalls, credit markets are looking at how well-defined core service lines are and whether revenue comes predominantly from high-margin lines—cardiology, oncology, orthopedics, neurology—because it's the high margins that sustain the mission and allow you to have access to capital," he explains.

On the other side of that coin is cost management and a comprehensive cost analysis by service line that clearly shows the cost of doing business, Young adds. "Hospitals have not had the kind of sophisticated ability to break down costs that the market required. It's only been in the last few years that hospitals have been able to examine vulnerable cost exposures and utilize strategies and methods of measurement and benchmarking so there will be no surprises to them or to bondholders."

The fragile nature of many hospitals' operating margin dictates that top executives and boards comprehend cost issues. "It's not good enough to sit at the hospital board meeting and point to the six areas that almost every trade journal identifies as cost sensitive. Management and boards must understand how these areas are going to affect the bottom line and ultimately the bondholder by having a method that benchmarks them on an ongoing quarterly, if not monthly, basis," Young advises.

In a nutshell, says Scrine, "hospitals, at the end of the day, have to generate capital internally from operations; so the first focus is to get their shop in order and their cost structure in line. Hospitals need to restructure their portfolios of assets, their cost base, and operations before they can look to the debt markets."

Once they enter the debt markets, hospitals have to be especially careful about covenants because lenders have been narrowing borrowing requirements to give bondholders a superior position. In fact, observes Young, "You're apt to find today that covenants have been tightened to a point that they can inhibit an institution's ability to access capital further down the road."

Covenants that can get a hospital in trouble are the ones that mandate coverage ratios or the amount of reserves related to the amount that's been borrowed, says Martin Klein, trustee of Mount Auburn Hospital, Cambridge, Massachusetts, and president, Institutional Strategy Associates, Inc., Belmont, Massachusetts. "There may be things associated with debt service that will be difficult to live up to three to five years down the road. If things go a little bad, you want to be sure you're not in a position that you come perilously close to the ratios in your bond covenants," he advises.

So although many hospitals have been refinancing in the last few years because of low interest rates, the bond industry sees not-for-profit hospitals as risky because balance sheets are increasing in leverage and core service lines are vulnerable. Executive leadership and boards consequently need to concentrate on the fundamentals— core business, cost management, and covenants. Says Young, "Hospitals have to tell their story to debt holders and bondholders, and it's not the story they put in high-gloss community reports."

What Makes a Winner?
Key Characteristics of
Peak-Performing Hospitals

By Nathan S. Kaufman

Last year, approximately half of U.S. hospitals had profit margins below 3 percent, and one-third actually lost money. During this same period, a select group of hospitals produced profit margins in the range of 5 to 8 percent. Of particular note is that many investor-owned hospital systems have achieved exceptional performance over the past year as evidenced by the doubling of their share prices in 2000.

Although profit margins of private not-for-profit systems eroded by 1.2 percent to 2.2 percent, the margins of for-profit hospitals rose by .7 percent to 3.5 percent. There is no evidence that the relatively poor-performing hospitals can be excused by their "mission activities." And because the not-for-profit systems operate in the same markets as investor-owned systems, one cannot blame performance erosion on environmental factors such as reimbursement, nursing shortages, and so on.

Nathan S. Kaufman is senior vice president for health care strategy, Superior Consultant Holdings Corp., San Diego. He can be reached at (858) 487-9771.

A hospital's performance is contingent upon three factors:

1. Franchise location or reputation. Principles of supply and demand apply to the health care business. Rarely can hospitals achieve peak performance if they are located in an area with a declining population, where people have poor access to the institution, and/or are in a market with excess hospital capacity.
2. Policy and culture established by the board. The board has the critical role of approving "the flight plan" of a hospital and hiring the "pilot," that is, the CEO. Peak performance is never achieved if the flight plan takes the hospital in the wrong direction.
3. Management's effectiveness. Given clear direction from the board, it's management's responsibility to execute the policy and ensure the delivery of cost-effective, high-quality care.

Within these three areas, peak-performing hospitals have eight characteristics in common:

1. Their market share within the primary service area is in excess of 45 percent.
2. They have a balanced, well-informed board and effective management.
3. They close redundant facilities and consolidate select services into state-of-the-art disease management programs.
4. They consolidate support services.
5. They manage by nonnegotiable budgets.
6. They demand reasonable reimbursement rates from payers.
7. They have a collaborative but "arms-length" relationship with their physicians.
8. They continue to implement cost-effective information technology strategies to facilitate their peak performance in all of the above areas.

Market Share

In markets where there is excess capacity, physicians and payers play one system against the other. This results in lower reimbursement rates and an "arms race" for employees and equipment, which escalates cost. Once a hospital reaches more than 45 percent market penetration, it can no longer be excluded from health plans and can negotiate for higher rates. Achieving such market penetration does not occur by chance—it's a function of merging with or acquiring facilities in the primary service area.

On the other hand, merging or acquiring facilities *outside* the primary service area has actually detracted from a system's performance. Because physicians primarily control referrals, merging with a hospital outside the primary service area rarely results in an increase in market share. Most people in health care have assumed that when two facilities merge, there are significant economies of scale. But in order to achieve major cost savings, it's essential that clinical services be consolidated into a single facility. Because it is politically impractical to close and consolidate services in most health systems, the primary benefit of a merger is the ability to negotiate better reimbursement rates.

If the merged facilities are not located in the same primary service area, the amount of incremental negotiating leverage gained by the merger may be limited. At the same time, the overall costs within the system may escalate as a new level of "system" management evolves. It should come as no surprise that 70 percent of hospital mergers fail.

Well-Informed Board and Effective Management

Given facilities with similar market positions, the single greatest determinant of a hospital's performance is the quality of the board's decisions and the ability of management to implement those decisions. Boards of peak-performing hospitals are informed, objective, and do their homework. They base their decisions on an in-depth understanding of the issues. They establish the tone for the organization through a clear, proactive policy focusing on improving the quality of care and financial performance of the system. This minimizes board politics and the personal agendas of individual trustees (both of which are the Achilles' heels of many not-for-profit hospitals).

Boards of peak-performing health systems oversee management's performance without meddling but are prepared to take quick action when they observe a pattern of underperformance. It is interesting to note that most investor-owned hospitals have a small "advisory board" composed primarily of physicians. Policy is set by the regional management and the corporate office. The CEO of an investor-owned hospital does not need to care for, nurture, or "manage" a board and thus has significantly more time to devote to working with the medical staff and employees to improve the hospital's performance.

Senior executives of peak-performing hospitals are perceived as generally fair and competent. They are accessible to employees and the medical staff. They routinely review operational details and immediately address underperformance. Most important, the CEO's focus is targeted on improving the system's performance. This can only occur if he or she is not hampered by well-meaning but uninformed trustees, board politics, and meddling—situations common to poor-performing systems.

The board and senior management must develop a solid working relationship with the medical staff. There is, however, a delicate balance between open and inappropriate communication with the medical staff. It's essential that the board provide a forum where physicians can be heard; trustees need their vital insights on both the quality and cost of care provided in the system. At the same time, physicians can leverage their personal relationships with board members inappropriately to gain individual advantage and/or promote a personal agenda not shared by the medical staff at large. Finally, peak-performing hospitals have medical staff members on their boards of trustees.

An April 2000 *Forbes* magazine survey of the "nonfinancial" assets that contribute most to the success of an organization determined that "innovation" and "the ability to attract talented employees" are key. Peak-performing hospitals recruit, train, and retain high-quality management talent and deliberately focus on creativity and innovation. Both physicians and executives are assigned specific responsibilities to develop new clinical capabilities and innovative management systems.

The study of nonfinancial assets reveals that attributes that contribute least to the success of the organization include customer satisfaction and "brand investment." These attributes are necessary but not sufficient. That is, if patient satisfaction is high but the organization is not innovative and/or cannot retain talented employees, it can't achieve peak performance.

Even though subjective indicators are useful, the ultimate measure of a CEO's performance is meeting or exceeding specific economic and quality performance measures. Historically, quality has been based on the subjective perceptions of the medical staff and patients. However, quality can now be objectively measured by such indicators as length of stay, medication errors, infection rates, and mortality and morbidity data. In addition, there are benchmarking systems for determining "best practices" of hospitals down to the department level. A key responsibility of the board is to monitor the system's performance against quality and economic benchmarks and not tolerate negative variances.

Consolidating Clinical Services

Peak-performing hospitals consolidate clinical programs to eliminate duplication and achieve clinical excellence. For example, rather than a system's offering two marginal open-heart surgery programs, the programs are consolidated in a single facility. This reduces duplication costs and improves staff proficiency because physicians can perform more procedures.

Peak performers deliberately recruit physician stars to direct their "institutes." These institutes become incubators for clinical innovation, such as new surgical devices and medications.

A common mistake made by health systems is an attempt to centralize clinical services management. For example, some health systems have established a central radiology manager for several hospitals. In most cases this does not reduce cost, but it does reduce management's effectiveness to solve problems. Clinical services must have a manager on-site so that issues can be addressed immediately, not when the central manager happens to be available. Similarly, the CEO and CFO functions should not be consolidated in a multifacility system. Each facility needs strong management and financial leadership.

Consolidating Support Services

However, in order to reduce cost and improve performance, peak-performing hospitals do consolidate such support services as information technology and business office functions. The key characteristic of a successful regional support service is the competency and status of the manager responsible for implementing that regional strategy. Regionalization of support services fails when a midlevel manager, inexperienced in running large regional support centers, is assigned this responsibility. In order to navigate across the organizational structure, the leader of the regional support center must have the prestige of a senior executive in the organization with the authority to implement necessary changes. Because experienced talent for regionalizing support services is scarce, more hospitals are considering outsourcing as a viable option for select services, such as IT.

Nonnegotiable Budgets

According to the Healthcare Advisory Board, Washington, D.C., there is a difference of approximately $2,000 in admission costs between hospitals that are "cost disciplined" and those that are "cost challenged." Given that much hospital reimbursement is fixed, it's essential that leaders be obsessed with reducing costs. Peak-performing systems maintain staffing levels at or below 44 percent of net revenue. They keep their supply costs below 11 percent of net revenue. They collect the appropriate copayment at the time of service and aggressively manage accounts receivable. Physician directorships are reviewed routinely to ensure that the institution is receiving value for its fees.

Finally, the hospital's performance at the department level is regularly compared with benchmarks based on best practices, and no excuses are accepted for deviating from those benchmarks. The key to reducing costs is a routine focus on the details and taking action when there is a pattern of underperformance.

Demanding Reasonable Rates

Peak-performing hospitals offer significant discounts to payers only when the hospital is guaranteed a measurable benefit in exchange. All others pay "retail." The hospital industry is one of the few where discounts are provided without a guaranteed return benefit. Under most circumstances, peak-performing systems refuse to gamble on risk contracting. These systems realize that capitation is bad business and demand a fee for each service they provide. Finally, peak-performing hospitals analyze their pricing versus reimbursement to determine optimal "line item" pricing.

Striking the Right Note with Physicians

Few systems have succeeded at owning and operating physician practices. Thus, boards and executives of peak-performing hospitals and systems focus their relationships with physicians on:

- Retaining high-quality physicians in the market
- Using the physicians' expertise to improve the quality and cost of service
- Recruiting clinical stars to enhance quality and services throughout the system

These hospitals recognize that in order to ensure an adequate supply of physicians it may be necessary to employ them, but they prefer to work with established physician practices and use income guarantees and loans. When employment is the only option, smart organizations have a highly structured model. The employed physicians join a "medical division" of the hospital, which is run like a group practice. Their compensation is based on individual productivity and group performance. These groups are run by a highly qualified and experienced physician practice administrator, who has the trust of both the hospital administration and the physicians.

Hospitals are now recruiting physicians to run specific departments (e.g., radiology, cardiology, etc.). Many radiologists are far more experienced than hospital administrators at running outpatient radiology services. In order to improve the quality and financial performance of outpatient radiology services, some hospitals are joint-venturing this service with their radiology group and/or signing a management services agreement with their radiologists to manage the hospital's service.

Peak-performing hospitals also recognize that they cannot reduce costs or improve quality without the cooperation of the medical staff. These hospitals are using members of their own medical staff to lead initiatives in several key areas:

• Development of an in-house hospitalist program to significantly improve the quality and cost of care to critically ill patients
• Establishment of an inpatient formulary combined with information technology to reduce medication errors and improve the cost of care
• Development of standardized inventories to avoid the cost of stocking multiple equivalent devices
• Standardizing departmental protocols, such as in the cardiac cath lab, in order to ensure that the highest quality care is provided by all users

Investing in Information Technology

Information technology (IT) is one of the most critical and expansive investments being made by health systems. Not actually a separate category, IT is the common thread among the characteristics of peak-performing systems that makes the achievement and maintenance of quality, fiscal, and compliance goals possible. With the costs of hardware, software, and implementation declining, the cost-benefit of IT services should be increasing exponentially. In the future, the cost and quality of care provided by a health system will be heavily influenced by the system's ability to digitally transform its business, operational, and clinical processes. The IT strategies of peak-performing health systems have the following characteristics:

• They enable management to track and monitor revenue and its associated costs at all levels in the organization and provide "real-time" reporting on performance.
• They track and facilitate the management and collection of accounts receivable.
• They enable physicians to gain easy access to clinical information while protecting patient confidentiality and complying with HIPAA regulations.
• They enable monitoring and measurement of clinical quality and promote patient safety (e.g., by reducing medication errors).

- They reduce waste caused by duplication of administrative services and supply-chain processes.
- They provide the community with a resource for information.

Conclusion

A health system's performance is not a function of chance. Although there may be various causes for a system's failure to distinguish itself as a peak-performing organization, the following are the most basic: a weak franchise, in which case the system needs to merge and consolidate with another facility in its primary service area; ineffective implementation of the system's policies; and/or ineffective boards where the trustees distract the CEO from focusing on the hospital and market, do not monitor his or her performance, or set inappropriate policies. If you're trying to determine the underlying factors contributing to, or detracting from, the performance of a health system, the first place to look is the boardroom.

Best Financial Practices for Trustees

By James S. Vaughan
and Catherine J. Robbins

As not-for-profit health care organizations get bigger and more complex, they begin to look more like businesses. That means that trustees will be held to the duty of care and the duty of loyalty just as their for-profit siblings are. It also means that health care trustees may likely be more vulnerable to personal liability.

The duty of care generally requires trustees to perform their duties with the reasonable care, diligence, and skill that an ordinarily prudent person in similar circumstances would use. The duty of loyalty requires trustees to exercise their powers in the interest of the corporation, not in their own or another entity's or person's interest.

At the same time, state attorneys general, who are beginning to exert more active oversight in the wake of health system bankrupcies and near bankruptcies, will be more likely to second-guess trustees' decisions on behalf of the organization's charitable mission. In carrying out their duties of care and loyalty, trustees can

James S. Vaughan is a principal, and Catherine J. Robbins is vice-president, of Cain Brothers, a health care industry investment banking firm in New York City. They can be reached at (212) 869-5600.

expect to be judged by creditors and others against standards increasingly like those applied to for-profit directors. However, the same is not true of the third duty of not-for-profit trustees, the duty to mission. Whereas the best interests of their shareholders can guide for-profit directors, trustees of not-for-profit organizations must actively pursue the mission of their organization as defined in its articles of incorporation and/or bylaws.

There may be tension between the need to meet the standards of loyalty and care that creditors expect and trustees' unique responsibility to community mission. We are starting to see that boards face a greater risk of personal liability because of their oversight responsibilities. For example, trustees and officers of AHERF were sued for $1 billion for breach of fiduciary duty, among other things. However, the public will strongly resist actual judgments against individuals who volunteer their time as trustees.

Fortunately, there are some commonsense tactics trustees can employ to protect themselves and their organization. They must start by being involved in and attentive to governance and management oversight processes and by accepting the full scope of their responsibilities. Then, always within the context of organizational mission, they must:

- Adopt a business model of governance structure and reporting
- Manage the assets and liabilities of the whole organization, not just clinical operations
- Oversee the organization's financial status and take action in time of trouble

The Governance Business Model

The following guidelines will help trustees adopt a business model of governance:

- Reconfigure the board and its committees to a workable size with a structure—including the finance, investment, and audit committees, which periodically exclude management representatives—that ensures effective oversight and communication.
- Change membership, if necessary, to get needed business expertise on the board and ensure that those who serve are actively

pursuing their fiduciary duties. Design board terms to balance the need for continuity with desired membership change over time.

- Educate trustees and management about their obligations and personal liability. The New Jersey Office of Attorney General, for example, has considered requiring 20 hours of continuing education a year as a minimum for trustees.
- Ensure that board members assert their responsibility to challenge management when necessary, and seek periodic independent expert counsel on organizational effectiveness. Best practices suggest the board and/or its committees establish routine, documented opportunities for the organization's outside advisors and auditors to speak openly with independent board members in executive session. In some cases, trustee groups may want to retain their own, independent accounting advisors.

  Not burdened by the desire to preserve a long-term audit relationship, independent advisors can provide an objective opinion on questionable practices. In a similar vein, trustees may want to retain independent legal counsel in some cases, as the mutual fund industry has already done, for example.
- Ensure that the board is receiving regular monthly reports on key financial and operational measures of the hospital and health system. These reports should include cash flow and compare activities and budgets to the previous year. Boards must be able to intelligently review these reports and take action if results are not appropriate. Boards should analyze management's explanation if reports are not available on a timely basis and consider an outside review of the situation if they are not satisfied with that explanation.
- Develop policies on financial conflicts of interest for both board members and management. If trustees or their employers do business with the hospital or system, they must ensure proper disclosure and standards of care. Policies should require direct trustee review of executive compensation, low-interest loans, and withdrawals from deferred compensation plans.
- Assess the organization's directors' and officers' liability insurance. Update it if possible and as necessary.
- Boards must educate themselves about reporting requirements and penalties for noncompliance in the following areas:
  1. Donor restrictions, particularly in a health care system
  2. Reporting requirements of the Financial Accounting Standard (FAS) 124 that requires not-for-profit organizations to

report investments at market levels, and FAS 133 that defines and requires reporting of derivative instruments and hedging transactions

3. Quarterly financial reporting and significant event disclosures, the latter increasingly required to maintain municipal bond investors' interest in the organization's bonds and to allow the organization access to capital over the long term

4. Bond covenants, particularly in a system where obligated groups for financing represent only a portion of the not-for-profit organization

Managing the Assets and Liabilities of the Organization

Trustees who work in business are often skilled at making prudent financial decisions on behalf of their company. They may be quite comfortable with the principles of reducing risk and increasing return by creating a diversified portfolio of investments and matching the duration of assets and liabilities to expected uses. Each corporation may differ in its tolerance for risk as aligned with expectations of return, but leaders of these businesses know that they cannot serve the interests of their shareholders without managing these moving parts. However, for reasons of history, culture, and custom, it is not uncommon, when these same people serve as trustees of a not-for-profit hospital, for them to leave these principles behind.

Historically, a trustee of a small freestanding hospital did not really have to worry about asset and liability management. With most hospital assets invested in buildings, equipment, and accounts receivable, and with little debt and a modest operating cash flow, focusing on medical staff relations and clinical operations often best met community mission. Hospitals saw themselves first as public charities. In these circumstances, trustees usually followed management's lead and focused on operations. It was not uncommon for one or two trustees who possessed some financial expertise to review big transactions on an ad hoc basis with the full board affirming their actions.

This is no longer the case. Many hospitals are part of complex systems; hospitals are often highly leveraged, and more hospitals have become dependent on nonoperating sources of income to achieve still-shrinking margins. It is exactly this kind of environment that should motivate hospital management and trustees to put more effort into actively managing all of the assets and liabilities of the organization in order to meet community need. State laws now fully support this activity through the prudent business person principle. Trustees, in turn, may have to worry about accusations of wasting organizational assets if they avoid the challenges of actively managing all of the organization's assets and liabilities.

Trustees and administrators can, however, effectively manage assets and liabilities. The board should develop and adopt financing, risk, and investment guidelines and objectives. Policies should clearly delineate expectations for management action, empower management to act within those policies, and identify the parameters under which direct board review and/or approval is required. The board should also consider hiring outside investment counselors while maintaining solid trustee oversight. Systems may find that developing in-house financial expertise can bring sophistication unavailable to stand-alone hospitals.

One reason that trustees must act on these issues is that most hospitals generate comparatively low operating margins and have therefore become increasingly dependent on investment income to provide organizational resources. The tables (page 247) from Moody's Investor Service show trends in excess (i.e., total) margins over the past five years, separately identifying what portion of that margin comes from operations compared with all other sources, including investment income.

The tables show that, although total margins have been cut in half since 1997, the decline has mostly been in operating margins, whereas the remaining components of excess margins have remained relatively steady. Table 2 shows that operating margins have decreased from 60 percent of excess margin in 1995 to only 17 percent in 1999. The implication of this is huge for trustees: hospitals have become far more dependent on nonoperating sources of margin. Further, this has occurred in a very good climate for both equity and fixed-income investments. Trustees need to consider financial management strategies that will position their organization to cope with an unpredictable future.

Trustees must also be aware that the risks related to many hospitals' increased levels of debt can and should be managed. For example, a debt structure with a 100 percent long-term fixed rate probably does not make sense in all circumstances. By contrast, a judicious amount of variable-rate debt, either issued directly or created through interest rate swap transactions, can significantly reduce the overall cost of capital. Trustees need to consider carefully the kinds and amounts of risk that make the best sense for their organization.

Trustees who venture to understand the asset side of a hospital's balance sheet are most likely to ask how to reduce days in patient accounts receivable and how to understand the cash situation. Hospital management often behaves as if once a building or program is in place, questions about it will never be raised again. A responsible trustee should always be asking questions such as, "Should we continue to own this building?" or "Does an asset's financing arrangement continue to make sense in light of the current environment?" All assets and liabilities should be reviewed continually. Timely restructuring of certain assets and/or liabilities may provide opportunities to develop more resources to meet the organization's mission. But remember, the best time to ask these questions and analyze opportunities is before the organization falls into financial difficulties.

Table 1. Total Hospital Margins

	Operating Margins	Other, Including Investment Income
1995	3.3%	2.1%
1996	3.3%	2.7%
1997	3.3%	2.8%
1998	1.6%	3.1%
1999	0.5%	2.5%

Source: Moody's Investors Service, Hospital Medians. Reprinted with permission.

Table 2. Sources of Excess Margins

	Operations	All Other
1995	60%	40%
1996	55%	45%
1997	54%	46%
1998	35%	65%
1999	17%	83%

Source: Moody's Investors Service, Hospital Medians. Reprinted with permission.

Overseeing Financial Status and Taking Action in Time of Trouble

Hospital and health system trustees have an obligation to understand the organization's financial statements. It is imperative that financial problems be identified early before significant deterioration takes place.

A comprehensive board-level plan to regularly review the total financial health of the organization should include:

- Understanding how the local health care system works, including how costs and cash compare with competing peer groups of similar organizations. To do this will require comprehensible, timely reports from management.
- Ensuring that trustees with business experience conduct detailed financial and audit reviews for the organization
- Requesting management analysis of problems and recommendations for solutions
- Implementing periodic outside reviews by independent, reputable financial/strategy advisors

Trustees should be familiar with warning signs that point to financial stress (see the box on the next page). If these signs do arise, they need to be investigated and discussed openly at the board level in a timely manner. When it becomes apparent that, despite your best intentions and efforts, your organization's financial obligations cannot be met, you should keep in mind the following:

- Operating priority should focus on cash—increasing its incoming flow through realistically valuing accounts receivable and paying attention to the business office while stemming outgoing flow in such discretionary areas as capital expenditures, travel bonuses, and, occasionally, retirement fund contributions.
- Recognize that if creditors see the board and management as full partners in a shared problem, such as seeking to develop an equitable payment plan, they are more likely to be flexible about options for the organization. If, however, creditors perceive that the board and management have a bunker mentality against

them, they will be more likely to sue, potentially making claims against trustees personally.

- Because asset values will be higher prior to a bankruptcy filing, trustees will often have more flexibility at that time to develop sensible restructuring and a process that brings higher values to all parties. Trustees should look at exit strategies early on while options and time to conduct a process exists.
- There is a greater opportunity to preserve mission while pursuing prudent business principles prior to a bankruptcy filing. Trustees need to carefully assess the local and state government oversight environment early in a restructuring or bankruptcy process. Based on that assessment, trustees should take steps to avoid a conflict over mission that could tie their hands and create delays. Delays usually destroy residual asset values that otherwise might be available to the community.

Warning: Financial Danger Ahead

Warning signs that may signal financial trouble include the following:

- More accounts receivable and/or accounts payable
- Shrinking operating margin
- Less cash
- Decreased market share
- Loss of key admitting physicians
- Organizational inability to measure monthly financial and operating performance and report it in a timely manner to the board
- Negative variations from approved budgets
- Organizational inability to respond to regulatory actions
- Advisor turnover (especially legal or accounting advisors)
- Rating agency debt downgrades and/or change to negative outlook
- Violations of restrictive covenants in borrowing and credit enhancement agreements
- Executive compensation and benefits packages that are controlled by management and not the board
- Management recommendations to diversify in order to increase revenue when internal operations are not well controlled

---

- Boards may want to consider retaining outside legal counsel and financial advisors with experience in restructuring.
- The board may want to form an independent committee that can devote its full energy to coping with the bankruptcy/restructuring process. This committee should maintain open and frequent communication with the full board.
- Trustees should expect intense public and creditor scrutiny of all actions that they and management have taken in the past and will undertake during a bankruptcy/restructuring process. For example, favoring creditors with whom there is a perceived or real conflict with board members must obviously be avoided.

Conclusion

The health of not-for-profit health care organizations is dependent on the willingness of talented community and business leaders to accept governance responsibility. At the same time, the board's job has been made more challenging by the need to balance society's increased willingness to hold trustees accountable for stricter standards of care and loyalty, with an equally increased willingness to call them to task on mission. Trustees must be willing to accept more personal responsibility in these circumstances and adopt more rigorous governance practices within the context of organizational mission.

Ten Financial Components of a Successful Hospital/System

By R. Brent Hardaway

Although trustees are not accountable for the day-to-day activities of their hospitals, they have the formidable responsibility of establishing policy, assuring the community of quality patient care, and providing leadership for organizational planning and management. Entrusted with the fiscal health of a hospital or system, many trustees contend with poor financial performance and associated bond downgrades resulting from several contributing factors. It is popular to say that the primary reason for these problems is the Balanced Budget Amendment (BBA). However, our experience has shown that the BBA is merely one factor—and not even the primary one. Instead, we believe that poor financial performance is chiefly attributable to the following four factors.

The Four Main Problems

1. Inadequate Financial Information

It is standard operating procedure that all health systems provide trustees with quarterly, sometimes monthly, hospital or systemwide

---

R. Brent Hardaway is an associate partner of Phase 2 Consulting, Austin.

income statements, balance sheets, and cash flow statements. However, it is month-by-month financial reporting and cost accounting systems reported at the cost center or business unit level that offer the most accurate and significant financial performance data.

Trustees should be given data on the cost centers' or business units' individual performance, as well as reports on their aggregate performance. If trustees continue to receive only aggregate information, the economic performance—gains or losses—of a cost center will be buried in the health system's operating statements, which could very well interfere with their ability to render knowledgeable decisions.

2. Managed Care Pricing and Payment

Everybody likes a bargain. Trouble is, many competing systems have agreed to very low per diem rates (some are far below average per diem cost) in order to secure managed care contracts. To make matters worse, the same managed care companies have increased claim denial rates and delayed payments—tactics that only serve to harm a system's declining cash position. Hardly a bargain.

A trustee must be aware that marginal cost pricing simply does not work. Managed care contracts must be renegotiated or, if the situation warrants, terminated. Hospitals should never subsidize below-cost contracts.

3. High Costs of Core Businesses

The cost structure of most hospitals is significantly above the managed care market price. Although this fact may justifiably alarm some trustees, steps may be taken (besides renegotiating or terminating managed care contracts) to realize notable margins on all payer types.

- *Staffing Levels:* Although the heart and soul of health care is undeniably its highly trained workforce, many hospital departments are staffed well above national benchmarks for comparable facilities. An optimal staffing level must be found and be complemented with optimal work processes. Staffing productivity standards remain uneven, with staffing not adjusted for patient volume fluctuations.

- *Supply Costs:* Supply costs per case, especially in cardiology and surgery, have increased with little remedial action.
- *Benefit Costs:* To ensure a viable, steady workforce, many systems have plumped up employee benefit packages but have failed to manage or market them effectively, inadequately promoting cost-saving cafeteria plans.
- *Position Control:* Far too many hospitals allow department heads to hire additional full-time, part-time, or temporary employees, as well as to authorize overtime, regardless of budgetary concerns.

4. *Aggressive Implementation of a High-Growth Integrated Delivery System Strategy*

A system's core business is providing hospital services. That sounds logical enough, but most health systems have expanded services and ambulatory care sites, acquired physician practices, purchased or developed risk-based HMOs, and capitated risk contracts—to the potential detriment of their core business. These enterprises have generated significant, sometimes catastrophic, financial losses because system management lacked the experience and know-how to develop and operate noncore businesses.

Management and the board must focus on providing hospital services. Too many health care systems have become financially overwhelmed by noncore business venture losses.

Components of a Successful Hospital/ Health Care System

Stewardship of your hospital or system requires many skills and personal characteristics, including dedication, a great deal of time and energy, common sense, financial acumen, integrity, and leadership. As a leader, you should also be aware of 10 components that define a successful health system—and of your attendant responsibilities.

1. *Monitor Accounts Receivable Reserve Levels*

What used to be considered simple tasks (such as verifying that accrued patient revenue is actually tied to patient cash collected) are rendered far more difficult by the intricacies of managed care pricing and contracting. Frequently, account reserves are understated, with more revenue being recognized monthly than the system is entitled to or can realistically collect. As a result, the system's true financial position is obscured.

Trustees must be able to monitor the reconciliation of accounts receivable (AR) reserve levels to actual cash collections for each business unit. Reviewing a quarterly report (with unbundled accounting practices for not only Medicare and Medicaid but also managed care contracts and self-pay) is the most efficient way to ensure that AR reserve levels are appropriate and sufficient.

2. Ensure Appropriate Pricing of Managed Care Contracts

Strict attention to negotiated managed care contract rates is essential. In the heated spirit of competition and because of inadequate or inaccurate cost accounting information, many systems have accepted dangerously low payment rates. This capitulation to managed care contractors can be devastating as contract rates fall well below hospitals' average total costs, jeopardizing their ability to generate profits.

Trustees should review, on a quarterly basis, the hospital's average per-day reimbursement as compared with its average total cost per day for each major payer. This review is designed to reveal which services have contracts that are being reimbursed below cost.

3. Ensure Billing and Collections Procedures in Practice

In virtually every hospital and system, billing and collections remain a significant problem. Delayed payments (or nonpayment) from managed care companies, incorrect billing practices, lack of experience, and faulty monitoring all play a part in the millions of dollars hospitals lose each year.

Trustees must be aware that the problem exists and, in turn, be willing to ensure that an adequate billing and collections process is in place. They must then monitor monthly reports of AR collections and reserve ratios, guaranteeing accurate reports that ensure proper collections, and correctly report reserve factors.

4. Be Willing to Close Noncore Components Immediately

Most "integrated systems" are little more than successful hospitals that own unsuccessful noncore businesses—a sad, but true, commentary. And just as unfortunate, without vast amounts of capital, turnarounds are not likely. As the noncore entities continue to incur losses, both financial resources and management's time are diverted trying to improve their performance. Unfortunately, there is neither enough time nor money to fix these businesses.

Management must assure trustees that each business entity is reported separately and be convinced that each product line has intrinsic value. For instance, if an ambulance service is unprofitable, it would better serve the hospital to investigate competitive services and to examine the defensive strategy: What is the overall value of this service? Does it attract profitable admissions? Does it eventually add revenue to the bottom line?

Trustees must also be willing to recognize the folly of entering the integrated delivery service game without a substantial cash reserve and to close noncore, operating margin-draining components immediately.

5. Assess Profitability of Product Lines

Product line analysis is critical, especially when a hospital or system experiences a financial crisis. It is a trustee's duty to periodically assess the viability and profitability of a product line's revenue, profits, and costs in order to determine which ones are losing money and why. In order for trustees to evaluate product lines, it's essential that the hospital or system have a state-of-the-art cost accounting system in place.

6. Monitor Productivity of Staffing and Budgeting

Managing variable costs—those costs that change with volume, such as labor and supplies—is critical. Line managers need volume-driven information delivered to them in a timely manner in order to monitor performance and be able to take corrective actions expeditiously.

Although not involved in the cost management process, trustees must monitor the productivity of staffing and budgeting, ensuring that budgetary projections are met.

7. Inquire About Cash-on-Hand

Cash is king. Trustees should heed this truism because overspending is an all-too-common downfall of many hospitals and systems. Ask management how much cash is received and dispersed for every business unit on a weekly basis, and compare the closing cash balance with the cash forecast. Weekly monitoring is a powerful tool to generate predictable cash flow, as it shortens management's response time to performance shortfalls, thereby ensuring that money not on hand is not spent.

8. Scrutinize Percentage of Self-Pay/ Uncompensated Care

Every hospital, no matter the size or ownership, expends resources for which there is no associated revenue. Uncompensated care—the amount written off by hospitals—represented 6 percent of operating expenses of U.S. hospitals in 1998.

While demanding assurance that management is seeking efficient methods of controlling and/or reducing uncompensated care costs, trustees must continue to scrutinize the expense as a percentage of total operating expenses. A good rule of thumb is to manage self-pay volumes to 10 percent or less of the hospital's total business.

9. Monitor Nondirect Fixed Costs

Nondirect fixed costs should average 40 percent of a hospital system's expenses. Unfortunately, many hospitals focus exclusively on variable, direct costs, which may serve only to reduce quality of care, customer service, and the ability to grow.

Trustees should be aware that certain actions will help reduce nondirect fixed costs, including eliminating or consolidating hospital/system functions, increasing spans of control (i.e., more staff reporting to a manager), reducing medical directorships, pooling support personnel, and reducing levels of management. This means that some managers will have to take on more responsibility so that the management pool will need to be highly talented, highly skilled, and very flexible professionals.

10. *Planning the Future*

Predicting hospital financial futures is simple: Health care expenditures will double within the decade, with ever-increasing pressures on the price of health care.

Hospitals exist to provide acute care services. It makes sense: In the acute care marketplace there are fewer competitors, and there hospitals enjoy their greatest product differentiation and reputation. Acute care services also produce the greatest profit margins.

The duties and responsibilities of health care trustees are not simple, nor are they always obvious. Entrusted with fiduciary responsibilities and assigned the duty of leading management, trustees are the vital link between the hospital/system and the community.

Achieving Peak Performance through Strategic Visioning

By Nathan S. Kaufman

In little more than a year, the disparity between peak-performing hospitals and their peers has widened. Even though the American Hospital Association warns that "many American hospitals are sitting on the edge of fiscal viability," ("State of Hospitals' Financial Health," 2002) many investor-owned hospital systems are reporting growth in profitability. Tenet recently reported a record 13 percent operating margin, and HCA reported its 20th quarter of double-digit growth in earnings. Many of these record earnings can be attributed to a focus by these systems on peak-performance status.

Capital and Financial Solvency: A Primary Mission

Hospitals have an insatiable appetite for capital. Facilities and equipment become obsolete within 5 to 10 years. New technology, rising construction costs, and the need for comprehensive information systems are all driving the need for capital. In most cases,

Nathan S. Kaufman is senior vice president for health care strategy, Superior Consultant Holdings Corp., San Diego. He can be reached at (858) 487-9771.

hospitals with access to the least costly capital will dominate their markets. Thus, understanding and meeting the funding criteria for low-cost capital is paramount for sustaining peak performance in a health care organization. The capital markets use the following quantitative business criteria to determine the availability and cost of capital for a hospital: amount of debt; funds in reserve; and cash flow.

Strong financial performance ensures that relatively inexpensive funding will be available to upgrade and expand a hospital. Weak financial performance will result in depleting reserves, high capital costs, eroding quality, and eventual hospital closure or sale. In 2001, an estimated 35 tax-exempt hospitals were sold to investor-owned systems because of their poor financial performance. Regardless of sponsorship, hospital trustees must recognize that one of their primary missions is to guide the hospital to achieve exceptional financial performance; that is, having an operating margin of 5 percent or better. High profitability enables the hospital to treat the medically indigent and provide other mission-related services.

Developing a Performance Culture

Peak-performing hospitals have a performance culture characterized by the establishment of quantitative benchmarks that require commitment and effort to reach. Once established, these targets are non-negotiable. Performance is evaluated within the organization based on achieving these benchmarks. Should the hospital underperform, management is required to take immediate action and bring the organization's performance back to an acceptable level. Finally, if the hospital continues to underperform consistently, personnel changes need to be made. For managers, the risks within a performance culture are high, but so are the rewards—high-performing managers receive significant merit-based compensation.

Strategies to Achieve Peak Performance

Peak-performing hospitals and systems employ three key management disciplines: portfolio management; focus/resolve to achieve quantitative benchmarks; and informed, objective decision making.

Portfolio Management

Portfolio management is defined as the right hospital with the right services in the right place. This major driver for peak performance rarely happens by chance. Both HCA and Tenet have adopted a strategy of regional dominance: neither company will enter a new market unless it believes it can capture a critical mass; that is, a minimum of 20 percent of that market. Specific tactics for managing a hospital portfolio include the following:

- Sell, merge, or close hospitals with weak market position and poor performance. These hospitals are a major drain on scarce capital and rarely turn around regardless of the dollars invested. HCA cut its losses in Atlanta by closing Parkway Regional and West Paces Ferry Hospitals. Tenet closed St. Luke's in Pasadena, California. A system should not suffer when the community is unwilling to support one of its facilities.
- Limit management focus to the core business. A hospital is one of the most complex businesses to operate. Related, but noncore services, such as home health care, skilled nursing care, and health clubs operate at a deficit, dilute management focus, and ultimately hurt the hospital's ability to access less expensive capital. If a peripheral service is operating at a deficit, in most cases the hospital should eliminate it. Instead, the hospital should promote the delivery of peripheral services by other niche providers and coordinate care with those providers.

Focus/Resolve to Achieve Quantitative Benchmarks

Pricing and expense control are the primary tactics here. Occupancy rates for hospital beds bottomed out in 1997 through 1998 and are now rapidly increasing. Diminishing capacity in the system is exacerbated by the shortage of both ICU beds and key hospital personnel (e.g., nurses, physical therapists, etc.). This has created an extremely favorable environment in which hospitals can demand the prices they need to achieve peak performance.

In 2001, HCA and Tenet combined achieved a 7.8 percent increase in net revenue per patient day. This increase could have only been achieved by double-digit increases from commercial and managed care plans. Anecdotal information and personal experience with tax-exempt hospitals support the premise that any hospital with a strong regional presence that is willing to walk away from a payer offering a bad contract can achieve significant rate increases.

Hospital supply and personnel costs are escalating at 5 to 10 percent per year. Medicare rates are only increasing by two to three percent. Aggressive pricing is the only option a hospital has to maintain consistent revenue and profit growth.

A common rationale used for pricing hospital services below their cost is "contribution margin." Some believe that it is good to accept any revenue from a payer that covers the variable costs of providing care and, thus, "contributes" to the fixed costs of the facility. The airline industry has used contribution margin pricing for years, and it has not worked successfully. Eventually all customers migrate to pricing based on the contribution margin, and no one pays full price. Hospitals that are losing money on Medicare/Medicaid payments (which usually represents at least 50 percent of the hospital's revenue) must cover their total costs (and more) with payments from commercial payers and, thus, should not price their services based on contribution margin.

Expense discipline is the other tactic necessary to achieve quantitative benchmarks. All expenses within a hospital must be benchmarked and measured routinely. By adopting the culture of performance, department managers understand that their job is to run the department within nonnegotiable financial parameters. In addition, the medical staff leadership must work to reduce supply and personnel costs. It is critical that physicians see the fruits of their labor in the form of increased capital expenditures for the facility.

Decisions Based on Objective Information

Hospital trustees are faced with extremely complex decisions that rarely have obvious, simple solutions. Decision making becomes easier once trustees accept that the success of a hospital over the long term depends on the hospital's performance as a business.

Key elements to make appropriate decisions are the following:

- Place the greatest weight for making any decision on financial analysis that is based on reasonable assumptions.
- Avoid theoretical, qualitative rationales; for example: "We may lose money, but ultimately it will be better for the patients." In other words, if you can't prove it, don't believe it.

Strategic Vision

Critical Performance Indicators (CPI)	Possible Target
Operating margin	>5%
EBDITA (Earnings Before Depreciation, Interest, Taxes, and Amortization)	>15%
Personnel expense (i.e., salaries, wages, benefits, agency fees)	<45% of net revenue, 5.0 employee per AADC (Adjusted Average Daily Census)
Supply expense	<16% of net revenue
Annual growth in net revenue, per adjusted patient day *[A calculation that converts outpatient visits to equivalent inpatient utilization]*	>6%
Annual growth in net revenue	>8%
Inpatient surgeries per 100 admissions	>28
Bad debts as a percent of net revenue	<8% of net revenue
Accounts receivable	<65 days
Annual growth in emergency department visits	>3%
Other key services	To be determined
RN turnover	To be determined
Employee turnover	To be determined
Patient satisfaction	To be determined
Quality indicators	To be determined

Note: Targets can be modified slightly to reflect market conditions.

Source: Nathan Kaufman & Superior Consultant Company, Inc., 1993–2002. All rights reserved.

- Mission is not an excuse for poor performance. The financial impact of mission-related activities must be quantified and controlled. For example, losing a predetermined amount of money on a free clinic is a rational decision; claiming mission as an excuse for out-of-control supply costs is not.
- Focus on essential hospital services. Hospitals are highly complex organizations requiring intensive management focus. Hospitals that deliver services that are outside their core competency dilute scarce management resources and capital. Hospitals must focus on essential hospital services, especially the emergency department, the intensive care unit, inpatient surgery, and cardiology. These are essential hospital services and require the majority of the organization's capital investment and management attention.

Strategic Visioning

Most hospitals have developed qualitative mission and vision statements (e.g., "to be the provider of state-of-the-art quality services"). These mission and vision statements serve little purpose if they do not tie into the hospital's operations and if they cannot be quantified (thus they will not be achieved).

Strategic visioning is a process of defining the future vision of the hospital using measurable critical performance indicators (CPI). These indicators are based on an objective assessment of the environment, which identifies what the hospital must do to capture market share and achieve the necessary financial performance.

The CPIs provide the hospital board with a framework for regularly assessing the hospital's performance. When a hospital underperforms with respect to its critical performance indicators, it is a warning that it will not be able to achieve its strategic vision. Thus, an action plan must be initiated to bring performance in line with the CPIs. The above chart provides an example of the types of CPIs that make up a hospital's strategic vision.

The community has entrusted hospital boards with the awesome responsibility of governing their local hospital. Financial performance is a significant measure of the board's stewardship. Understanding the drivers of peak performance and using strategic visioning to guide the institution are essential tools of hospital trustees.

The Capital Conundrum: Balancing Needs under Pressure

By Jeff C. Goldsmith

Many hospital trustees may be feeling better about their institution's future prospects than they did three years ago. Thanks to improved Medicare funding rates, increased private insurance reimbursement, and a lot of hard work on the part of administrators and boards to reduce costs, hospitals' financial performance is on the upswing. And for the first time in more than a generation, many hospitals find themselves needing more beds to accommodate increased demand. Extrapolating the past two years of increased inpatient utilization over the next decade, the Healthcare Advisory Board, Washington, D.C., recently forecast that hospitals will have to increase their bed capacity by a stunning 40 percent to meet projected demand by 2010. Ambulatory care capacity continues to lag behind demand, while hospitals face insatiable demands from their medical staffs to upgrade radiology and laboratory equipment (major profit sources).

Jeff C. Goldsmith is president of Health Futures, Charlottesville, Virginia. He can be reached at (434) 979-9524 or www.healthfutures.net.

The author wishes to thank Tony Speranzo, CFO of Ascension Health, St. Louis, and Don Ammon, CEO of Adventist Health System West, Roseville, California, for their comments and advice on this article.

At the same time, it is increasingly clear that needed operational improvements—ranging from better revenue cycle management to improved patient safety—will not be possible without major investments in information technology (IT). Hospitals stand on the brink of being able to eliminate paper records and orders, as well as radiology film and pathology slides. They will also be able to replace telephone-based scheduling and ordering with computerized order entry.

These improvements are vital not only to reducing medical errors, but also to improving working conditions for physicians, nurses, and other scarce clinical personnel. Through The Leapfrog Group, businesses have already made it clear that they want their employees to use hospitals that have made the digital "leap." Yet computerizing hospital operations is very expensive and will draw on the same limited stock of capital as all other improvements.

Trustees thus face a major dilemma: How should they allocate the organization's limited capital between upgrading facilities and information technology? How boards resolve this dilemma may be one of the most difficult challenges they face over the next 10 years—perhaps second only to finding sources of capital in the first place.

Boards need to plan for the next 10 to 20 years, not just address immediate needs. To do this responsibly, trustees should ask some hard questions. One of the toughest: How enduring is the current surge in inpatient utilization likely to be? Is the increased demand of the past two years (against a backdrop of 20 years' decline) the result of relaxed managed care restriction or the long-anticipated influx of the aging baby boom population?

A Contrarian View

Contrary to much popular sentiment, this current surge is not about the aging of the baby boomers. Demographics are a glacial force—powerful but *very* slow moving. The modal baby boomer turns 47 this year, and the youngest is in his or her late 30s. The real impact of baby boomers on inpatient demand is at least 10 to 15 years off.

Moreover, the current upswing in inpatient care cannot be traced to new technologies that require a patient's hospitalization. In fact, the long-term technological trend is toward reduced hospitalization for increasingly complex conditions. Surgery, in particular, continues to migrate into the ambulatory setting.

I believe the current surge of hospitalization stems from the collapse of health plan oversight for physician and hospital use. Not only have managed care restrictions been successfully overridden by state and federal regulatory changes, but many strictures have been abandoned by the plans themselves because their administrative costs outweighed the savings they were intended to create. Physicians, in turn, have reacted to the end of managed care's "gatekeeping" technique by pushing the envelope of the level of care they can provide to patients.

For example, a recent Centers for Disease Control and Prevention (CDC) analysis showed national Caesarean section rates of almost 25 percent, a level not seen in a decade. Federal and state legislative overrides of managed restrictions in the late 1990s sharply increased lengths of stay for obstetrical deliveries. There are also more medical admissions from the emergency department (ED), possibly because physicians are directing more chronically ill patients to the ED rather than treating them in their outpatient settings.

How Will Payers React?

Hospitals can count on a strong payer reaction to this cost surge. Hospital utilization increases, as well as prescription drug spending, are sparking a stunning resurgence in health costs after a decade of relative quiet. Employer health insurance renewal rates have increased 20 percent for large groups and twice that for smaller groups.

Therefore, although it is good news in the short term for hospitals, the current surge in hospital utilization has sown the seeds for a powerful health insurance counterreaction. As employers tire of large premium rate increases, they will place tremendous pressure on health plans to rein in health costs.

Health plans have already begun to respond—by significantly increasing employee cost sharing as well as by moving to multitiered provider networks, with higher cost sharing for patients who use more expensive facilities and services. This will have the immediate effect of increasing hospitals' bad debts and encouraging patients to postpone or avoid hospitalization.

In the likely event that these efforts fail to slow the cost surge sufficiently, health plans will return with a vengeance to the provider bargaining table and demand significant price concessions from hospitals. Such concessions will not be achieved easily, particularly in highly consolidated hospital markets. Like many hospitals in the western states today, their beds will be full, but they will not be able to generate an operating margin.

Will the Current Demands Continue?

How sustainable current inpatient demand is may depend on the individual institution and its market position. For some dominant institutions, such as major teaching hospitals and regional referral centers, current utilization growth is probably attributable, at least in part, to market share gains (measured by growth in hospital admissions and procedures). These gains may well endure.

On the other hand, some hospitals' utilization increases may be the result of deteriorating internal controls. This is particularly true for ICU beds, where lengths of stay (and resource use) may vary by as much as three times for patients with the same severity of illness, depending on their physician. This variability, as well as many questionable ICU admissions, often disappears once ICUs become staffed by intensivists (another of The Leapfrog Group's primary criteria).

There is also significant variability in how operating suites and procedure rooms are used, as well as the rate of bed turnover. Bed shortages may be a result of deteriorating scheduling, poor internal communications, and poor information systems support. If hospitals are experiencing LOS increases (in addition to admission increases), trustees and management may be able to trace them to reduced clinical discipline and poor communication or coordination of services inside the hospital.

It is also important for trustees to ask how much of current inpatient pressure for beds is driven by "outliers"—preventable infections, readmissions, and other quality problems. Recent CDC analyses found that hospital-acquired septic infections are growing annually by 17 percent, resulting in almost 100,000 deaths (many of which are preventable) and billions of dollars in avoidable medical costs.

Analytic tools exist to help hospitals examine variations in clinical resource use and to determine if they have a basis in clinical severity. These tools enable management to determine how much capacity could be freed by more effective internal utilization systems.

Good analysis, however, requires good clinical data and reporting systems. As long as clinical records remain in paper form, it will be difficult to evaluate and control variations in hospital usage. There may be a direct trade-off between clinical IT spending and expanding the physical plant.

Precisely to avoid unnecessary operational spending, hospital trustees should have as great an interest as health plans in reducing variation or clinically questionable use of their hospital's resources. Trustees should satisfy themselves that the hospital is making the most effective use of its existing capacity before adding new beds.

Can the Hospital Staff More Beds?

Many hospitals are unable to fill all their licensed beds because of nursing shortages. It is a questionable use of scarce capital to build additional capacity you cannot staff or can staff only by driving up operating costs, thereby cutting into operating profits.

Nationally, hospitals are experiencing a nurse vacancy rate of more than 12 percent and have resorted to mandatory overtime, as well as engaging expensive temporary agencies to fill the gap. Reasons for the shortage are complex and will likely endure for many years. (See "Nurses Needed STAT!" in the June 2000 issue of *Trustee,* and "In Our Hands," an AHA report available on the AHA's Web site, www.aha.org. Click on "Workforce" in the center column, first page.)

Although many hospitals have stepped up recruitment efforts, adequate staffing ultimately depends on improved retention and job satisfaction among current skilled workers.

Can the Information System Support Capacity?

As suggested previously, capacity use and information systems are intimately linked. Information technology, particularly the electronic record, as well as supporting scheduling systems, can play a major role here. Automating clinical systems may markedly improve productivity, while reducing medical errors, and facilitate higher clinical personnel retention rates.

Many hospitals continue to support clinical care with information technologies more appropriate to the precomputer era than to a modern enterprise. Paper records, curly fax paper, telephone message slips, paper scheduling systems—all are incontrovertible evidence of an early 1970s information environment. Effective internal scheduling, care coordination, clinical profiling and utilization control, patient safety, and improved efficiency and morale on nursing units all depend on the quality of clinical and administrative information.

If overutilization can be attributed to clinical variation, poor scheduling, and coordination and quality problems rather than to sustainable gains in market share, then the board should give funding priority to IT for clinical and administrative programs rather than to new construction.

But IT that enables these programs to function at maximum efficiency first requires a willingness to reexamine care processes and workflow. However, such reexamination will likely expose clinicians and administrators to countless "Who Moved My Cheese?" (in the words of best-selling author Spencer Johnson, when referring to the resistance to changing comfortable routines) moments. Trustees must insist that improving care and service go hand in hand with IT investment.

Ask the Tough Questions

Trustees should consider the following before they approve a major capital spending plan, either for the physical plant or for IT:

- *What is the return on proposed capital investments?* Trustees should insist on a rigorous analysis of the investment return on their limited capital dollars. These analyses should apply to all forms of capital investment—plant, equipment, and IT infrastructure. Although some essential capital investments may not generate identifiable returns (e.g., replacing existing beds; correcting building code problems), they may be unavoidable if the hospital is to remain in business.

  However, for major capital expenditures, all other things being equal, trustees must be willing to give higher priority to capital expenditures that can generate higher rates of return. If operating savings are projected from a capital investment (facilities or IT), there should be an explicit responsibility assigned for realizing them, and trustees must be willing to hold management accountable.

- *How sustainable is demand and financial performance?* The strong likelihood of health plan and employer reaction to the present cost explosion makes it dangerous for hospital managers and boards to assume both continued volume growth and continued robust operating margins. One or the other will probably suffer within the next 18 months to two years as payers respond to employer outrage over rising costs. For this reason, simply projecting today's demand and payment rates over the next 10 years on a straight line is not prudent planning.
- *What is the quality of increased demand?* One advantage of being at full capacity is the opportunity/necessity of making choices about who uses the hospital and for what purposes. Trustees should ask management whether bed requests are coming from market share gains or from slackening clinical discipline and resource use variation. Trustees should also ask if increased utilization is coming from the hospital's leading clinicians and clinical programs or from its marginal practitioners and programs. Are the clinicians who are creating utilization pressures the same physicians trustees and their families are likely to use for their own medical problems? Building new capacity to accommodate physicians or programs that trustees do not have complete confidence in is not responsible investment strategy.
- *How ready is the hospital to use clinical IT?* Some hospitals that need modern clinical information systems do not possess the management depth or physician support to manage the installation effectively. Does the hospital have the managerial and medical staff commitment and understanding to actually change clinical care processes? Can its IT staff ride herd on the vendors and ensure "value for money" in the IT installation process? Getting the return on an IT installation is a complex, demanding task—one which trustees should not take for granted.

Hospital and system trustees face difficult challenges in the coming years to make the best use of limited capital. Setting the right balance between investments in the physical plant and in IT infrastructure may be their most difficult challenge. There is no magic formula that will work for every institution. To find the right balance will require not only rigorous analysis but sound, prudent judgment by trustees and managers.

PART SIX

Quality

Quality:
The Key Issue
for the Board

By A. Thomas Hollingsworth
and Dwain Harper

Although the fiscal viability of a health care organization may be the board's first priority, long-term viability results from many inter-related factors, one of the most important of which is the institution's quality of care. With the recent reports from the Institute of Medicine and employer coalitions such as The Leapfrog Group (see the article "Raising the Bar" on page 278), which is using its purchasing power to influence hospitals' practices, quality has become a front-burner issue for many health care providers. The Leapfrog Group is trying to make quality an explicit way to differentiate hospitals.

Crossing the Quality Chasm, the Institute of Medicine's second report, issued last March, proposes six key facets to improving health care: patient safety; effectiveness (the avoidance of both service under- and overuse); patient-centered delivery that reflects patient preferences; timely service delivery; efficient resource use;

A. Thomas Hollingsworth, Ph.D., is professor of management and dean of the School of Business, Florida Institute of Technology, Melbourne. He can be reached at (321) 674-7327. Dwain Harper, D.O., is a health care consultant with Contemporary HealthCare Associates, Stuart, Florida. He can be reached at (561) 225-6222.

and equitable delivery so that all patients receive the same high level of care.

Stating the Commitment

First and most important, the mission and vision of a health care organization must clearly and unequivocally specify its commitment to a strategy and vision that emphasize quality.

The following mission statement exemplifies this point:

> The mission of Hospital A is to improve the health status of individuals within the community through prevention, education, and delivery of the highest quality health care services. We are a community-owned and governed organization committed to the principles of quality, value, and service without regard to financial status.

Fulfilling the Commitment

Ensuring that processes are in place to fulfill your hospital's or system's commitment to quality means that staff must measure quality indicators, correct for variances from acceptable results, and track corrective actions. Ultimately, this process will lead to the development, use, and continuous refinement of best practice models, not only in clinical areas, but throughout the hospital.

To ensure that CQI has a high priority in the hospital and that staff are given the resources necessary to conduct it appropriately, the board should create a standing committee (see "Board Quality Committee Description," page 275) comprising trustees, medical staff leaders, and key administrators to review variances in quality indicators each month. Also, a member of the organization's quality assurance department should report regularly to this standing committee's meetings. Finally, a member of the board's executive committee, who can report to the whole board at each meeting, should chair this quality review committee.

Trustee members of the board's quality committee should regularly attend medical staff quality and executive committee meetings. Because the board has the final responsibility for the quality of care delivered in its institution and for credentialing the medical staff, it's a trustee's duty to attend these meetings and be involved in all aspects of the quality process.

The Process

Continuous quality improvement does not have to be complicated. It requires establishing performance benchmarks and giving clinicians feedback on their practices relative to the benchmarks and to their peers in the institution. Departmental quality committees and the risk management department will review these data and report any significant variances to the medical staff quality committee with suggested actions needed and/or taken. Depending on the severity

---

Board Quality Committee Description

1. The committee continually assesses the organization's quality of care. It will review performance improvement plans and make appropriate policy recommendations to the full board.
2. The committee monitors the risk management program. It will review legal activity from incidents involving patients, visitors, or personnel and make policy recommendations to the board.
3. The committee participates in developing policies to contain costs. It makes reports to the board concerning local, state, and national policies and issues that affect the cost of delivering health services and makes appropriate recommendations.
4. It will adopt and periodically review a written plan to safeguard patients, visitors, and personnel in the event of an internal disaster such as a fire and ensure that all key personnel rehearse drills to comply with JCAHO standards.
5. The quality committee shall also adopt and review a written plan for the receiving, care, and evacuation of mass casualties, and shall ensure that such a plan is coordinated with inpatient and outpatient services. Key personnel should rehearse the plan in accordance with the JCAHO standards.
6. The committee will review all physicians who are under investigation by the medical staff executive committee.
7. The committee will review quality issues presented by the medical executive committees, departmental quality committees, risk management, and service line directors.
8. The committee will review all service line and departmental quality improvement plans and cost containment plans on an annual, or as-necessary, basis.

of the variance, it would then be reported to the medical staff executive committee and the board quality committee for appropriate actions.

Generally, two pathways would be necessary—one for physician-related incidents and the other for nonphysician incidents. Again, this is an oversimplification; in actual practice, the role of each committee has to be defined carefully.

Patients and the Quality Process

A variety of instruments exist for measuring patient and family perceptions of quality and satisfaction and for comparing those perceptions with satisfaction data from the best institutions of similar size and location. Your board should also monitor both positive and negative letters from patients and family members.

Because of reduced lengths of stay, patients and/or their caregivers must be given postdischarge instructions for their home care in a timely manner. Case management procedures therefore play an important role and should track patients from the time they leave the hospital until they are fully recovered.

Specific Quality Issues

The quality evaluation process should look at both iatrogenic (that is, occurring because of an action or procedure performed in the hospital) and nosocomial (occurring while the patient is hospitalized) illnesses. Mortality and morbidity should also be reviewed closely. Is your institution making people well or making them sicker? There must also be provisions in your quality system for monitoring "near misses" without staff fearing a threat of punishment. Root cause analysis of a near miss is much better than analysis of a sentinel event. This is a proactive part of the quality process that prevents problems from occurring in the first place.

Achieving high-quality care has always been providers' primary goal. Very few hospital staff perform badly on purpose. In many cases, hospital systems are at the root of medical errors. That's why the board must ensure that caregivers are given the assistance and resources necessary to provide the highest possible quality of care.

Quality Quiz for Trustees

The following quiz should give you insight on how good a job your board is doing in managing your institution's quality. All questions can be answered "yes" or "no."*

- Does your hospital's mission statement and strategic plan state that the board is unequivocally responsible for your institution's quality?
- Do you rate your hospital high to excellent for patient care quality?
- Are you satisfied with the methods that you use to derive this rating?
- Does the board receive regular quality reports on all aspects of hospital operations?
- Does the hospital have a separate quality department?
- Does your board have a standing quality committee?
- Do trustees regularly attend quality committee meetings?
- Are mortality and morbidity reviewed monthly by a committee of the medical staff?
- Can you demonstrate your hospital's level of quality to an outsider?
- Is your board aware of all quality problems within the hospital, and does it address them efficiently?
- Are you satisfied that your institution handles patient chart completion and discharge summaries accurately and efficiently?
- Do you rate the quality of case management services in your organization as high to excellent?
- Does your organization have a process that tracks patients from the time they leave the hospital until they are fully recovered?
- Are you satisfied that your organization's physician credentialing and recredentialing processes ensure the highest level of quality in your institution?

*If you cannot answer all of these questions with a "yes," your institution may well face a quality crisis in the near future.

Raising the Bar

Purchasers and Providers Must Work
Together to Meet
the Quality-of-Care Challenge

By Karen Sandrick

For business leaders like Bruce Bradley, director of managed health care initiatives for General Motors, "The current health care environment is untenable. There's just too much waste in the system—and we're not talking about tongue depressors here. We're talking about injuries, disabilities, and lost lives from medical errors." Bradley brings the statistics from the Institute of Medicine (IOM) report on medical errors down to life on the assembly line: "If you extrapolate the IOM data, which said there were 98,000 preventable deaths per year, to the total 250 million U.S. population, you get about 39 preventable deaths per 100,000. GM covers a million and a quarter lives. So every single day, we could be losing between one and two employees as a result of a medical error."

That's why Bradley, one of the founding members of The Leapfrog Group, wants to create a new climate that will lead to incentives for hospitals to use resources efficiently and effectively through targeting quality and patient safety. "We're looking for breakthrough improvements in quality and safety that can have a

---

Karen Sandrick is a health care writer based in Chicago.

huge impact on injury and disability and the number of lives saved," he says, adding, "These are our employees who [may] get less than optimal care, and this is our money."

"Employers and business coalitions have been concerned about getting value for their health care dollars for many years—and quality plus patient outcomes, including safety as well as cost, have been part of the value equation," says Gregg Lehman, president and CEO of the National Business Coalition on Health (NBCH), Washington, D.C.

Until recently, employers worked through managed care plans. But, says Becky Cherny, CEO of the Central Florida Health Care Coalition, Orlando, "The health care delivery system couldn't respond to anyone other than the health plan, and employers didn't talk to anyone other than the health plan. It was just like having one huge wall up between us."

Employers and business coalitions are now working directly with providers—and they're flexing their muscles. With declining Medicare payments, the business coalition community is becoming the key customer for many health care providers. "Since we're the largest purchasing group nationally, we believe we have the right and the responsibility to be monitoring the health care delivery system and demanding improvements," Cherny says.

At the national level, NBCH and Leapfrog act as clearinghouses, reviewing best clinical practices and establishing basic purchasing tenets, serving as catalysts for reform in local markets, identifying standards of patient safety, and rewarding hospitals that meet them. Locally, individual employers and business coalitions are engaging providers in disease and quality management projects and comparing hospital data on quality, safety, and outcomes. And business leaders are inviting hospital and health system trustees to help in their efforts by calling for long-term strategic plans for quality and safety, challenging capital budgeting priorities, advocating quality improvement, urging investment in often costly automated quality data systems, and encouraging public accountability.

The Purchasers' Perspective

Purchasers are part of the problem, Bradley acknowledges. "We historically have not done a very good job of even saying that quality is important, much less measuring it and then recognizing and rewarding better performance."

But purchasers are becoming more sophisticated customers—and they want to partner with providers. "We have to leave our guns at the door," says Lehman. "We have to stop being adversaries and saying that hospitals are at fault because they're raising their prices when we're not sure the outcomes are good. We have to listen to providers who say, 'Why should I invest in a long-term strategy if you shift your business every year and stop sending your employees to us?'"

The Leapfrog Group consequently is hoping to create a new relationship among health care purchasers, hospitals, and consumers, explains Suzanne Delbanco, the group's executive director. "Leapfrog primarily is about putting information in the hands of consumers so they can make more informed health care decisions, and an important part of that is highlighting hospitals that have put very effective patient safety practices in place," she says.

The Leapfrog Group came together almost three years ago "to send a strong signal to the health care system that breakthroughs in quality and safety are valued," she says. Founding Frogs, as they are called, including the Buyers Healthcare Action Group, GE, GM, Verizon, Pacific Business Group on Health, the U.S. Health Care Financing Administration, and the U.S. Office of Personnel Management, established a set of purchasing principles that would launch a voluntary effort among purchasers to start "buying right." The Frogs secured the support of the Business Roundtable, the national association of Fortune 500 CEOs, to encourage businesses to adopt the Leapfrog principles.

Leapfrog already has 84 purchasers on board that represent more than 26 million people and spend $45 billion on health care a year. In keeping with the purchasing principles, members have agreed to use performance measures from the Joint Commission on Accreditation of Healthcare Organizations, the National Committee on Quality Assurance, and other recognized groups to rate providers' performance and show employees how they can use these comparative ratings to choose high-quality providers. In turn, employers will reward providers that rate highly by working to increase their patient volume and pricing levels and recognizing them for outstanding performance.

How Is Your Hospital Responding to Business Coalitions' Concerns?

Business leaders suggest that trustees query their CEOs about three principal areas: their relationships with purchasers; how they collect quality and safety data; and their quality and safety practices in general.

Relationships with Purchasers

- Has your hospital talked to local business owners to see what their priorities are for reducing medical errors and improving quality and patient safety?
- Is the hospital aware of Leapfrog, the National Business Coalition on Health, and local business coalition efforts to improve quality and safety?
- Is your hospital committed to, or has it established, concrete plans to develop safety standards, such as a computerized physician order-entry system, volume thresholds for specific clinical care programs, or placing a certified critical care physician in the ICU?

Data Collection

- How is the hospital measuring, and demonstrating responses to, variations in clinical care delivery?
- Is your hospital reporting on a balanced set of quality and safety indicators, including process, structure, and outcome measures for major service areas?
- Does your hospital compare its performance measures against national and regional benchmarks?
- Do the hospital and its purchasers look at the same measures of quality and safety performance?
- How does your hospital demonstrate the value of services from both the cost and quality sides of the equation?

Quality and Safety

- What specific plans does your hospital have to address medical errors?
- What is your hospital doing to improve quality and safety?
- Has your hospital measurably improved health in your community?

—K.S.

Frog members are holding providers' feet to the fire by insisting that they adopt three standards employers believe will produce substantial patient safety gains:

- Computerized physician order entry
- Evidence-based hospital referral
- Intensive care units that are staffed by certified critical care physicians

These "leaps in patient safety" were chosen because they have been shown to improve patient outcomes and reduce complications and risk of death. According to Leapfrog research, the standards could save more than 53,000 lives and prevent nearly 522,000 serious medication errors every year. "We weren't reinventing the wheel; the leaps are evidence based," Bradley says. In addition, the "leaps" are easy to document. "You don't need a lot of in-depth research to know whether or not hospitals have programs in place that predict better outcomes and lower mortality. We know, yes or no, that a hospital has a full-time intensivist in the ICU, meets the minimum number of coronary artery bypasses or deliveries of low birth-weight babies, or has a computerized physician order entry system," he adds.

Particularly important for employees, "the leaps can be understood by Mom," Bradley says. "The average person can understand that by having a computerized system, you get rid of sloppy handwriting and institute some checks to make sure patients are getting the right drugs. [And] it's not hard to understand that practice makes perfect, so hospitals that do higher volumes of procedures do a better job, or that an intensivist with a concentration in critical care does a better job than physicians who run in and out of the ICU all the time."

Finally, Leapfrog's safety standards have a significant long-term economic impact. "There's a huge payback in terms of reducing the cost of adverse drug events, preventing complications, and cutting length of stay and inappropriate ICU admissions," Bradley explains.

Leapfrog initially is focusing on acute care providers in Atlanta; Seattle, Tacoma, and Everett, Washington; St. Louis; in eastern Tennessee; and throughout California, Michigan, and Minnesota. It is asking providers in these regions to complete a four-page survey declaring whether they will be committing to the purchasing principles in the next two years. Leapfrog will use the survey results to educate employees about patient safety and the group's three safety standards, as well as to recognize and reward providers that meet the standards.

NBCH, which includes 90 member coalitions representing 8,000 employers and 30 million people under its umbrella, likewise advocates the Leapfrog safety standards. In January 2000, its National Advisory Council also identified five strategic steps purchasers should take to address patient safety:

- Raise consumer awareness about safety.
- Encourage and support voluntary and mandatory provider reporting on quality and safety concerns.
- Create innovative financial models that reward providers for high-quality, safe, and affordable health care.
- Identify a variety of safe practice indicators utilized by health care organizations.
- Incorporate safety standards in contracting.

NBCH nevertheless leaves specifics about community-based quality and safety initiatives to local coalitions. "The approach we try to stress is to sit down at the table with providers to figure out what it will take in any given market to come up with solutions that are workable and really will have an impact on health care quality," Lehman says.

For instance, when Healthcare 21, a four-year-old business coalition in Knoxville, Tennessee, discovered that beta blockers were not being used as often as they could be by those with heart disease in the region, it gathered all stakeholders together to devise preventive health strategies. As a result, health plans have designed cardiac case management systems that remind physicians when to consider prescribing beta blockers, and employees have learned how to better manage cardiac disease, says Jerry Burges, Healthcare 21 president.

Lehman sees the effort extending beyond individual employers and providers and into the community at large to reach the uninsured and medically underserved. "Both groups need to help each other determine the strategic plan for their markets: where they want to be a year from now and three years from now, with programs that have traction and improve overall quality, the health of the employees, and the productivity of the workforce," he says.

For employers, the partnership helps ensure that providers keep their high-risk, chronically ill members healthy. The counterpoint on the provider side is to be assured that employers will steer employees and their families to hospitals and systems that achieve good outcomes.

What This Means for Trustees and Execs

According to the NBCH's National Advisory Council, support for patient safety at both the hospital and community level starts with boards of trustees, who can pressure health care organizations to change.

"Trustees are the eyes and ears of the marketplace. They are in the enviable position of representing the concerns of employers and hospitals as well as concerns related to the health of the community," says Lehman. Trustees also wield considerable influence on hospital leadership. "CEOs use trustees as a sounding board for new programs and ideas and obviously tweak the programs they are offering or change course based on what they hear from their boards," Lehman adds.

Board members should have a thorough understanding of safety issues, business leaders say. Trustees should be motivating their hospitals to nurture a culture of quality and act as champions of safety.

"One role trustees can play is to encourage, if not compel, management to begin making investments in quality from a philosophical standpoint in terms of encouraging continuous quality improvement, education, and systems thinking. They also should be making the hard-dollar investments that are required to adhere to standardized measures of quality," says Chris Queram, CEO of The Alliance, a business coalition covering a 12-county area in and around Madison, Wisconsin.

Bradley stresses the importance of trustees setting priorities for capital budgeting. He acknowledges that many hospitals are financially strapped and balk at spending millions of dollars on computerized physician order-entry systems. But, he says, "it's upsetting to purchasers when hospitals say they can't afford to [institute] a computerized physician order-entry system and yet they are about to

[add] a new wing or atrium. It's the board's responsibility, in no uncertain terms, to seriously challenge capital budgets so that hospitals put money into the kinds of things that will save people's lives."

Health care boards also need to be attuned to safety issues in their communities and question adding new clinical programs that cannot attract sufficient volume. According to Leapfrog research, coronary artery bypass programs that treat 500 or more patients a year tend to achieve superior outcomes. "The evidence that there is a relationship between volume and outcomes is powerful," Bradley says. "It's unconscionable to see new programs proliferating where they are not needed or low-volume programs that dilute other clinical areas. Trustees need to reflect the public's trust and have the courage to shut down programs that do not meet the kinds of standards of care that are possible," he adds.

Queram believes trustees should help hospital management accept public accountability for clinical performance. "Health care has been slow to embrace the idea of measuring clinical care, partly because it was too amorphous or too variable," he says. "Although that attitude is changing, there is still a tendency to want to hide information from the public, either for fear of liability or for fear that health care professionals will not be comfortable having their performance compared and judged in an open way. But the health care industry has to take a giant step forward to make data transparent, and trustees can play a critical role in helping to create a culture that embraces accountability," Queram says.

Health care institutions have to take a critical look at themselves and determine how they stack up against their own internal measures of quality and patient safety as well as against other hospital systems at the benchmark level, says Jim Hunt, CFO of Walt Disney World and a board member at Orlando (Florida) Regional Health Center.

Hunt also advises hospitals to take advantage of data collected by business coalitions "to see how they can use the information to continue on their journey of continuous improvement of quality patient care." As Lehman points out, business coalitions commonly aggregate data by procedure and disease and compare outcomes against best practices.

Health system and hospital chief executives need to understand that employers will insist on becoming more knowledgeable purchasers of health care services and therefore will be looking for detailed information, observes Dale Collins, president and CEO of Baptist Health System of East Tennessee in Knoxville.

As an example, in 1990, the Central Florida Health Care Coalition asked all 17 hospitals in its area to install a computer-based system that measures patient care quality. This system allows the coalition to have a common set of metrics with which to assess providers communitywide and make purchasing decisions, says CEO Cherny.

In East Tennessee, Healthcare 21 will publish a purchasing guide for its members that measures hospitals' performance against outcome criteria, such as mortality and morbidity, length of stay, and cost. As one of seven regional pilot areas for Leapfrog, the coalition will tie this information to volume and other important safety data.

This fall, The Alliance is releasing findings to coalition members and providers in its region from its first quality report on hospital performance in specific clinical areas—surgery, nonsurgical acute care, hip and knee replacement, cardiac care, and maternity care— that apply quality measures developed by the Agency for Health Care Research and Quality, data collected and maintained by the state of Wisconsin, and discharge data from providers in the 12-county area to compare performance among hospitals.

So, as Baptist's Collins notes, "Hospitals have to understand that, whether or not they agree with information about their performance, it is going to be published. They need to be part of the [quality and cost] debate to make sure that such information is as accurate as possible."

For trustees, that means encouraging their CEOs to "value the idea of transparency and share information with the community about their safety practices. Hospitals that are willing to get out early and share information about themselves ultimately will be in a winning position later," says Leapfrog executive director Delbanco.

Business coalitions are reviewing extensive data to examine clinical practice variation and to rate providers on their patient outcomes. Says Central Florida's Cherny: "Hospitals that try to say, 'We don't have those data' will be left behind, because the technology is available, and the purchasers will be taking advantage of it. Successful providers are the ones that stay ahead of the curve by continually assessing themselves internally and providing that information externally."

Focus on GM

In addition to its involvement with other employers in the national Leapfrog Group and the National Business Coalition on Health, General Motors has developed several of its own community initiatives to improve the quality, safety, and cost-effectiveness of health care in those markets with major GM employee concentrations: Anderson, Indiana; Flint, Michigan, and northeast Ohio.

In each area, GM creates coalitions of business leaders, consumers, insurers, labor unions, government agencies, philanthropic groups, the media, and health care providers to decide how to best improve the health status, not only of GM employees and their dependents, but the community as a whole, says Tony Stasunas, director of Flint's Community Initiative. The Community Initiative in Flint, for example, addresses the needs of the 430,000 residents in Genessee County as well as GM's 126,500 health plan enrollees.

Since it began in 1994, Flint's Community Initiative has produced criteria checklists to help providers select the most appropriate candidates for cardiac catheterization; encourage consumers to get more involved in fitness programs; and help diabetics manage their disease more effectively. In its first two years, the catheterization effort produced a double-digit decrease in the number of cardiac procedures, without increasing hospital admissions for myocardial infarction. The fitness campaign seeks to reduce the number of county residents who do not exercise from 55.4 percent to 49.8 percent by the end of 2001. Finally, the diabetes effort, which promotes annual hemoglobin A1c testing, has established the goal of decreasing diabetes deaths in Flint, which are currently 35 percent more common than the national average.

Says Stasunas: "Our principal interest is in improving the quality of health care. We feel that high health care costs are a symptom of poor quality and that, as a byproduct of improving quality, we will see our costs go down."

—K.S.

Above all, say business leaders, health care executives and trustees need to realize that employers are delivering a consistent message: We have a legitimate concern about quality and safety, and we expect health care organizations to meet common sets of expectations. "Providers are starting to see that the business community is firmly of the opinion that quality and cost are inextricably tied together," says Queram.

"If the business and provider communities work together to develop appropriate measures of quality and safety and make that information available to the public, we might change people's perceptions and utilization patterns," he continues. "The business case for quality is emerging in a way that's different from any time in the past."

Six Sigma:
Adapting GE's Lessons
to Health Care

*How Virtua Health Applied
a Quality Technique
from Manufacturing*

By Walter H. Ettinger, M.D.

All health care stakeholders, from the board on down, want to find ways to make their organization perform better. Increasingly, health care leaders have also realized they must reevaluate their institution's culture, along with their overall management strategies, to maintain a competitive edge and keep pace with an evolving industry. They're recognizing that managers must be encouraged to move beyond accountability for simple technical knowledge of specific functions and seek a results-focused, interdepartmental way to target the root causes of quality and efficiency problems. Having tried and failed to find the Holy Grail within their own industry, providers are now looking beyond the health care field to other industries for best practices in managing both cost and quality. The transportation, retailing, hospitality, and manufacturing industries, among others, offer valuable case studies for change. Arguably among the most successful approaches in any industry has been the General Electric Company's application of Six Sigma, with its related management methodologies.

Walter H. Ettinger, M.D., is executive vice president, Virtua Healthcare, Marlton, New Jersey.

Achieving high levels of quality, productivity, and financial resilience has been an evolutionary process at GE. Understanding that yesterday's top-down management approach would not work in a new, fast-paced environment of technological change and international competition, CEO Jack Welch set out to lead a series of initiatives to make GE a more agile and dynamic organization. For the last five years, GE has led an aggressive campaign to cultivate the use of the Six Sigma quality improvement process throughout the company. The results have been impressive: over $3 billion in savings and a 20 percent gain in productivity. It has been so successful, in fact, that GE's customers, including health care providers, have asked the company to help them adapt Six Sigma to their own organizations.

Translating the Six Sigma method to health care has been key to the success of an ongoing quality and culture change at Virtua Health, a four-hospital system in New Jersey. Created in 1998 through the merger of West Jersey Health System and Memorial Health Alliance of Burlington County, Virtua has become the dominant provider in the New Jersey suburbs of Philadelphia, bringing together four hospitals, two ambulatory surgery centers, two long-term care facilities, a health fitness center, and a home health company. And although most indicators showed that the system was performing at an average level, the board and senior executive team decided this was not good enough.

Through Six Sigma, Virtua sought to fundamentally change its management and operating culture and become even more competitive in its market. But could a management approach developed by a large international manufacturing company be applied successfully to an integrated health system? Absolutely. Not only that, but the implementation of Six Sigma also provides a case study in how our health system is leveraging the enthusiasm and commitment of its trustees to obtain system-wide quality improvement. To understand how we used Six Sigma for our purposes though, we first need to explain what it is and how it works.

Six Sigma at a Glance

Sigma is the Greek letter assigned to represent standard deviation; that is, the amount of variation within a given process. The higher the Sigma level, the lower the number of defects, and achieving a

Six Sigma level of quality equates to a mere 3.4 defects out of one million opportunities, or nearly error-free performance (see "Sigma Levels" below). The "Comparison of Industries" chart below illustrates various industries and medical services with their corresponding sigma levels. Clearly, health care has ample room for improvement.

Sigma Levels

Sigma	Defects per Million Opportunities (DPMO)
1	690,000
2	308,537
3	66,807
4	6,210
5	233
6	3.4

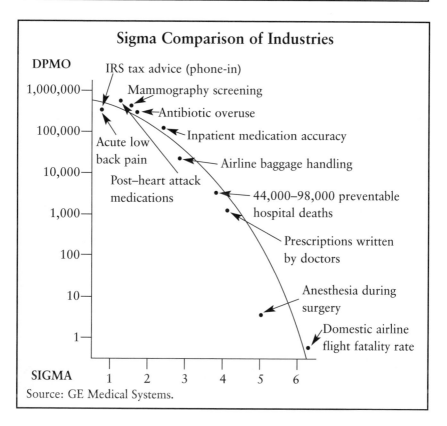

Sigma Comparison of Industries

Source: GE Medical Systems.

As a quality methodology, Six Sigma isn't complex, and it isn't a magic elixir. In fact, it shares similarities with other programs familiar to providers, such as total quality management and continuous quality improvement but with several key differences (see "Ensuring Quality: A Comparison," page 298).

Six Sigma can blend with or be the next initiative after a hospital's existing quality program, but it definitely goes beyond either homegrown efforts or external initiatives. It's a rigorous, statistical approach to problem solving designed to help organizations significantly reduce the defects that drive up costs and diminish quality of care. With Six Sigma, you don't go on to the next step until you've proven empirically that you're ready. GE's approach to Six Sigma helps to clearly define, measure, analyze, improve, and control (DMAIC) quality in every product, process, and transaction (see the DMAIC chart below). It has essentially changed the company's "DNA" and is now the way it works and designs all products.

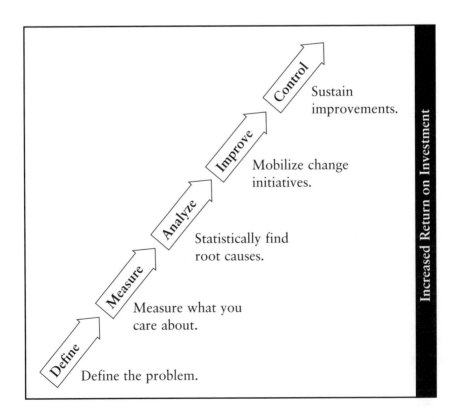

The Genesis of Six Sigma at Virtua

The senior executive team of Virtua held a retreat to create the long-term vision and goals for the health system and make a single, high-performance, blended "Virtua culture" out of two very different cultures. At that time the system was about a year old, and the initial integration of West Jersey and Memorial had taken place. The health system had one governing board and a fully integrated management team.

The team identified three measurable goals: to be recognized among the nation's top health systems; to win the New Jersey Governor's Award for Performance Excellence; and to be in the 90th percentile or above for overall patient satisfaction in all Virtua's clinical facilities.

To get there, we developed a cultural transformation program called the STAR Initiative, whose first aim has been to focus all the work of the health system on creating an outstanding patient experience, as measured in five domains:

- Excellent service
- Highest clinical quality
- A caring culture
- Best employee practices
- Resource stewardship

STAR's second aim is to transform Virtua into a high-performing organization, which we have defined as an organization that makes quick decisions, removes bureaucratic barriers for employees and physicians in order to create an outstanding patient experience, and is driven by valid measurement and accountability for results.

To quickly implement the STAR Initiative, we realized we needed a process that created a framework for setting goals, that defined the work needed to meet those goals, and that established measures of those goals; and we needed a common language—a road map and a mirror to hold up to ourselves. Investigation led to a relationship with the Healthcare Solutions Group of GE Medical Systems, based in part on its success in achieving its own goals of growth, quality, and customer satisfaction over the past 15 years.

Virtua's CEO, Rich Miller, has been the sponsor and champion of the STAR initiative. It is imperative that the change initiative be "owned" by the CEO. This sends a strong message that it cannot be ignored.

My role in STAR and Six Sigma is to oversee their implementation, monitor their progress, and work with the various other leaders in the organization to make sure we are doing what we have committed to do. I am the senior executive who oversees collaboration with GE.

Working with GE gave us the ability to implement proven strategies and tools built around Six Sigma methodology. These tools have allowed Virtua to successfully institute the STAR Initiative. And we also gained some valuable assets never fully realized through previous quality or process improvement efforts. Because Six Sigma has built-in skills and monitoring capabilities, Virtua can now use this approach to achieve balanced results that don't unravel over time.

Applying Six Sigma at Virtua

The partnership between GE and Virtua began in earnest in September 2000. Several planning meetings were held between representatives of the Healthcare Solutions Group of GE Medical Systems and Virtua senior management, leading to the development of a detailed plan for the partnership, the essence of which was an agreement for GE Medical Systems representatives to teach Virtua the Six Sigma tools, including two key components, the Change Acceleration Process (CAP) and Workout.

A Workout does what its name implies—it gets extraneous work out of a process through a session led by those closest to the process or problem at hand. It uses brainstorming and a focus on the overall process of the work to remove barriers between departments and generate action steps, with management approval and a rapid implementation time frame.

The Change Acceleration Process, or CAP, which encompasses a range of management tools to help drive strategic change, is based on the understanding that most initiatives (62 percent by some calculations) fail because they are not accepted by key stakeholders. The CAP techniques have all been applied to health care and are being used at Virtua. Our Six Sigma team is finding that the process actually helps to break down existing silos and get everyone speaking a common language. We expect Virtua Health to become self-sufficient in using these techniques over the next three years.

Six Sigma in Action—Reducing Length of Stay for Medicare CHF Patients

To understand how Six Sigma works, it's helpful to follow a case study project from conception to completion, looking at how Virtua identified and addressed a particular problem.

Step 1: Project Selection

Last year, as Virtua began the process of selecting a project linked to its key organizational objectives, senior execs decided to focus on reducing length of stay and denials of payment by Medicare and managed care companies—one of the areas we'd targeted for improvement. The project we chose involved reducing Medicare patients' lengths of stay for congestive heart failure (CHF). We needed to understand through empirical evidence what factors were extending care unnecessarily. We had to look at the sequence of events that might prevent one patient from returning home sooner than another.

This particular project was determined during the Define and Measure phases of Six Sigma training, because we knew we had access to an appropriate amount of data and could track the information through several key elements, including diagnosis, physician, and hospital. These phases of the project took about four weeks to complete and involved gathering the right data and using them to point our efforts in the right direction. We used the Pareto analysis initially, which led to identifying the CHF DRG as having significant impact and room for adjustment. The analysis also led to our decision to concentrate on one hospital in the system to achieve the greatest improvement.

Step 2: Looking for Clues

With the target identified, we formed a multidisciplinary team to tackle the project. The chief operating officer became the project's sponsor, and the assistant vice president for case management was the person responsible for implementing the necessary changes in procedures. The team also included case managers, clinicians, and a data analyst—about 10 people in all. We used the existing steering committee already formed to review length of stay and resource use.

Continued →

In the Analysis phase, we used data and statistical tools to help us take a closer and more accurate look at core elements of the process. It's important to note here that Six Sigma also involves a pattern of "train and do, then repeat." Instead of being abstract, the training is tied to an actual project, and concepts are reinforced as they're applied to actual challenges.

To help the team uncover reasons for variation in lengths of stay and bring some controls into care processes, we looked at various factors that might contribute to CHF length of stay. We used a "fishbone" diagram to help the team delve into cause and effect, looking for those critical factors or "X's" (i.e., determinants of length of stay) that would yield the best measurement and results. Many "X's" floated across the lens, and as we continually refocused, we analyzed and correlated such factors as different physicians, shifts, and days of the week for admission. This led to exploring issues of testing and physician availability on the weekends, which proved to be important.

Step 3: Changing for the Better

Armed with statistical evidence, we moved into the Improve and Control phases of our project. Applying what we'd learned throughout the process, we were actually able to implement improvements that led to a reduction in length of stay from 6.2 days to 4.6 days for CHF patients. Our success came from making the following changes:

- Early dissemination of discharge information

  Through our analysis, we found that one of the barriers to reducing length of stay was patient and family expectations. To improve this communication, we developed a handout and instructions for patients and family as early education and expectation-setting tools.

- Achieving process-of-care improvements with staff

  The CHF project team used the DMAIC process and GE best practices (including CAP and Workout) to achieve improvements with the staff and clinicians. The changes they put in place allowed them to accommodate the variables inherent in a complex care situation.

Continued →

- Development of a specific protocol for nurses

  To reduce variability and standardize the care patients receive when they have CHF, the team developed a specific protocol to follow. Analysis illustrated that the sequence of tests and treatments the majority of patients require must be done quickly to minimize waste and maximize benefit.

- Distributing information on posthospital care

  Patients with congestive heart failure tend to be older, and for a variety of reasons—from germ exposure to unfamiliar surroundings—hospitals can be hazardous to them. It's important to discharge them expeditiously once appropriate treatment has been given, and then to focus on the importance of posthospital care.

  Our team found that some discharge delays were the result of uncoordinated postdischarge services. To improve this situation and help the patient and family make appropriate preparations, we assembled a variety of useful information and made it available to patients early, so they would know what options were available with respect to home health, physician follow-up visits, and other services.

Throughout every phase of this project, we relied heavily, not only on the data, but on the leadership of Virtua Black Belts and participating physicians, because they drive the clinical decisions for the organization.

Testing also affects how efficiently CHF patient treatment and discharge happens, so we held a workout session to identify and address issues concerning accurate and efficient test results. The group identified ways to improve report turnaround time, an issue that can affect not only length of stay but also resource use, patient satisfaction, and clinical outcomes.

Once the initial plan was developed, our leaders designated six full-time "Black Belts," chosen from among the organization's best managers, to learn the Six Sigma tools and lead performance improvement throughout Virtua. Black Belts and coaches run the program internally and are trained by GE. Management identifies a problem or issue, and then Black Belts and clinicians manage the process and involve other stakeholders as needed—from nurses to

Ensuring Quality: A Comparison	
Standard Quality/ Consulting Initiatives	GE's Approach to Six Sigma
Lack of real training or mentoring that can be applied to any project or problem	In-depth coaching and skills transfer that give teams and individuals the power to lead sustainable change
Methods not tied to organizational objectives	Relevant, critical projects incorporated into training and tied to overall vision
Solutions often based on hypotheses or assumptions; data are sometimes questionable	Strongly evidence based: Improvement phase follows goal definition and data are used to measure and analyze contributing factors
Lack of control mechanisms to sustain change	Six Sigma is an ongoing process incorporating a stringent control phase to ensure lasting results
Perceived as "flavor of the month" programs	Process can actually change the culture and become the method organizations use to solve any problem
Little or no attention is paid to the "Acceptance" side of the equation (Quality × Acceptance = Effectiveness)	Drives ownership, accountability, and leadership support to build buy-in

materials managers and finance directors to medical directors. From the identification of a problem or defect to the correction, the process remains consistent. Instead of stakeholders being left to solve problems in their area by themselves, and perhaps not getting the support and resources needed to be successful, they can count on the support of the Black Belts, who truly represent the entire organization. This support system draws the entire organization together, and Virtua has seen an improved corporate culture as a result.

Black Belts will lead Six Sigma projects and performance improvement for two years and then will return to their former management jobs in the organization. This process serves two purposes: provide a critical mass of individuals leading the Six Sigma process and train potential leaders of Virtua in advanced management techniques.

Six Sigma projects have been developed to improve patient satisfaction in the emergency room and medical/surgical units; improve throughput (i.e., the number of cases per day) in two of the system's busiest operating rooms; find a way to rapidly hire the best employees; improve employee retention in such critical areas as nursing; improve the revenue cycle; improve the efficiency of home health nurses; reduce errors in the use of high-risk medications; and reduce length of stay for elderly patients with congestive heart failure (see "Six Sigma in Action," pages 295–297, for a step-by-step example of how Six Sigma was applied to solving this problem). In addition, over 30 other Workout projects have been successfully undertaken throughout the Virtua health care system.

Virtua has also trained 60 coaches who are experts in CAP and Workout techniques. These part-time coaches are taking on at least four Workout or CAP sessions each year, helping to solve a wide range of problems throughout the organization and leading change. This represents an investment in our employees. Enabling our entire organization through these skills is one of the hallmarks of Six Sigma.

Although there is a beginning to the Six Sigma process, there is no end, as we've come to expect from other quality assurance approaches. After people are trained internally and management or employees identify a problem or a hospital service that needs to be improved, the Black Belts sit down with the people responsible for those areas and evaluate the problems using the Workout or CAP methods.

Speaking Their Language: Six Sigma and the Board

Perhaps the most important result of the STAR and Six Sigma implementation is that it has given our trustees "tangibles" they can get their hands around. Most trustees are businesspeople who understand, and are comfortable with, income statements and balance sheets. They want clarity, hard facts, and numbers. Other change initiatives are often vague and lack the kind of goal setting, progress, and tracking measures on which the Six Sigma process depends.

The Six Sigma methodology provides detailed measures allowing trustees to:

- Be generally informed about the project, process, and projected outcomes in all domains of the health care system
- Participate in goal setting
- Understand how to interpret quality
- Base their directives on hard information
- Evaluate progress and judge success

One of the board's most important roles is to ensure that the health system is serving the community. The evidence generated by Six Sigma gives trustees the ability to show the community an unwavering commitment to both quality and fiduciary responsibility. The process provides them with proof that can be shared with the community and takes trustees out of the boardroom to understand what is happening on the front lines. Without such a program, trustees have a difficult time obtaining the information they need to make good decisions and convey results with confidence.

The Trustee's Role in Implementing Six Sigma

It is the board's responsibility to convince the leadership team to try these new methods to achieve proven results. To get the ball rolling toward Six Sigma implementation, the board should proactively encourage the CEO to champion the cause.

At Virtua, trustees quickly recognized that the structure provided by the STAR Initiative and Six Sigma technique would give them a strong framework for understanding the initiative's goals, process, and evidence. Indeed, Six Sigma's highly structured approach has given trustees and senior management a common language and focus to help the board evaluate matters linked to their fiduciary responsibility.

From Manufacturing to Medicine: Translating the Concept of Six Sigma into the Language of Health Care

Though it originated in a world of machines and assembly lines, with slight adaptations, Six Sigma is applicable to virtually any industry, including the delivery of health care. The underlying premise is that to improve a process and eliminate mistakes, you have to create a process that defines your goal, determines what is most critical to the process, puts improvements in place, and then monitors the results for long-term gain.

There is a strong rationale for using Six Sigma to improve health care. Providers are grappling with a host of challenges including increased competition, reduced reimbursement, and the need to provide safe and effective care. Every business must control quality, but defects in patient care delivery are perhaps more critical than in any other error-potential arena. Following the release of a report in November 1999 by the Institute of Medicine estimating the number of medical errors in the United States, increased attention has been paid to establishing better controls and minimizing patient safety risks.

The difference between Six Sigma and other quality approaches is that Six Sigma is based on very rigorous statistical methods and provides a robust implementation process. It also goes well beyond dispensing advice and actually transfers valuable skills to hospital personnel. It provides an extremely detailed, measurable, and sustainable methodology, giving it an edge among physicians and health care executives over other approaches to quality and process improvement. Appropriately implemented, Six Sigma can improve performance throughout the hospital—process by process, and department by department. Examples of its current application in health care range from a reduction in patient waiting times to faster medical report turnaround time to fewer errors in pharmacy and lab procedures.

The Virtua board has been closely engaged in forming the health system from its two predecessors. They understand what everyone wants to accomplish and exactly how it's going to be done. Interestingly, as we've broken down the STAR Initiative into five points, certain trustees have picked out aspects they're really interested in—clinical quality in particular. Suddenly, we found our trustees telling us that although they understood issues around finance very well because of their own business backgrounds, they wanted help understanding quality, so they could judge whether we were delivering it to our community.

Virtua trustees are not just witnessing cultural change; they are very much a part of it. They're using STAR and Six Sigma to help create a great health care system for the community.

Accounting for Success

Several key factors account for the success of the STAR Initiative's implementation and of the Virtua-GE partnership thus far:

- The ability to obtain endorsement of, and commitment to, the process from the system's boards, senior management team, and medical leadership
- Day-to-day support for the process from senior management, including the CEO
- A delineated vision and goals for the organization
- Commitment of resources to support the process
- A systemwide communication plan to spread the initiative and its tools throughout the 7,000-employee organization
- A strong commitment to meeting deadlines and creating measures of success
- Creation of a plan for self-sufficiency to ensure that training in management techniques will continue beyond the three-year contract between GE and Virtua
- A focus on specific projects that are critical to the organization's success

Virtua's experience with GE's approach to Six Sigma demonstrates that it is quite possible to take the best techniques and strategies from other industries and apply them to health care. It also offers a valuable lesson on how best to leverage the enthusiasm and commitment of a health system's trustee leaders in helping their organization move toward new levels of accountability for quality of care, service, and stewardship of resources. We are optimistic that use of Six Sigma will continue to reap rewards for the system and that Virtua might offer a model for leadership and process development for other patient care organizations nationwide.

Quality and Value: Overcoming Barriers

By James E. Orlikoff
and Mary K. Totten

After 20 years of working with quality improvement
issues and processes in health care, I am convinced
that poor quality is not a technical issue
nor the fault of poorly performing individuals. . . .
It is the product of an insular,
individually focused, blame-oriented culture.
—Martin Merry, M.D.,
American Governance Leader April 2001

When we anticipate the next big "breakthrough" in health care delivery, improving the quality and value of care and service delivery should be at the top of the list. Patients, purchasers, and health care practitioners are all demanding a renewed commitment to quality improvement from health care organizations and hospital and health system leadership. Patient safety concerns and the need to reduce error rates and adverse patient care events are further stimulating renewed quality improvement action.

James E. Orlikoff is president of Orlikoff & Associates, Inc., Chicago. Mary K. Totten is president of Totten & Associates, Oak Park, Illinois.

Although recent quality improvement initiatives have identified the positive characteristics of quality care and what it takes to ensure continuous monitoring and improvement in health care organizations, the weight of history is still an obstacle not easily overcome.

Milestones in the Quality Journey

Although the board's accountability for quality care is a relatively recent responsibility, quality concerns date back thousands of years and still influence how health care organizations and practitioners currently view quality: malpractice prevention and avenues of redress for patients who claim malpractice against a physician; quality as the responsibility of the individual physician or practitioner; different standards of health care applying to different patient populations; and defining quality as the absence of negative outcomes rather than the recognition of positive attributes.

Despite the work of Florence Nightingale in the 1850s to establish standards for ensuring quality and the efforts of innovators like Ernest Amory Codman, M.D., to apply these practices to improving hospital care in the early 1900s, the notion that physicians, not hospitals, were responsible for patient care quality persisted until the mid-1960s. The landmark court decision in *Darling v. Charleston Community Memorial Hospital* made the hospital, and therefore its board, accountable for the first time for the quality of care delivered in the hospital by its staff and physicians.

After the *Darling* decision, hospitals and their governing boards began to take seriously, not only their legal and regulatory responsibilities for ensuring quality care, but their fiduciary obligations as well. As overall resources and payments to hospitals tightened, health care organizations and their boards began to focus on the positive impact that good quality care could have on their institution's reputation and financial health. Data showed that people's perceptions about quality of care influenced their choice of hospital, and that poor-quality care cost the hospital more to deliver than high-quality care. This information, along with growing patient and purchaser demands for increased quality and value made oversight and continuous quality improvement a key governance concern.

Yet the quality assurance processes used in hospitals often provided the board with an incomplete and inaccurate picture of the care and service actually being delivered. Quality assurance processes that focused on analyzing incidents of poor quality typically identified problems in some, but not all, areas of the hospital. And when quality problems were identified, the blame often fell on individuals.

Many hospitals had also not developed a definition of quality that encompassed clinical, patient, purchaser, and other important perspectives that could provide a more comprehensive framework for analyzing and improving quality. Hospital leaders began to realize that even though the clinical quality of their care might be excellent, if service quality or other areas of patient satisfaction received low ratings, the hospital's reputation and market share would suffer.

This incident-oriented, individual- and blame-focused approach to ensuring quality, so reminiscent of Hammurabi's code, remained largely unchallenged for almost 4,000 years. Then, in the 1980s and 1990s, experiences from other industries and research on health care quality began to show that most quality problems in hospitals were not the result of individual error. Rather, the majority of quality problems were caused by breakdowns in processes and systems of care that were often complex and involved many people, work units, and disciplines within the organization.

Questions for Discussion

1. What is your hospital's definition of quality?
2. Does your organization's medical staff participate in quality improvement activities?
3. Do your organization's quality improvement activities focus on systems and processes of care rather than on individuals?
4. Are your hospital's quality improvement processes integrated with other quality-related activities?
5. Do your hospital's quality improvement activities actually improve quality organizationwide? How do you know?

Quality: A Systems Issue

The *Harvard Medical Practice Study,* published in 1991, called for health care leaders and practitioners to rethink how issues of poor quality were being addressed in their organization. In this major study, a group of Harvard researchers reviewed 30,121 randomly selected medical records from 51 randomly selected acute care hospitals in New York State. They found that almost 4 percent of hospitalizations had resulted in adverse patient events or injuries. Of these adverse events, about 1 percent were due to staff or physician negligence. Three percent were caused by "other errors."

These findings were consistent with previous research, such as the *California Medical Insurance Feasibility Study* of 1977. They also were further supported by research published in 1995 (Bates, et al., *JAMA*, 1995) concerning drug administration errors. That study found that errors in drug therapy result in more than 200,000 injuries to hospital patients each year. Almost a third (28 percent) of these are preventable as are 42 percent of life-threatening adverse drug errors (ADEs). Significantly, in no case was a single physician or nurse responsible for a pattern of these errors. Further, the cause of all preventable ADEs was systems errors—breakdowns in several steps of the drug therapy process.

Additional study of the same data showed that preventable ADEs cost twice as much as nonpreventable ones and that the average cost of a preventable ADE was $4,685. Hospitals in the study lost $2.8 million each year from errors that could have been prevented in drug therapy administration.

In 1999, the Institute of Medicine looked at these and other studies and determined that errors cause between 44,000 and 98,000 deaths each year in U.S. hospitals. This means that hospital errors rank between the fourth and seventh most common cause of death in the United States.

What all of these data tell us is that we have yet to achieve levels of care and service quality that are acceptable both to those who deliver and those who receive health care in this country. Further, we know by looking at other industries that health care quality ranks substantially below many others. Many airline, publishing, and manufacturing companies, for example, have adopted the Six Sigma approach to quality assessment and improvement and have achieved high levels of quality (4 to 6 sigma) by significantly reducing defects and errors in their systems and processes. (See chart of sigma levels in the previous article, page 291.)

For instance, the airlines have reached quality levels above six sigma, with 0.43 deaths per million passengers. By comparison, most of the health care quality outcomes that have been measured fall in the two to four sigma range.

Why has health care quality lagged behind other industries in quality levels? The bad news is that health care continues to perpetuate, through training and in practice, a largely physician-driven, insular culture of individualism and autonomy in decision making rather than a multidisciplinary, team-oriented culture that values and draws on the best skills and experience available within and outside health care. In addition, many health care organizations still lack the information systems and architecture necessary to provide the kinds of data that are essential to understanding quality, which would provide the framework for ongoing monitoring and improvement.

Testing for System Breakdowns: An Exercise

One way organizations can assess the integrity of their systems and processes is to periodically test how well they function. Try this test of your organization's medical staff credentialing system and then discuss the results with the board.

Have a physician schedule a surgery that he or she does not have privileges to perform in your hospital. For example, a surgeon with privileges to perform abdominal surgery schedules herself to do a laparoscopic procedure for which she does not have privileges. Then, assess how far the process proceeds before the error is caught. Consider the following questions in your analysis:

1. How was the error identified?
2. At what point in the process was the error identified?
3. Who brought the error to the physician's attention?
4. If the physician took issue with "the messenger," was the messenger supported by the organization and its leadership?
5. What do these test results indicate about the integrity of your credentialing system?
6. What changes need to be made?
7. How were the results of this test shared within the organization?

The Good News

Although we still have significant barriers to overcome, the good news is that we understand where the majority of errors originate. Therefore, we can draw on modern quality improvement techniques, such as continuous quality improvement and total quality management, to monitor and improve the complex systems we use to deliver care and service.

We are also beginning to frame our concept of quality in positive terms that enable us to take specific steps for building it into our systems and processes. Rather than viewing quality as merely the absence of problems or negative outcomes, we are beginning to talk about essential characteristics of quality care and of environments that promote good outcomes.

The 2001 Institute of Medicine (IOM) report (see pages 310–312) outlines several steps for redesigning our nation's health care system to remove barriers to high quality and to promote those conditions that support quality and value in health care service delivery. Motivated by the recent IOM report, 60 large American companies have banded together to force hospitals to reduce medical errors. The Leapfrog Group—which includes companies such as AT&T, Delta Airlines, General Electric, and General Motors—provides health benefits to more than 20 million people and spends more than $40 billion on health care annually. The group plans to steer its employees to hospitals that conform to its evidence-based hospital referral system. The group will send employees to hospitals that:

- Have computerized physician drug order entry systems that The Leapfrog Group says could avoid more than 500,000 serious medication errors each year
- Perform high volumes of specific high-risk surgeries, thus saving about 2,500 lives per year
- Staff their critical care units with physicians who are intensive care specialists, which the group says would prevent about 50,000 deaths annually

For more information about this group's efforts, visit its Web site, included in the box on page 313.

IOM 2001 Report Recommendations

In March, the Institute of Medicine released its much-anticipated report outlining steps for redesigning the nation's health care system. *Crossing the Quality Chasm: A New Health System for the 21st Century* outlines an agenda for change based on the following recommendations.

1. All health care organizations, professionals, and purchasers adopt as their explicit purpose to continually reduce the burden of illness, injury, and disability, and to improve peoples' health and functioning.

2. All health care organizations, professionals, and purchasers pursue six major aims: that health care should be safe, effective, patient centered, timely, efficient, and equitable.

3. Congress should appropriate funds and the Department of Health and Human Services (HHS) should establish monitoring and tracking processes for evaluating how success in these six aims is progressing. The HHS Secretary should report annually to Congress and the president on the quality of care.

4. Purchasers, health care organizations, clinicians, and patients should work together to redesign health care processes according to the following rules:

   - Care based on continuous healing relationships
   - Customization based on patient needs and values
   - The patient as the source of control
   - Shared knowledge and the free flow of information
   - Evidence-based decision making
   - Safety from injury caused by the health care system
   - Clarity of information for patients and families to aid informed decision making
   - Anticipation of patient needs
   - Continuous decrease of waste
   - Cooperation among clinicians

Continued →

5. The Agency for Healthcare Research and Quality (AHRQ) should identify at least 15 priority health conditions, "taking into account frequency of occurrence, health burden, and resource use," and work with key stakeholders to develop ways to substantially improve quality for each of the conditions over the next five years.

6. Congress should establish a Health Care Quality Innovation Fund to support projects that help achieve the six aims or substantially improve quality for the priority conditions. (The report suggested a commitment of $1 billion over three to five years.)

7. The AHRQ and private foundations should convene a series of workshops involving representatives from health care, other industries, and the research community to identify and implement state-of-the-art approaches to address:

   • Redesign of care processes based on best practices
   • Use of information technologies to improve access to clinical information and support clinical decision making
   • Knowledge and skills management
   • Effective team development
   • Coordination of care across patient conditions, services, and settings over time
   • Incorporation of performance and outcomes measurements for improvement and accountability

8. The Secretary of HHS should be given the responsibility and resources to establish and maintain a comprehensive program that makes scientific evidence about treatments more useful and accessible to clinicians and patients.

9. Congress, the executive branch, health care organization leaders, purchasers, health care informatics associations, and vendors should build an information infrastructure to support health care delivery, consumer health, quality measurement and improvement, public accountability research, and clinical education that should result in the elimination of most handwritten clinical data by the end of the decade.

Continued →

10. Purchasers should examine current payment methods to remove barriers to quality improvement and build stronger incentives for enhancing quality.

11. The Health Care Financing Administration and the AHRQ should take the lead to develop a research agenda to better align current payment methods with quality improvement goals.

12. A multidisciplinary summit of health profession leaders should develop strategies for restructuring clinical education consistent with the principles of the 21st-century health system envisioned by the Committee on the Quality of Health Care in America and assess the implications of these changes for provider credentialing programs, funding, and health profession educational program sponsorship.

13. The AHRQ should fund research to evaluate how the current regulatory and legal systems facilitate or inhibit the changes needed for the 21st-century health system and how they can be modified to support achieving the six aims.

Health care organizations can also draw on quality improvement systems from outside the field, such as the ISO 9000 (see "High Standards," in the February 1999 issue of *Trustee*, available in the archives on *Trustee*'s Web site—www.trusteemag.com) and the Malcolm Baldrige quality award criteria (see the box on the next page) to adapt and apply new approaches for improving quality.

In fact, experts suggest that the talent and expertise needed to convert health care into a high-performing, quality-focused industry is likely to come from outside health care. And one of the most important, accessible links a health care organization has to other industries is its governing board.

There are several steps board members can take to both increase their understanding of barriers to quality that may exist in their hospital and to provide assistance and resources that can lead to significant quality improvements.

Quality-Related Web Sites

http://www.asq.org: The site for the American Society for Quality. Includes the latest news on quality practices in the United States and how a variety of businesses have benefited from these practices.

http://www.ihi.org: The home page for the Institute for Healthcare.

http://www.leapfroggroup.org: Information about the initiatives and plans of the Washington, D.C.–based Leapfrog Group.

http://www.quality.nist.gov: This site provides information about the Malcolm Baldrige National Quality Award and showcases past award winners.

Quality Improvement Tips for Boards

1. The board should ensure that quality improvement is a core organizational strategy and that quality improvement activities are closely linked to the organization's strategic priorities.
2. At every meeting, the board should receive a focused report addressing the quality and outcomes issues of greatest interest to the hospital, its patients, and the community.
3. Accountability for improving identified deficiencies in outcomes or quality of care should be assigned to specific individuals and groups within the organization, including the governing board.
4. A portion of the top management team's compensation should be based on achieving quality and outcomes objectives.
5. Board members should personally participate in quality improvement teams and ensure that the board participates in processes to improve both individual trustee and full board performance.
6. The board should ensure that sufficient financial resources have been allocated to support continuous improvement of quality and outcomes, including adequate support for information system upgrades.
7. The board should regularly monitor and oversee the organizationwide quality improvement process and ensure that it focuses on systems improvements, not on individuals.

8. Board members should work with local, state, and national groups to develop a legal, regulatory, and reimbursement environment that supports continuous improvement of quality and outcomes of care.
9. Individuals with experience in continuous improvement processes in health care or other industries should be recruited as new board members.
10. The board should ensure that lessons learned from the hospital's quality improvement activities are disseminated throughout the organization.

Conclusion

Making significant improvements in quality and value is the next competitive challenge facing the health care industry. Understanding that quality is a systems issue and employing the best of what modern quality science offers will help hospitals and systems use resources most productively. Board members have an obligation to understand the level of quality and service that their organizations deliver. What can your business or another organization you help govern teach your health care organization about improving quality and value? What have you done to facilitate this transfer of knowledge and skills?

PART SEVEN

Patient Safety

Ending the Culture
of Blame

A Look at Why Medical Errors Happen—
and What Needs to Change

By Laurie Larson

The blunt statement that as many as 98,000 Americans may die every year from medical errors, largely as the result of an increasingly complex and fragmented health care system, justifiably grabbed headlines when the Institute of Medicine (IOM) released its watershed report last November. But perhaps what is most shocking and groundbreaking about the report is not what it says—it is the willingness to say it.

Medical errors have been a problem as long as hospitals have existed. They may be increasing as a result of exploding technology combined with stressed and financially strapped delivery systems. But what has surely grown, at least as large as the mistakes made, is the fear of their being discovered. Medical errors most often happen in haste, in ignorance—and, finally, in silence.

"The culture is an impediment to acknowledging error," says Kenneth Kizer, M.D., president and CEO of the National Forum for Health Care Quality and former head of the Veterans Administration. "Peer group pressure is the biggest impediment to talking

---

Laurie Larson is the staff writer for *Trustee*.

about it—what your peers will think of you for making a mistake. You are taught that losing your credibility is the worst thing that can happen to you."

The medical profession demands perfection and punishes imperfection. In such a culture of blame, then, who will step forth to admit a mistake? And without full knowledge of what the mistakes are, how can we learn how to stop making them?

Among dozens of professional and academic groups studying these questions, the John F. Kennedy School of Government at Harvard University has been working on the problem for three years. The Harvard Executive Session on Medical Error Reduction comprises close to two dozen health system CEOs, government officials, and academic thought leaders, who meet formally twice a year to talk about their own experiences, share potential solutions, and take them back home to try out.

Stating their purpose to "create a kind of national board of directors whose boundaries extend beyond the domain of any single institution or agency," attendees are all senior leaders in their institution, positioned to define the issues facing the field as well as to implement novel strategies. All discussions are confidential. Practitioners rather than academicians set the tone.

"We choose people to be members who can actually make changes. Who you invite is critical—you need creative thinkers," says Saul Weingart, M.D., one of the chief organizers of the medical errors executive session and part of the faculty of general medicine at Beth Israel Deaconess Medical Center in Boston.

Those thinkers include, among others: former VA chief Kizer; Lucian Leape, M.D., an international expert in error reduction; David Lawrence, M.D., chair and CEO of Kaiser Permanente; Robert Waller, M.D., president emeritus of the Mayo Foundation; Gordon Sprenger, CEO of Allina Health System; James Reinertsen, M.D., CEO of CareGroup health system; and Dennis O'Leary, M.D., president of the Joint Commission on Accreditation of Healthcare Organizations.

In its four meetings to date, the executive session has inventoried its collective expertise, looked at case studies of error reduction in other industries, gone back and personally investigated an error in their own organization, and come up with some ways to implement patient safety initiatives.

The ultimate goal: to change the medical culture from one of blame and punishment to one intent on working for the higher—and safer—good.

"The health care system is complicated and Byzantine—I've spent the past five years making people aware of errors and how to solve this," says Leape, adjunct professor at the Harvard School of Public Health. "We've come up with three basic concepts: error is not a sin; it's caused by system failures; and it's a managerial problem. We have to redesign the whole system of health care in many different places and on many different levels."

Program organizers describe the sessions as a series of ongoing demonstration projects—"a big conversation over several years" with each CEO realizing in his own way how system change must happen.

"We've learned a lot, and the harder we look, the more disturbing information we find," says Don Berwick, M.D., one of the organizers of the Harvard sessions and president and CEO of the Institute for Healthcare Improvement (IHI) in Boston.

"Through IHI I've also worked with 100 various health care organizations to see how to do best practices. I've learned that people really do want to make improvements as long as executives will support them and that there are many simple things to do to reduce error."

Although the session's purpose is not to issue formal recommendations or a report, it has identified a list of barriers to error reduction, many "so embedded in the professional culture of medicine, organization of hospitals, and behavior of regulatory agencies that they have become structural impediments to change," according to a recent session summary. These include inadequate reporting, as a result of the punitive nature of reporting; tolerance of error, as part of the complexity of health care; "blame and shame" responses to error as well as financial disincentives; punishment of faulty institutions rather than error correction; and legal obstacles through a tort system focused on individual accountability for error and financial compensation for injury. Because there is an overlap between the membership of the Harvard Session and the IOM researchers, many of the group's comments and suggestions have turned up in the IOM report, participants say.

Reducing complexity has been a recurring theme, Berwick says. Recommendations include standardizing equipment and procedures;

computerizing patient records, including medications and as many other aspects of care as possible; and making sure that each person to whom the patient is "handed-off" during the sequence of care has the same body of information about his or her care.

"That's where error happens—in the hand-off," he says. "People need to understand each other's jobs more—to say, 'This is what I do; what do you do?' It's team-building." Along these lines, he thinks patients need to speak up more in those hand-offs as well, learning and asking questions about their care and being informed enough to be able to share the basics of their own medical records.

VA Leads the Way

The VA has been ahead of its civilian counterparts for some time now in making improvements on medical error, perhaps because of the more open public scrutiny to which military culture is exposed. Former chief Kizer's creation of the National Patient Safety Partnership in 1997 has paved the way for many of the ideas incorporated into the IOM report as well. Although the system has long had an internal confidential registry for adverse hospital events—a "quality assurance review"—it is now investigating errors in greater depth.

Currently being piloted in Florida, this new, third revision of the VA's reporting system follows the recommendations of Kizer and the VA's new chief executive, James Bagian, a physician, engineer, and former astronaut who investigated the causes of the Challenger space shuttle explosion. Any adverse event goes under a "prioritization tree," which asks how rare an event it is, how likely it is to recur, how likely it is to have an impact on patients, and how severe it is. The questions asked are designed to force people to think of better systems or procedures that would fill in where people are most fallible, such as repetitive tasks. In the first half of 2000, this analysis is expected to roll out to the rest of the VA.

In one highly effective example, patients now wear bar-coded wristbands, read with a handheld scanner that gives their name, basics of their record, blood type, and medication dosage and frequency. One of the VA's hospitals has seen an 80 percent reduction in medication errors from the use of the wristbands, Kizer says.

The VA also has a computerized order entry system for prescriptions and electronic medical records. Such standardizations, including computerized physician order entry (CPOE), is one of the Harvard group's most enthusiastic endorsements.

"Electronic records have to be the norm soon—we have to bite the bullet," Kizer says. "Yes, there are costs with that, and there is physician reluctance to do it, but at the VA, they [doctors] have all eventually come around" over a two-year period.

Lessons from California to Minnesota

To shed light on new ways of thinking about errors at Kaiser Permanente, CEO David Lawrence sends out an electronic newsletter to all Kaiser facilities called "CEO Journal," in which he shares summaries of some of the lessons learned from the Harvard sessions.

In return, he asks for annual quality reports from all Kaiser member CEOs to the Medical Directors Quality Committee, a "built-in key component" that Kaiser has implemented for many years and that follows and investigates problems from surgical infection rates to sentinel events. Kaiser uses the adverse drug event prevention recommendations of the Institute for Healthcare Improvement (IHI) to educate its doctors, nurses, and pharmacists. Lawrence says he thinks Kaiser doctors stay up to date on patient safety issues because they work in groups and take a team approach to clinical care, a method shown to greatly reduce error.

Examining how error is dealt with in the larger context of the industry was a major "ah-ha" as he describes it, for Gordon Sprenger, CEO of Allina Health System, based in Minneapolis, Minnesota. "I had compared our incident rates, infection reports, [and so on] for years with other institutions and felt we were doing okay. It was complacency," Sprenger says. "But now I have taken this information from the context of my own organization, and I'm seeing . . . the magnitude of the problem. This has forced me to step back and listen to others and see the big numbers. It hits you between the eyes."

Each Allina facility has specific, measurable safety goals set for this year. The system has further declared that verbal medication orders are to be avoided if at all possible and repeated back twice if they must be given. More pharmacists will review patient drug and dosage charts at nurses' stations and use "big red dot" warning labels for look-alike and sound-alike drugs, as well as for flip-top bins (like bread boxes) to single out especially lethal medications.

Allina has further partnered with the locally based headquarters of 3M, having its safety engineers come through the hospital to "look at processes and see potential problems with different sets of eyes," Sprenger says.

What CareGroup Did

Jim Reinertsen, M.D., who is CEO of Beth Israel Deaconess Medical Center as well as the six-hospital CareGroup system to which Beth Israel belongs, has also been very active among Harvard executive session members in initiating concrete error reduction changes. Jeanette Clough, president of CareGroup's Mt. Auburn Hospital, is point person for the system's quality and medication error reduction goals.

Clough explains that each of the six hospitals in the system puts together a team comprising the CEO, a pharmacist, a physician leader, and a nurse leader to look at how medications were administered in their facilities. "Each organization could see the complexity of delivering meds to patients," Clough says. "There was lack of automation in the system and in the units. Different parts of the hospital handled medication dispensing completely differently, and day and night procedures were very different."

Next, the teams looked at where the majority of medication errors were occurring—and found that approximately 40 percent of errors happened when the order was handwritten as a result of bad penmanship, misinterpretation, and other pitfalls. Finally, errors were ranked as a Level 1–4, with 4 being the most serious. Each hospital has shared with the others all the details of at least a Level 3 drug incident, an "open guts look," as Clough describes it, of a medication mistake.

"It was the first time we began to get comfortable talking about an error. If we can't get comfortable, how can others?" she asks. From what they learned, CareGroup has made several significant changes, all based around automating as many of its medication procedures as possible, including development of a computerized physician order entry system and a "Pyxis 2000 Med Station," an advanced system for controlled med dispensing in the nurses' stations that does "drug profiling"—tracing medication orders from the pharmacy to the patient floor.

Within the CareGroup system there is now an intranet executive information system that immediately shares red alerts of medication errors or near misses as soon as they happen. Invariably, Clough says, there is not one single mistake but a "chain of events" leading to the error. Across the CareGroup system, there is an expectation of reporting errors as a professional responsibility. And trustees and senior management are expected to "triage" the resources, both in the reporting and the solution, which they do with "a wholehearted effort" Clough says.

"When you start to unravel some of these stories, you realize that fail-safe mechanisms are very much needed," Clough says. "The big reason mistakes happen is that there are not systems to prevent them. We are much too reliant on humans to pick up error. There have not been great systems yet."

"There is an underlying mismatch between health care delivery and science and the technology available," Lawrence says. "Science is too complex for the mainstream delivery chassis of primary care medicine to carry out. The problem is likely to increase because science and technology are exploding—the health care system cannot deliver care safely and reliably enough to keep up."

"There is a delusion of technology," Kizer says. "The public thinks health care has gotten better because of advanced technology, but the reality is that [technology] is part of the reason errors are more common."

Mandatory versus Voluntary Reporting

Publically acknowledging these difficulties brings up the most controversial section of the IOM's report—mandatory error reporting. The report urges that all hospitals participate in a "nationwide mandatory reporting system that provides for the collection of standardized information by state governments about adverse events that result in death or serious harm." Voluntary reporting for less serious injuries "should be encouraged," the report states. Many health care executives and officials fear that mandatory reporting will promulgate continued secrecy about error and will leave hospitals even more vulnerable than they already are to lawsuits—the harshest aspect of the stoic medical culture.

"Changing the culture of blame means that you need explicit boundaries on how far legal discovery can go in investigating [medical] problems, 'in the name of investigation,'" Lawrence says. "If all the potential problems relative to safety issues could be discovered by lawyers, fishing expeditions would abound. You've got to create 'cones of protection' around reporting near misses and safety improvements such as other industries have."

Lawrence, however, favors mandatory reporting to learn in depth how to correct mistakes. "The only way to see if we are making improvements is to collect information systematically," Lawrence says. "Otherwise, it's too vague. [Reporting] can be used to leverage the rapid improvements needed in health care." In addition, he describes voluntary reporting as "a treasure trove" of information for near misses and dangers, provided it too is confidential.

Leape believes the risk of litigation is "a red herring." Almost all states have peer review statutes that protect against legal discovery for quality improvement, he says, but the real key is making health care professionals feel that sharing errors will not only be safe but that it will truly make a difference.

"One of the little secrets in the hospital is that doctors, nurses, and pharmacists are very interested in ways to make fewer mistakes and do better," Leape says. "There is an incredible resource in people that we have to unleash by removing punishment and giving them the opportunity to practice how they want to practice."

Changing Culture from the Top

Forcibly or voluntarily, Harvard executive session participants agree that medical error reduction starts at the top—and is a crucial leadership issue.

"CEOs and boards need to make [error reduction] personal and their own," Weingart says. "They need to place medical safety among their top priorities. The pace of change is directly related to how much attention it gets." Safety needs to be reviewed at every board meeting, he says, to keep changes progressing. There needs to be a nonpunitive environment around discussing error, and that message has to get out to the front lines past bureaucracy and hierarchies. He suggests that the way to do this is by example; for instance, using a high-profile case of an error showing tolerance and a nonpunitive approach to getting the details—which are vital to correcting the mistake.

To send the message that patient safety rests firmly and finally on leadership's shoulders, Kaiser will begin basing at least part of its executive performance-based pay on meeting specific patient safety goals, starting this year. Each executive is asked to define a patient safety issue that he or she wants to focus on and establish a safety baseline for that issue. A baseline is also set to determine how "blame-free" errors really are for that safety concern; that is, how conducive the environment is for reporting safety mistakes. An explicit intention statement will then be drawn up to work on the problem and track results.

Allina has similar goals. "What I've been trying to do is develop a blameless culture and system," Sprenger says. "My interest is to ask, 'What happened?' not 'Who did it?' We have to make sure the caregiver is given support when the error is made. . . . We have to start sharing stories nationally across the health care system to build this culture."

"It starts with education, and the CEO has to say what's important," Kizer says. "He or she should ask, 'What can we do immediately to improve safety? What costs money and what doesn't? How can we put safety into our strategic planning process?' And, finally, [the board and CEO must] work out the capital budget, funding those changes that will require money."

Financial reports and quality reports should be given equal weight at each board meeting. "There should be the same level of scrutiny and detail for quality and patient safety as for financials," Kizer says. "At every meeting the board should demand to see the numbers. As far as the long-term viability of institutions, [looking at quality] will be critical, based on what's coming down the pike from the government—reporting and safety performance measures. The landscape will change very quickly. Quality will be the Holy Grail of the 21st Century."

Weingart sums it all up: "The recurring theme is that change needs to be comprehensive—the root of the way medicine is practiced. We have to keep repeating that message through multiple channels of communication. We have to come at the problem from multiple directions."

The greatest achievement in reducing and eliminating medical errors to date may simply be daring to talk about it. But that breakthrough may be the floodgate to a healing long overdue.

Industrial Strength

*Patient Safety Means Leading
Preindustrial Health Care
into a Postindustrial World*

By Chuck Appleby

When Gail Wolf observes the swirl of activity on hospital floors in Pittsburgh, she sees automobiles being made. Toyotas, to be exact.

No, she's not a patient on the psychiatric ward. As senior vice president and chief nursing officer at UPMC Health System, a 16-hospital integrated delivery system based in Pittsburgh, Wolf is applying the Toyota industrial model to analyze and reengineer traditional health care processes. And it has begun to shape everything she does.

"When we're designing pieces for the electronic medical record, I find myself thinking like Toyota, eliminating unnecessary steps in work. Some people say you can't apply car manufacturing [techniques] to health care. Basically, we said, while we don't make cars, we certainly have a lot of processes screwed up," Wolf says.

In taking lessons from non–health care industries, UPMC is in the vanguard of providers seeking a systems approach to ensure quality and safety for its patients. Figuring into that new global view is the organization's involvement in the Pittsburgh Regional Healthcare Initiative (PRHI), a community-based coalition of employers, providers,

---

Chuck Appleby is a writer based in Benecia, California.

and other community representatives. PRHI's overarching goals are clinical improvement and patient safety.

Out of the Box

Alcoa, based in Pittsburgh and a key member of the coalition, adopted the Toyota production principles in 1996. Although Alcoa already had an exceptional safety record, the new Alcoa Business System, based on Toyota's principles, further enhanced safety practices— since 1997, Alcoa has achieved a 68 percent reduction in lost workdays. In 2000, only 48 employees out of more than 100,000 missed a workday because of injury at its plants around the world. Former Alcoa chairman and CEO Paul O'Neill convinced health care members of PRHI, such as UPMC, to adopt these quality and safety standards.

In so doing, health care providers and their boards are not only thinking outside the box; they're breaking the box wide open to find solutions that eliminate medical errors and improve patient safety. The days of executives and boards concerning themselves strictly with financial matters and leaving clinical outcomes to physicians are disappearing fast.

"Health care is headed into the era of clinical accountability," says David Classen, M.D., vice-president of First Consulting Group, based in Long Beach, California, and a patient safety expert. "Clinical performance will be as important for hospitals' financial future as the ability to send a bill."

Martin Merry, M.D., a senior advisor for medical affairs to the New Hampshire Hospital Association and a former industrial relations specialist, offers a historical perspective: "Quality is [achieved] differently in a postindustrial society than in health care, which remains in a preindustrial craft era. Clinical care has been independent of management resources, and clinicians have been isolated from any administrative system," he explains.

Bark and Bite

But not for long. Blame the change on three Institute of Medicine reports issued since 1999 that unveiled shocking medical error statistics to an increasingly educated and demanding consumer marketplace. Ironically, the third report, *Envisioning the National Health Care Quality Report* (www.iom.edu/IOM/IOMHome.nsf/Pages/Recently+Released+Reports), issued in March 2001 with the least fanfare of the three, will probably have the greatest impact because it actually has some teeth, according to Classen, who was a member of the committee that issued the IOM's *National Report on Healthcare Quality*. New standards from the Joint Commission on Accreditation of Healthcare Organizations (JCAHO), which went into effect in July 2001, emphasize patient safety programs, safety reporting metrics, sentinel event (i.e., medical errors, such as wrong-side surgery) disclosure, patient/family involvement, and proactive redesign of high-risk clinical processes. And starting in 2003, Congress has mandated the federal government to create an annual report that contains health care statistics analogous to the leading economic indicators.

Perhaps the *coup de grace* for the old order was the seemingly overnight emergence of the Leapfrog Group forged by 70 of the largest U.S. employers as a driving force for health care quality. (See the article "Raising the Bar" starting on page 278.) Through Leapfrog and other business coalitions, employers are now negotiating directly with providers, demanding specific strategies that providers should follow to ensure the clinical safety of employees. But many providers disagree with the Leapfrog standards.

Leapfrog seized leadership of the patient safety issue after what it perceived as decades of health care industry inaction. In this new information era, in which consumers scour Web sites for comparative quality data about hospitals and physicians, health care trustees will be held just as accountable for clinical quality as they have been for financial performance.

"Quality and safety will never be assured if the board doesn't take a leading role in demanding accountability and measurement in those areas," says Classen. "It should be as important to the board as the financial metrics reported to them."

"An Irresistible Moral Spearhead"

"For a long time, board members deferred the product [i.e., clinical care] to the experts, the medical staff," says Mark Laskow, a member of the UPMC board's executive committee and CEO of a Pittsburgh-based investment consulting firm. "The first IOM report was a lesson that that approach no longer works. The medical community has had 50 years of academic research on this subject and has done nothing but a lot of throat-clearing. They can no longer say to us 'butt out.'" That's why Laskow's involved in the PRHI coalition and its emphasis on Toyota's production process. Applied to health care, the process relies heavily on executive involvement—starting at the patient's bedside.

"It's one of the most fascinating things I've ever seen," says Laskow, who was at first skeptical of what seemed to him another in an endless succession of trendy and superficial quality initiatives. However, "[Alcoa's] O'Neill was very persuasive" and convinced him to use patient safety as "an irresistible moral spearhead" to introduce the Toyota principles into the delivery of health care.

Laskow, who decided 12 years ago to focus his governance attention solely on health care after serving on boards in other industries, is convinced that patient safety and quality of care translate into good business. "It costs hospitals money to cause errors because they're usually the result of [inefficient] processes. They're not limited to just the cost of cleaning up the errors afterward," he explains.

One at a Time

Enter the Toyota principles, which stipulate that all work be highly specified and that there is only one way to do any given task. The only way to modify a process is to offer a testable hypothesis for change and then implement only one change at a time.

"You're actually able to solve problems because you're only [handling] one at a time—isolating a task instead of trying to change the entire system in one fell swoop," Laskow says. "It gets at very complex problems and lets the process redesign itself. And it appeals to health care professionals because it is utterly based upon the scientific method. You don't use Pareto charts [a special form of vertical bar graph that helps you determine which problems to solve in what order] or 80/20 priorities. You stand there, look at a patient, and solve the first problem."

That's exactly what Wolf has done at UPMC, which has adopted PRHI's two specific clinical goals:

1. Eliminate medication errors
2. Eliminate hospital-acquired infections

Using the industrial concepts, UPMC established four "learning lines," or system-redesign groups, focused on medication improvements. Since then, they have also established a learning line for hospital infections.

Wolf is enthusiastic. "Toyota's strategy is complex in its simplicity. What I love about it is that it puts change in the hands of employees." The approach involves taking a problem step by step back to its root cause.

For example, while once observing hospital patients receiving medications, she noticed that a 9 A.M. medication had not arrived on time. Wolf went to the pharmacy and through a logical series of questions found that the medication was not on the shelf because it was an unusual drug that the pharmacy technician didn't know they hadn't restocked. Unlike most drugs, this one lacked its own storage bin, which when empty would have signaled the need for reorder. The solution: create a bin for every medication the hospital needs to stock.

"It's little things like that that combine to create a solution. You keep asking, 'Why did that happen?' until you finally arrive at the root cause of the problem. The principles are so basic. We've been able to make huge progress in a relatively short period of time," Wolf says.

Employing such a strategy has enabled UPMC to cut missing medications by 55 percent in just 30 days. In another case, a learning line found that the 8 A.M. medications at one of its hospitals were always late. It turned out that the pharmacy delivered them late because the hospital's two pharmacists, oblivious to the situation, didn't arrive until after 8 A.M. The nurses were so used to getting medications late that they just accepted it, without anyone exploring the root cause of the problem. When apprised of the issue, the pharmacists changed their schedules to accommodate the 8 A.M. medications. Problem solved. Wolf says hospital processes are riddled with such seemingly illogical and counterproductive habits, which often go unchallenged for years because of entrenched habit.

"Until you observe and start asking questions, you don't realize all that's going on. It's not rocket science. Unlike TQI [total quality improvement], this technique helps identify and change work processes on a very small level and just keeps improving them until you get it right," says Wolf.

Improving clinical processes using industrial models can go a long way toward reforming a system that leads to medical errors, but it's not the whole story. Changing physician culture so that it embraces a protocol—an IT-based approach to patient care—is also critical to care quality.

Immeasurable Perfection

Joseph Bujak, M.D., vice president of medical affairs at Kootenai Medical Center in Coeur D'Alene, Idaho, and a frequent national speaker on board-physician leadership, says one of the obstacles to implementing patient safety is that physicians convince themselves that everything they are doing is perfect and that patients expect perfection.

"If your starting point is perfection and someone presents you with data that say you're less than perfect, you either discredit the data by responding that no health care data are good enough to meet the scientific method, or you justify the data by saying 'my patients are uniquely different,'" Bujak says. He adds that a third option is to "shoot the messenger" by questioning that person's ability to provide medical service.

Also, physicians typically perceive any attempt to change what they're doing as financially motivated; that is, "I'm perfect, and you're asking me to do less, to cut corners." Bujak attributes such attitudes to the "expert culture" that physicians inhabit, based on their individual skill, energy, and aptitude. "Experts always view the world from the perspective of 'What's in this for me?'" Bujak says. "They lack a collective identity."

These attitudes have led to a punitive culture that covers up errors. "Ours is a culture of personal accountability, so when someone says we have an adverse or sentinel event, we can always find someone in the chain to blame. We always 'assign blame and then train.' We never implicate the processes," says Bujak.

Near Misses Ignored

Bujack has a favorite analogy when it comes to medical errors: earthquakes. "Near misses"—medical errors that do not result in harm to anyone—are like small earth tremors that never rise above a certain Richter-scale level and never become public, he says. But unlike those small earthquakes that are used by scientists to project trends, near-miss medical errors that could highlight trends are often ignored and eventually lead to more serious errors. For example, when a patient allergic to penicillin is inadvertently given the drug and survives, the error usually goes unreported because there is no systematic process to deal with such problems. "One in 100 patients dies of a mistake, but all errors happen because of bad processes. That bad process puts 100 patients at risk," Bujak says.

Besides trying to shift to a focus on process instead of personal liability, Kootenai is also emphasizing changes to institutional structures and systems:

- Decentralized pharmacy—Put the pharmacists in the clinical units, positioning them between the prescribing doctor, whom they can teach, and the nurse, with whom they can communicate. "That will have a huge impact," says Bujack, adding that eliminating dosing errors, duplicate prescribing, and adverse drug interactions will more than offset any extra costs.
- Electronic order entry—This will eliminate overnight errors made from misinterpreting poor handwriting, such as drug interactions and incorrect dosages, by automating the process and providing alerts.
- Bar coding—This helps ensure that nurses give the right drug in the right dose to the right patient at the right time. Bar codes can be added to the patient's identification bracelet and to the drug. Not only would bar codes eliminate administration errors, but the data gathered could keep a tally of near misses and allow for ongoing process improvements.
- Drug indication—The indication states why a doctor orders a certain drug. It helps avoid confusion between drugs whose names are similar such as Prevacol (for high cholesterol) and Propanalol (for high blood pressure).

More Bar Codes Coming Up

Of course, obstacles hinder even the most logical processes, but at least one of those obstacles will be resolved soon. Assistant U.S. Health & Human Services (HHS) Secretary Bobby Jindal announced at the American Society of Health Systems Pharmacists meeting, December 4, 2001, that HHS is proposing that all drugs be required to carry bar codes by sometime later this year.

In another IT approach, Kootenai launched a pilot project for physicians to prescribe drugs using portable, handheld computers. But the whole idea of automated prescribing may be moot given an Idaho law that requires all prescriptions for controlled drugs to be written on a physician's personal prescription pad.

At the least, however, Kootenai's board of directors fully supports these efforts. "We made patient safety an organizational goal and presented it to the board," says Bujak. Kootenai has also partly decentralized its pharmacy, putting pharmacists on its cancer unit and transitional care floor. So far the strategy has enabled Kootenai to cut its adverse medication events to one in 500 from a previous rate of one in 300, according to Bujack, who acknowledges that initiating change may be the most difficult part.

"The problem is how do you create a starting point? Once you get it up and running, you look worse," because errors that were previously covered up are now being reported, he says.

Toolkits and Webinars

A starting point is exactly what Child Health Corporation of America (CHCA) has fashioned for its members in an attempt to systematically measure and manage patient safety. CHCA, a business alliance of 38 children's hospitals based in Overland Park, Kansas, in conjunction with First Consulting Group, developed a tool set to help members and other health care organizations respond to the JCAHO's new standards. The Patient Safety Solution Set has three components:

- Patient Safety Assessment—an online survey to evaluate an organization's JCAHO and patient safety readiness and identify targeted areas for improvement. The assessment is based on a four-stage model developed by First Consulting Group (see the box on pages 334–335). Boards and senior management must provide leadership to navigate their organization through these stages.
- Patient Safety Toolkit—a set of procedures, templates, frameworks, and sample tools to help organizations meet the new JCAHO patient safety standards

- Patient Safety Webinar—a Webcast review of the assessment and toolkit, their objectives and benefits, and how they have been used at other organizations, including an interactive question-and-answer session

Step Up to the Plate

First Consulting Group's Classen says boards should first demand to see reports on quality and safety performance as often as they do financial reports. Such reports would include a combination of

How Organizational Approaches to Patient Safety Evolve		
The components of patient safety provide the basis for evaluating how well developed an organization's patient safety program is.		
Stage	Description	Characteristics
Stage 1 Awareness	Patient safety is one of many priorities. Structure and accountability for patient safety is not clearly defined, and reporting primarily involves individual incidents.	• Roles and accountability for patient safety are not clearly defined. • Departmental initiatives have no overall strategy. • Standard definitions, metrics, and regular reporting mechanisms for patient safety are lacking.
Stage 2 Organizational Learning	Patient safety is recognized as a strategic priority with executive ownership. A culture of safety is being created with a focus on a non-punitive environment. Clinicians, patients, and families are getting involved in safety.	• Roles of the patient and family in safety are clearly defined. • Organizational strategies for patient safety are defined. • Resources have been committed to patient safety initiatives. • Patient safety metrics are routinely measured and monitored. • Technology does not play a fundamental role in improving patient safety.

Continued →

quality measures (e.g., success rates for coronary bypass grafts and rates of adverse incidents associated with that procedure) and safety measures (e.g., drug interaction rates).

Second, the board should require that a member of the senior leadership team, excluding risk management, be appointed as chief quality and safety officer. Just as a chief financial officer is in charge of financial metrics, a chief quality officer would be responsible for patient safety measures and metrics. Unfortunately, Classen says, very few organizations have created such a position, choosing instead to disperse the responsibility throughout a department.

Stage	Description	Characteristics
Stage 3 Proactive Risk Mitigation	Patient safety is a strategic and tactical priority with increased use of tools and technologies to create an effective surveillance system and to reduce the risk of an event. There is movement toward proactive responses, including redesign of high-risk clinical processes.	• Role of technology is clearly defined with a strategic IT plan to improve patient safety. • High-risk clinical processes have been redesigned with active clinician involvement. • Technologies such as adverse drug event (ADE) surveillance, computerized physician order entry (CPOE), and bar code medication administration have been implemented.
Stage 4 High-Reliability Organization	Patient safety is everyone's priority with a focus on organizational learning and incorporating "lessons learned" into training. Sophisticated tools and learning technologies (e.g., simulation) are frequently employed. Proactive risk assessment at the individual patient and organizational level are routinely implemented and monitored.	• Patients are proactively assessed for probability of an event. • High-risk clinical processes are simulated to improve competency. • Criteria—(e.g., a risk-prediction model that shows whether a patient should undergo a procedure) are in place for determining when the patient care environment is "unsafe."
Source: First Consulting Group, Long Beach, California.		

Hospital leaders are beginning to realize that the quality and safety officer should be a high-level position filled by a member of the senior management team "who understands that quality and safety constitute the hospital's core mission and who will be rewarded for achieving it. We know that from studying safety in other industries," Classen says.

Third, the board should realize that safety is a long-term effort. Regulatory, market, and payer sectors are demanding it as the cost of doing business. Also, a board should insist that its organization go beyond minimum standards and distinguish itself in the marketplace. "The organization should be able to say, 'We do provide the best care, and we can document it,'" says Classen.

As part of its demand for performance metrics, a board should be informed about sentinel events and question how its organization is investigating them.

"The board needs to clarify the organization's approach to medical errors, because what we've learned is that the natural tendency is to blame frontline operators such as nurses and doctors. But all accidents have much deeper causes. The board should demand that there be a [safety] plan and demonstrate a capability for learning and transmitting that plan to the organization," Classen advises.

Boards also need to ask how the organization is educating patients and families about taking a role in their own care and how the employees throughout the organization are being educated about safety and quality.

Medical advisor Merry suggests that trustees start with educating themselves on this very complex subject. "They need to roll up their sleeves and become more knowledgeable about such factors as critical pathways and service-line management of hospitals," he says. Then it's important to give the quality and safety effort the necessary support and resources.

Says Merry, "Board members should encourage collaboration among clinical people and management people. This is a major shift in culture. But in the end, everyone ends up more empowered."

Creating the Patient
Safety Mindset

*Two Health Systems Explain How
They Are Making Safety Improvements—
and Proving Them*

By Laurie Larson

Is it dangerous to be a hospital patient today? It's often difficult to separate the attention patient safety has received in the medical and popular press from its actual condition. But can it improve? Always.

"It seems that the way you create change in a society is to first create fear," says Patrice Spath, president of Brown-Spath & Associates, Forest Grove, Oregon. "That's the cycle now [in health care]. But [safety concerns] are also a part of the public's anger toward managed care and the health care system."

In her work as a health care quality consultant, Spath often goes on-site to interview administrators and help them assess the safety of their institution (see the box on the next two pages). She always counsels that improvement in patient safety begins with an analysis of what a hospital will do *when* rather than *if* an unsafe event occurs. And she listens for three common statements that tip her off to an institution's need to become safer:

- *"It's never going to happen to us."* Hospitals that have never had a major sentinel event may say this, keeping them from identifying

Laurie Larson is *Trustee*'s staff writer.

What's Your Patient Safety Culture?

The statements below reflect how staff feel about various human factors that affect patient safety in your organization. Place a check in the appropriate box to indicate how strongly you agree with each of these statements.

People in this organization . . .

	Low	Medium	High
1. Are open to hearing how their actions affect patient safety.	☐	☐	☐
2. Can listen to feedback from others without getting defensive.	☐	☐	☐
3. Don't blame others for their mistakes.	☐	☐	☐
4. Don't retaliate against those who make mistakes.	☐	☐	☐
5. Believe that even competent, well-trained professionals make mistakes.	☐	☐	☐
6. Are willing to admit to patients that caregivers sometimes make mistakes.	☐	☐	☐
7. Cooperate with one another to resolve problems.	☐	☐	☐
8. Regularly report all patient incidents.	☐	☐	☐
9. Feel comfortable reporting unsafe conditions to their supervisor.	☐	☐	☐
10. Believe that there are things that can be done to reduce the likelihood of a medical mishap.	☐	☐	☐
11. Are willing to change some of their old habits in order to improve patient safety.	☐	☐	☐

Continued →

	Low	Medium	High
12. Believe that a medical accident could occur in this facility.	☐	☐	☐
13. Take time to discuss what went wrong when a significant patient incident occurs.	☐	☐	☐
14. Are willing to share information about errors they have made and the contributing factors.	☐	☐	☐
15. Believe that most patient incidents are preventable.	☐	☐	☐
16. Agree that patients play a role in preventing medical mistakes and mishaps.	☐	☐	☐
17. Believe that the organization's leaders are committed to improving patient safety at all costs.	☐	☐	☐

Sample tabulations of responses for each item, using percentages (not just raw numbers), will generally suffice. These can be indicated on a copy of the questionnaire, with percentages filled in where the checkmarks would go. Some results may be ignored later, but it is important to begin by tabulating everything.

The next step is cross-tabulation for items that may have some important relation to one another. For example, to determine whether the culture in particular patient units or among particular disciplines is more error-prone, one would cross-tabulate units or disciplines by the survey findings.

The exact form of the final survey report will depend on its purpose. If the data will be used to work on error-prone attitudes in small groups at all levels, the report should avoid inferences and conclusions. It should contain data grouped by unit, department, or division and be very clear, even to nonexperts. If senior managers and medical staff leaders will be using the data to formulate work culture improvement action plans, summary data and important findings may be more desirable. When preparing the final survey report, be sure to consider who will use it and for what purposes.

Source: Patrice Spath, *Patient Safety Improvement Guidebook*. Brown-Spath & Associates, 2000 (www.brownspath.com).

near misses and even smaller mistakes that may mean trouble down the road.

- *"We're no worse than anyone else."* This implies an "acceptable" error range, Spath says, which dismisses improvement as unnecessary. "If an airline said, 'We don't have any more plane crashes than anyone else,' that would not be okay," Spath says. "What we should have is zero tolerance. Even one error should be prevented."
- *"There's nothing we could have done about it."* Spath says she hears this statement most often. "If we continue to blame the patient or the system, it keeps us from being proactive," she says. Even though an error itself cannot be "taken back," it should not prevent investigating how to keep it from happening again.

"These attitudes are something trustees can [look] for when they [see] quality reports—they can read between the lines," she suggests.

"Generally, I find people want to have a safe environment," Spath says. "We've got low morale in hospitals because caregivers know where the problems are, but management isn't listening. If trustees see a high employee turnover rate, it's a sign that [staff] are sick and tired of trying to convince management that there is a problem. Look at your turnover rates."

Other warning signs of a poorly constructed or nonexistent safety program include low attendance at quality-related meetings, particularly low physician attendance, or not having a specific individual in charge of safety. Quality improvement projects that tend to focus on business over clinical processes, such as reducing patient wait times versus treating pain, are other signs of misplaced priorities.

How Intermountain Aims High

A health care system known for more than 20 years of making safety a cutting-edge priority, Intermountain Health Care (IHC), Salt Lake City, continually works on patient safety through clinical quality improvement.

"Every employee at all 22 of our hospitals is aware that he or she is responsible for clinical quality . . . and that a culture of safety is part of a culture of clinical quality," says William Nelson, IHC's president and CEO. As early as the 1970s, IHC's flagship, LDS

Hospital, innovated with its "Help System." Among many "prompts," this computerized medical data storage system combined lab data with patient information to flag contraindicated drugs on patient charts. It has since been replicated at the majority of IHC's other hospitals in Utah, Idaho, and Nevada, and will soon expand into its second incarnation, "Help II," a more thorough patient care management system. This prompting system will give electronic recommendations, make clinical suggestions, and generally help clinicians provide optimal care and reduce error rates. IHC hopes to initiate a pilot Help II within the next two years.

LDS Hospital has continued to lead the field with a recent study on prophylactic antibiotic treatment published in a peer-reviewed journal. Staff researchers found that giving patients antibiotics between one to two hours before surgery was an optimal time frame for preventing surgical infection. The procedure is now used in all system hospitals. Now IHC has stepped up its safety efforts.

"For the past two years, we've started focusing on specific patient safety goals as part of our annual strategic goals," Nelson says. In addition to its proven perioperative antibiotic initiative, which aims to be used on time in 90 percent of all IHC surgeries this year, the system has three other specific patient safety goals: eliminating adverse drug events (ADEs); preventing falls; and improving compliance for patient restraints.

The initiatives are led by a central operating group chaired by Nelson and divided into five geographic regions, three urban and two rural. In addition to a regional vice president leader from each region, this central group includes representatives from IHC's physician group, its health plan, human resources, legal counsel, and Greg Schwitzer, M.D., IHC's vice president of inpatient clinical programs and support services. The central group meets monthly and sets annual operations goals, which the IHC board must approve.

Standardized data gathered from all hospitals for each initiative are reported to a central operating group, which summarizes outcomes and sets patient safety objectives from the data gathered. Next, the system's professional standards committee, a system board subcommittee, reviews the central group's summarized findings and sends them quarterly to the full 27-member system board for review and approval.

Eleven Safety Practices Anyone Can Use

The Agency for Healthcare Research and Quality (AHRQ) recently issued an extensive report outlining several dozen health care practices that it endorses for improving patient safety. Of those recommendations, the following 11 procedures gave the strongest evidence supporting widespread implementation.

"No good system should fail to have these in place," says Brent James, M.D., vice president of research and education at Intermountain Health Care in Salt Lake City.

Safety practices are listed in order of proven efficacy and are geared toward care of the acutely ill.

1. Appropriate prophylaxis to prevent blood clots in at-risk patients
2. Preventive use of beta-blockers in cardiac patients before surgery to improve outcomes
3. Use of maximum sterile barriers while placing central intravenous catheters to prevent infections
4. Preventive use of antibiotics prior to surgery to avoid perioperative infections
5. Asking patients to recall and restate what they were told during the informed consent process
6. Continuous drainage of subglottic secretions to prevent ventilator-associated pneumonia
7. Use of pressure-relieving bedding materials to prevent pressure ulcers
8. Use of real-time ultrasound guidance to assist central line insertion to prevent complications
9. Appropriate outpatient self-management for warfarin (Coumadin) for effective anticoagulation without complications
10. Appropriate nutrition, particularly early enteral nutrition, in critically ill and surgical patients
11. Use of antibiotic-impregnated central venous catheters to prevent catheter-related infections

Source: Agency for Healthcare Research and Quality. Find the full report at: www.ahrq.gov

In his leadership position, Schwitzer takes prime responsibility for quality improvement and risk management for the system, monitoring patient safety goals and coordinating all IHC's patient safety initiatives systemwide.

"There's a high degree of variability among 22 hospitals, and it can vary within each hospital as well," Schwitzer says. IHC began all its initiatives with uniform definitions and baselines of where each hospital stood systemwide.

"It takes a multidisciplinary team of clinicians and administrators to set up the processes that will facilitate measurement and improvement," Schwitzer says. "There are four steps: define an area to pursue; make sure your definitions and measurements are commonly agreed upon; decide on your measurement tools; and get a baseline for the system."

He cautions that it takes six to eight months to find common measurement systems and definitions and tools, and six to eight more months to establish a baseline.

"You need at least two quarters of time or [ideally] a year to account for the seasonal variation of hospitals and establish a baseline," Schwitzer cautions. "Often analysis [estimates are] shot from the hip." He adds, "It's impossible to take a 'Big Bang' approach with patient safety. You have to evaluate and implement goals sequentially in a way that makes sense. What can you realistically do? Set a series of goals that can give you real benefit and are easily measured."

Resident Expert

Nelson acknowledges that one of the biggest reasons IHC has been ahead of the curve with patient safety was the foresight of its CEO in bringing Brent James, M.D., on board 15 years ago. Currently IHC's vice president of research and medical education, heading up clinical improvements, James was one of the authors of the groundbreaking 1999 Institute of Medicine report on medical errors. Consequently, he's quite familiar with how hospitals have handled safety problems historically.

Errors are typically reported in one of three ways, James explains. First, by voluntary reporting as injuries occur, which "tends to be underdetected," he says. Second, by detecting injuries

through retrospective chart review of procedures with a high probability of injury.

"This is bad because it's expensive, the information is received
well after any intervention opportunity has passed—and it misses a
third of actual injuries," James says.

The final way of detecting medical error, and what James defines
as "the gold standard," is through prospective expert review—or
detecting potential errors "ahead of time." One key component of
such a system is "data-based clinical trigger system responses," or
tracking typical ways errors are fixed. This is what the Help System
and Help II are designed to do.

For example, certain drugs are typically used to counteract over-
doses of opiates, he says. A tracking system designed to flag orders
for the antidote to that overdose would instantly question why it
was ordered, potentially catching a near miss. The same clinical trigger principle in an error detection system could detect many other
types of errors, both retrospectively, as in the above example, or
prospectively, flagging such problems as a too-high drug dosage
ordered for a patient's level of kidney function. Because 90 percent
of injuries come from six events (adverse drug events, hospital-
acquired infections, pressure sores, venous thromboembolisms,
patient falls and injuries due to bed rails and restraints, and inappropriate blood product transfusions and reactions), James says that
choosing what to watch becomes evident. IHC already tracks ADEs
and hospital-acquired infections and is developing systems for the
other areas.

Even with these systems, however, voluntary reporting still
requires ongoing staff education. James sees IHC's culture of safety
as being one where potential injuries are immediately regarded as
system failures, not professional incompetence. This attitude eases
fears of reporting mistakes, he says. But staff are reminded that they
are expected to report errors, both for legal protection and to establish a professional ethic.

"You need to make it easy to report," James advises. "Look for
where data bottleneck and target reporting there." He cites IHC's
Pixus system, a central patient prescription dispensing system at a
majority of nursing stations. The Pixus system identifies drugs
ordered for treating injuries. The computer then automatically asks
the orderer if that drug request is the result of an ADE. It is easy to

answer yes or no, and no individual name is attached to the response. James says reporting has increased "100-fold" since IHC implemented the Pixus flag.

How Baptist Created Its Own Council

Another system ahead of its time, Baptist Memorial Health Care in Memphis, did a benchmark study with VHA (a national network of community-owned health care organizations and physicians) hospitals on medication usage and decided to make changes—a year before the IOM report came out. "After the benchmark study, the board set an [overall] patient safety mandate," explains Stephen Reynolds, Baptist's president and CEO. "We took the recommendations of those closest to the patient, and they told us that [to meet the board mandate] we needed a safety council." The three making the recommendation were William Poston, M.D., Baptist's chief medical officer; Nancy Nowak, vice president of nursing; and Jule Keegan, system director of pharmacy. They in turn chose the other 11 members of what became Baptist's Safety and Quality Council.

"Trying to make changes across the system [is an enormous task], but if we were trying to do best practices at the flagship (Baptist Memorial Hospital in Memphis), we had to do them at all hospitals," Nowak says. Baptist has 17 urban and rural hospitals across Mississippi, Arkansas, and Tennessee.

Launched in April 2000, the council exists to provide organizational leadership for patient safety initiatives; establish a safety plan; oversee data collection and analysis; foster best practices implementation; and partner with patients and the community in care delivery.

In addition to Keegan, Poston, and Nowak, who chairs the council, members include Baptist's system director of clinical services, chief information officer, risk management director, and vice president of finance, among other leaders.

"These are the key decision makers across the system," Nowak says. "At this level, we can quickly bring information to senior leadership and make recommendations to systems operations and the board; it's easy to effect change quickly—there are key interconnections."

To get started, the council looked to national experts. "We looked at regulatory changes from the Joint Commission, the Health Care

Financing Administration, the Occupational Safety and Health Administration, and others to see where they were focusing their efforts [in patient safety], and we did the same . . . to see what initiatives were most important," Nowak says.

Baptist currently has 10 active safety initiatives: medication system variance (now called the medication use safety team); use of restraints; pain management; in-house resuscitation; patient falls; needle safety; mandatory physician handwriting legibility guidelines; moderate sedation; and the clinical pharmacist practice model.

Each initiative has a representative safety council member and a system team. Each hospital has an equivalent team. Similarly, safety councils that mirror the system council have been implemented over the past year at each hospital.

Every facility has a data "grid" for each of the 10 initiatives that it must fill out monthly for its system council. Each initiative asks for different types of data, but all hospitals fill out the same information for each. The chief nursing officer of each hospital is accountable for the reports. Nowak meets monthly with each of these nursing officers.

Just as system problems can be found this way, if an individual hospital finds an exceptional way of improving safety, its success can be shared systemwide.

Safety council structure is flexible within each hospital, depending on its size, but all include the chief nursing officer, a physician leader, and staff from medical records, risk management, and quality assurance.

Nowak and Poston report safety council activity at all system board meetings. "The data allow us to take snapshots [of how the initiatives are progressing] and keep drilling down, asking continually, 'Are we doing our best? Could we do better?'" Nowak says. At the annual strategic planning and budget meeting, all initiatives are analyzed for what they have achieved and what new goals need to be added. Nowak calls it "a project in motion.

"It can be overwhelming. You have to tackle each initiative one at a time," she says. "But once you get rolling, it becomes a partnership versus 'What piece belongs to me?' The philosophy is that all of us take care of patients no matter what we do and if we're all asking the same questions, we'll come to the same outcomes."

To lead by example, Reynolds writes a letter to each system board member weekly, always including a note on patient safety, and he encourages every CEO in the system to do the same. All medical staff meetings include quality reports, and the topic is covered monthly in the employee newsletter.

Zeroing In on Medication Safety

To date, Baptist has spent the most time and effort on its medication safety initiative. For the past four years, the system's pharmacy team has collaborated with the VHA and 33 other hospitals to benchmark medication use. From this, best practices have emerged, and the Baptist system's director of pharmacy, Jule Keegan, has been able to effect innovative change.

"We check all the drugs in our formulary to look for potential confusions between them," Keegan explains. "If we determine we need both/all drugs that sound or look confusingly similar, we try to add additional information to separate them further from each other."

Beyond this, Keegan's department has focused on three high-risk medications—heparin, insulin, and warfarin—and has significantly reduced associated ADEs. Preprinted physician orders are required for heparin, preventing handwriting problems. Nurses monitor the administration of all three drugs particularly closely, and additional lab tests are ordered to tightly track patient drug levels—a team effort.

"Health care teams have proven to have more positive outcomes than physicians alone," Keegan explains.

Similarly, Baptist's clinical pharmacy model safety initiative gives pharmacists more help—and more time to monitor drugs in patient units. A certified pharmacist assistant now performs the computer order entry of prescriptions, freeing clinical pharmacy specialists to make rounds, seeing patients for therapeutic drug monitoring, as well as getting more involved in patient education and discharge planning.

Like IHC, Baptist has gone to great lengths to make incident reporting and its perception more "blameless," starting with system-wide education for bedside staff. The clear message from the board on down is that the data collected will make care safer and that those filling out incident reports will not be held personally accountable.

Reports now have "action plans" on the back of them, where staff can address what they think would keep a problem from happening again. "It makes them feel more comfortable to be able to say, 'Here's how to fix it' and write it out," Keegan says. These changes

What's the Trustee's Role?

Beyond the data, models, and the teams in the field, trustees need to understand that the safety of their hospital is ultimately their responsibility.

"We approach the business of the hospital with the same degree of concern as we do our own personal business," says Watson Bell, trustee at Baptist Memorial Health Care. "You think of it as though you, or a member of your family, was receiving care." Bell also chairs Baptist's Joint Conference Committee, which meets quarterly with chiefs of staff at all the system's hospitals to review safety, among other clinical, operational, and strategic goals related to patient care. They look at performance improvement reports, discussing their experiences and ways to improve safety.

"Trustees should demand accurate safety reports and ask appropriate questions of management, such as: 'Why do our data show this increase [in falls, for example]?' 'Are they the result of more reporting or a bigger problem?' 'Are we adequately resourcing patient safety?' 'What resources should be given?'" explains Greg Schwitzer, M.D., Intermountain Health Care's vice president of inpatient clinical programs and support services.

Asking these types of questions creates a "culture change" that lets the CEO know that the board expects safety to be a top priority, says Patrice Spath, president of health care quality consultants Brown-Spath & Associates.

"Boards need to realize that they have to [get involved in patient safety] whether they want to or not—there's a national push in that direction," says Brent James, M.D., IHC's vice president of research and medical education.

"We [trustees] bring a lay perspective to the board and sometimes [that] perspective is a breath of fresh air," Bell says. He knows from listening to local residents, for example, that a patient judges good nursing care by how quickly a call button is answered rather than more technical skills. "We feel, as trustees, the hospital reflects upon us . . . so we take it very personally," Bell adds. "Safety is part of our fiduciary responsibility."

—L.L.

have increased the number of reports "by leaps and bounds," Nowak says, with more near misses versus incident reports. She says a follow-up survey is planned soon to determine if the staff now feels more comfortable with incident reporting.

Keeping Up with Change

Is patient safety in crisis? IHC's Schwitzer says that the acuity of patients has risen in hospitals—and it does make safety tougher. "[We] have a different kind of patient now," he says. "Historically, we had a large population of [relatively] healthy, alert inpatients. Now the majority is sicker, older, more disabled, and more medicated"—and more prone to patient safety problems. Staff are also more stretched, with a higher volume of patients needing more resources just when staffing ratios are tightening. Technology figures in as well.

"Every time you increase technology to save people, the care environment becomes more complex," Schwitzer says. "But if we're going to improve [care], we have to have technology. Extensive training and setting goals and monitoring them for realistic improvement is the answer."

Ultimately, action may count the most. Spath points out that as of July 2001, the Joint Commission requires all hospitals to target at least one high-risk procedure for improvement, and if hospitals aren't sure where to start, the most common sentinel events are listed on the JCAHO's Web site.

"Choose a high-risk process, go to the staff, and ask them about it," Spath suggests. "Use their input to choose one to two projects. You don't have to spend so much time analyzing . . . just do something!"

Although other industries offer great models for safety improvement that health care can learn from, it is still a field unto itself in many ways.

"We do not have the luxury of stopping our work to fix things—and we [treat] people [when they are] most vulnerable and sensitive," Nowak says. "We have to keep doing the work while we fix it."

The solutions are being discovered, as IHC and Baptist, among many others, are proving. And as more of these models are found and followed, the axiom "practice makes perfect" becomes a foreseeable goal.

Patient Safety:
It Starts with the Board

*When It Comes to the Fundamentals,
Patient Safety Tops the List*

By Shari Mycek

I was in Paris interviewing airline pilots for a travel story when the Air France Concorde crashed just minutes after takeoff. The crash killed all 109 people on board as well as four more people on the ground. Reaction from the pilots was one of shock, numbness, and disbelief. The Concorde, which flies at an altitude of 60,000 feet and crisscrosses the Atlantic in just three-and-a-half hours, had been considered among the world's safest planes. It had never been involved in an accident before. Immediately after the disaster, Air France grounded its five remaining Concordes until "passenger safety could be ensured."

In 1982, Johnson & Johnson quickly recalled 264,000 bottles of Extra Strength Tylenol from store shelves after seven Chicago-area residents died after taking the nonprescription pain medication. A probe revealed the product had been laced with cyanide, and the incident ultimately led to an FDA mandate that all over-the-counter pharmaceuticals must have tamper-resistant seals.

Shari Mycek is a writer based in Belle Mead, New Jersey, and a contributing writer to *Trustee*.

But the "celebrated" cases are not reserved solely for the transportation or consumer industry.

In 1995, two tragic medication errors at the Dana-Farber Cancer Institute in Boston rocked the health care industry. One of the errors resulted in the death of a well-known *Boston Globe* reporter; the other triggered a significant medical intervention.

"Not only was the attention of the public and the media riveted on the events, so were the eyes of the entire health care field," wrote Jim Conway in his introduction to *Strategies for Leadership: Hospital Executives and Their Role in Patient Safety*, published recently by the American Hospital Association. Conway is the chief operations officer at Dana-Farber and now a board member of the National Patient Safety Foundation and the Massachusetts Coalition for the Prevention of Medical Error's steering committee. "'What happened? Why? What can be done to be certain it doesn't happen again?' were questions we were asking ourselves," Conway adds.

Four years later, in 1999, health care leaders were once again troubled when the Institute of Medicine issued a groundbreaking report that as many as 98,000 Americans may die each year from medical errors. Although the IOM's most recent report, *Crossing the Chasm: A New Health System for the 21st Century,* addresses quality problems inherent in the health care system as a whole and doesn't single out patient safety, Don Nielsen, M.D., the AHA's senior vice-president for quality leadership, warns that health care leaders cannot relax. "The first report focused very much on medical errors; this one did not, but that doesn't mean there are fewer [errors]. Much work still needs to be done."

And that work starts with the board.

"Patient safety should be a standing item on the board agenda," says Nielsen. "It should not be an ancillary add-on item, but an item in which trustees should be asking questions of the organization's senior management as well as the clinical staff."

What exactly is patient safety? Kenneth Kizer, M.D., president and CEO of the National Forum for Health Care Quality and former head of the Veterans Administration, defines it as "continuously seeking to minimize hazards and patient harm. . . . [It is] shared responsibility for risk reduction . . . free and open communication . . . and facilitated reporting of errors . . . in a nonpunitive environment."

Brock Nelson, CEO of Children's Hospitals & Health Clinics in Minneapolis, says his organization is working hard to create a patient-safe culture. Children's operates from two sites, employs 1,400 professional staff, 3,500 total employees, and serves the entire state of Minnesota. More than half of the hospitals' patients are critically ill.

In September 1999 (two months before the first IOM report was published), the Children's board endorsed an organizationwide patient safety initiative as part of its overall strategic plan.

"No specific incident—wrong-leg surgery or chemotherapy case—[inspired] this effort," says Nelson. "There was just an awareness [of the importance of patient safety]. We had a new chief operating officer at the time who was very much [concerned about the issue] of patient safety, and our board leadership was also very familiar [with the area] and supportive as well. The chair at the time had a child who had died—not the result of a medical accident or error, the child had cancer—but he saw a lot of opportunities, during the course of his child's treatment, for errors to occur. Another board member was in the transportation business and was well aware of [the significance of] safety."

Following the board's endorsement of a patient safety initiative, focus groups were conducted with hospital staff, physicians, and parents, asking them what errors they had seen and what they believed could be a problem. As a result, patient safety courses have been conducted for staff, and a steering committee composed of physicians and parents has been established to oversee the patient safety program. Also, patient safety is now tied to compensation—for Brock, senior management, as well as departmental directors and clinical chairs throughout the organization. Board members receive dashboard-type key performance indicator reports, one quadrant of which covers patient safety.

"Now, [when] the board sees a financial report, it also sees a safety report," says Nelson. "Having a patient safety plan has made a big difference in terms of [getting] everybody's attention, but [ensuring patient safety] doesn't get easier; in fact, it gets harder."

For example, at this writing Nelson had just suspended a surgical program temporarily. Although he declined to elaborate on his reasons for doing so, he did note that no "incident" had prompted the measure but, rather, the potential for an error to occur.

"Physicians questioned my authority to suspend the program temporarily," says Nelson. "Why would I do that? We'd been doing [this procedure] forever—but it just came down to safety and whether or not we could guarantee it. A task force of physicians is now working on the issue, identifying what needs to be in place before we can resume—and we probably will resume [the program] in the very near future. Although their reaction [to the suspension] was negative, physicians are definitely part of the process—trying to figure out what needs to be done and making the necessary changes. And their buy-in is critical."

Indeed, physicians can make or break an organizationwide patient safety plan. According to Steven DeLashmutt, M.D., a trustee at St. Elizabeth Health Services in Baker City, Oregon, and chair of the AHA's Committee on Governance's patient safety committee, there are two partners in the "patient care business": the board/CEO and the medical staff. And the two must jointly commit to a patient safety plan "to successfully make the thing fly."

Certainly, that was one lesson learned at Dana-Farber. In the years following the high-profile medical errors there, COO Jim Conway has hit the lecture circuit, sharing with colleagues ways to guide their organization to a "culture of safety."

"Without voice, visibility, and commitment from the top of an organization, little progress is possible," says Conway.

But obtaining buy-in from boards, CEOs, and the medical staff is not as simple as it sounds.

"Most business partners try to work together because it benefits them both," says DeLashmutt. "But in a board-physician relationship, there's sometimes mixed direction. If the hospital does well, the board is happy. If the hospital does well, the physicians may or may not be happy. And so, if the business thrives, you have two partners—one of which will always be happy and the other who may or may not be—and that's a funny [kind of] partnership.

"The question comes down to: How can the board motivate physicians to participate in a patient safety plan? And the key is that physicians, 100 percent of the time, are geared to getting the best care for their patients. The way to get physicians on board is to [say], 'We can take better care of your patients by implementing a patient safety plan. At the other end, we'll come out with fewer errors, less harm to your patients, and they'll be safer in our institution. But you have to help us do that. You have to be an integral part, an architect, of the plan.' The reward comes for the physicians when they see, in actual fact, that things have changed, that their patients are being taken care of better. All this takes time, of course—six months to a year minimum."

Getting started is often the most difficult step. Once the board has committed itself to making patient safety fundamental to the organization's internal strategic initiative, a patient safety plan—crafted with input from physicians—should be put in writing (see box below).

"There is no magic formula for creating a culture of safety," says DeLashmutt. "And it's also impossible to peg a number and say the overall hospital error rate should be .001 or .00001, because every hospital is going to have a different goal—and a different culture.

What Makes a Patient Safety Plan?

Steven DeLashmutt, M.D., trustee of St. Elizabeth Health Services, in Baker City, Oregon, and a member of the AHA's Committee on Governance, suggests the following elements be included in a patient safety plan:

- An outline of the patient safety officer position
- Quality improvement for patient safety
- Measurements to be monitored for patient safety (e.g., mortality and morbidity rates, length of stay, etc.)
- Details of error reporting and error assessment methods
- A comprehensive method for evaluating hospital and medical staff competency
- Outline of patients' and families' roles
- Qualifications of outside contractors
- Type and methods of ongoing education for all staff
- Type of data to be collected and to whom they will be reported internally
- How departments will collect and report data required by external organizations (e.g., JCAHO, the Institute for Safe Medical Practices)
- Brief description of the "culture of safety"
- How quality assurance will be built into the system
- Description of a "crisis team" comprising a cross-section of staff (e.g., social workers, nurses, physicians, etc.) and the training required for communicating with patients and families who have experienced a medical error
- Hospital's participation in patient safety research, if appropriate
- How often the plan will be updated, reviewed, and critiqued

Our hospital, for example, is small and rural. We don't do cardiac catheterizations or chemotherapy. So our rate of error will be different from that of a hospital doing more complex procedures."

To determine where patient safety problems may exist within an organization, DeLashmutt suggests a study of quality indicators. "There will be a problem area," he says candidly. "There's not a hospital in the United States that doesn't have a problem someplace, so if you pull up the right indicators for your institution, it will put you on the right trail to figure out where your challenge lies."

Quality indicators may include death rate; length of stay; number and type of malpractice cases; number of patient falls; number and rate of errors made; number and type of sentinel events; number and type of near misses; policy changes as a result of error analyses; reports to the board by performance improvement teams involved in patient safety via the quality committee; reported hours spent in training staff in patient safety; and patient assessments of their perceived level of safety.

"An interesting piece of patient safety is patient satisfaction," says DeLashmutt. "If all the wheels are turning right in the patient safety arena, then patient satisfaction should also be high."

DeLashmutt also suggests tying CEO compensation to patient safety—as has recently been done in conjunction with healthy community initiatives. "Linking patient safety to compensation shows the CEO that the board is serious about its commitment. If the hospital's error rate drops by 15 or 20 or 30 percent, then there should be a bonus for the CEO or senior administration."

Like the AHA's Nielsen, DeLashmutt advocates making patient safety a topic at every board meeting.

"Trustees, persistently and doggedly, at every board meeting must ask, 'How many medical errors have [we made] in the past month? How many near misses have there been? And what is being done about them?' And you hope the answer isn't, 'Oh, we fired the dude who did this.' You don't want to hear that," he says. "By and large, it is not the person who's at fault but the system.

"I once read a classic account on how to ride a dead horse," DeLashmutt continues. "Many strategies were offered. You could change the rider, form a team to discuss how to ride the dead horse. But, in the end, the only thing that made sense was to call it a dead horse and get off; figure out a different—and better—way to get where you need to go."

Strategies for Leadership in Patient Safety

Complete?
Yes   No

Personal Education

☐   ☐   Read *To Err is Human: Building a Safer Health System,* edited by L. T. Kohn, J. M. Corrigan, and M. S. Donaldson. Washington, D.C.: National Academy Press, 1999.

☐   ☐   Participate in external safety education programs, conferences, etc.

☐   ☐   Hold detailed conversations with in-house experts on our realities of practice.

☐   ☐   Walk my hospital with a human factors expert.

☐   ☐   Walk my hospital as a patient.

☐   ☐   Familiarize myself with enhanced JCAHO Patient Safety Standards (see "Patient Safety and the Joint Commission: The Latest News," page 27, in the March 2001 *Trustee*).

☐   ☐   View Bridge Medical video "Beyond Blame" and Partnership for Patient Safety video "First Do No Harm."

Call to Action

☐   ☐   Speak publicly to the following audiences on the unacceptability of the current state of, and my commitment to, patient safety as a personal and corporate priority, as well as including a safety focus in hospital publications, strategic plans, etc.:
- board leaders
- patients/consumers
- media

☐   ☐   Implement a proactive effort on patient safety design, measurement, assessment, and improvement. Include direct care, administrative and clerical staff, and patients and family members in all aspects.

Continued →

Complete?		
Yes	**No**	
☐	☐	Set the goal of establishing an environment of trust with a nonblaming, responsibility-based approach to the causation of incidents and errors; establish policy in this area.
☐	☐	Set the expectation for timely and interdisciplinary error and near-miss investigations with an emphasis on: patient/family affected by the error; the broader institutional implications of and learning from the error; and the support of staff closest to care.
☐	☐	Build quality improvement and patient safety policies into staff orientation and continuing education offerings.
☐	☐	Set the expectation for executive involvement in significant incident investigations.
☐	☐	Establish a policy to ensure patients/families are notified ASAP when an error affects a patient.
☐	☐	Establish effective grievance systems for patients/families who see themselves as "victims of error."
☐	☐	Establish mechanisms to train leadership and other experts in patient safety.

Practicing a Culture of Safety

☐	☐	Openly engage with medical staff, nurses, and other leaders in patient safety planning.
☐	☐	Continuously articulate the business case for safety improvement.
☐	☐	Personally participate in a significant incident investigation/root-cause analysis.
☐	☐	Tell "my story" around incidents/errors that I have been involved with and the systems improvements that could have prevented them.
☐	☐	Routinely involve myself, all levels of our staff, and our patients and family members in direct ongoing communications around the patient safety work of our institution and areas for improvement.

Continued →

Complete?
Yes   No

☐   ☐   Routinely probe staff perceptions of risk areas from existing or proposed systems and take immediate actions wherever possible.

☐   ☐   Openly support staff involved in incidents and their root-cause analysis.

☐   ☐   Ensure that there is ongoing prioritization and achievement of safety improvement objectives.

☐   ☐   Ensure that articles on patient safety matters regularly appear in my organization's communication vehicles.

☐   ☐   As part of annual budget approval, ensure resources are funded for priority safety areas.

☐   ☐   Ensure self-assessments from the AHA and others are completed and used internally for quality improvement activities.

☐   ☐   Cultivate media understanding of patient safety and my organization's efforts to improve safety.

☐   ☐   Ensure effective systems are in place to assess individual accountability and competence.

Advancing the Field

☐   ☐   Share my personal and the institution's patient safety learning outside of the organization.

☐   ☐   Participate in local, regional, and national conferences, coalitions, and other efforts to improve patient safety.

☐   ☐   Engage in initiatives to drive enhancements in regulatory, facility/professional licensing, and accreditation agencies that support safety improvement and cultural change in consort with the specific goals of the organization.

Excerpted from *Strategies for Leadership: Hospital Executives and Their Role in Patient Safety,* by Jim Conway, chief operations officer, Dana-Farber Cancer Institute, Boston. Reprinted with permission from the American Hospital Association, copyright 2001.

According to Nielsen, the journey must include a nonpunitive reporting mechanism. He advises that "trustees must ask what kind of data and information are being collected in regard to safety and the care being provided. They must ask how opportunities for improvement are being identified and what actions have been or are being taken to improve/rectify the situation. But before they can do any of that, they must ensure that people are reporting what may potentially be unsafe practices or practices that have already caused unfortunate outcomes. Everyone has an obligation to report 'near misses' or events they think are leading to unsafe care. And trustees must ensure that the reporting mechanism be nonpunitive and, at least at the beginning, confidential."

Unofficially and among themselves, physicians already do that. "Physicians are not hesitant to talk about mistakes [among themselves]," says DeLashmutt. "The idea is that if you can talk to somebody else and share what may have happened to you that was not good, it may prevent [your colleagues] from having a similar problem. But there's no systematic way to do that; there's no forum. Right now, it's just a matter of physicians bumping into one another and saying, 'Hey, guess what happened to me last week,' and sharing that experience."

But the trust necessary to share those experiences typically rests among physicians only.

It becomes a different story when another party, such as the board, enters the picture—to review competency, for example. On this issue, DeLashmutt humbly acknowledges he has limited advice.

"Part of any patient safety program has to include competency," he says. "You don't want people in the hospital who are incompetent taking care of patients. That's a no-brainer. But competency can be a dark can of worms. While the competency of hospital staff is relatively easy to corner and measure, [that of the] medical staff is very difficult to measure. Still, boards must address competency. And that's really tough. You go back to this strange [board-physicians] relationship where one partner [the board] is immune, but the other partner [physicians] has to go through some sort of competency evaluation, and that's a really funny business model. Hospital boards do—or should do—self-assessments every year on their effectiveness," DeLashmutt continues. "But that evaluation is a *self*-assessment. It is unusual for the board to have evaluations done by employees of the hospital or by the physicians. That's not to say it can't be done; it just isn't.

"The rules for physicians are different. While physicians also undergo an appointment/reappointment process that assesses their ability to practice medicine, new JCAHO guidelines now demand a program where staff members and other physicians can refer a physician to be evaluated for illness or impairment.

"So far, the hospital board is immune from a system of hospital staff or physicians referring a board member for evaluation of illness or impairment," says DeLashmutt. "The 'partners in quality' [i.e., the board and physicians] do not receive equal treatment under the new JCAHO guidelines.

"Plus, you have the egos of the physicians saying, 'What are you looking at me for? Obviously I'm an M.D. I've been practicing for years. So I'm competent. You don't need [to know] anything else but that.' The potential for tension is great."

Other stumbling blocks or "threats" to implementing a patient safety program do exist, according to DeLashmutt, but none of them "is a good enough reason not to implement an initiative."

Those threats may include:

- Board apathy
- A CEO who doesn't support a program
- A board that insists on starting a program before obtaining CEO buy-in
- Complexity of restructuring the reporting mechanism in order to channel patient safety data to the safety officer
- Public opinion and suspicion fueled by a lay press exposition of medical errors (e.g., the "celebrated" cases)
- The threat of litigation from discovery in an open, communicative environment
- Chronic history of denial by hospital administration, board, and physicians that errors occur
- Lack of awareness by the board and/or administration that a problem exists (i.e., poor information reporting)
- A traditional medical culture of individual responsibility and blame
- Inadequate allocation of resources for quality improvement and error prevention

- Inadequate knowledge by the board and administration about the frequency, cause, and impact of errors, as well as about effective methods for error prevention
- Belief that the current error rate is acceptable
- Notion that problems can be fixed as they happen (i.e., no proactive approach)
- The idea that patient safety is "a phase" that will pass if ignored long enough

CEO Brock Nelson, for one, begs to differ with this last impediment. "I've been around a long time," he says. "And, yes, a lot of things are fads that come and go. But patient safety isn't one of them. Those who view it as such are in denial."

And denial can be very costly—to an institution's reputation, to the hospital's bottom line, and, most important, to patients' life.

Patient Safety,
Thy Name Is Quality

By David Classen

When the *Journal of the American Medical Association (JAMA)* published conflicting arguments in July 2000 about the number of people who die each year from medical errors, it was just the latest media flare-up in what has become a seemingly unquenchable fire in the mainstream press. That fire was sparked by an Institute of Medicine report in November 1999, which claimed that as many as 98,000 people die annually from medical errors in U.S. hospitals, more than from car accidents, breast cancer, or AIDS. The more recent *JAMA* controversy pitted medical researchers who claimed the IOM report exaggerated the number of patient deaths against experts who argued the IOM figures were actually underreported.

In a typical media response, Katie Couric of NBC's *Today* show investigated the debate to try to nail down exactly which side held the correct numbers.

The answer, of course, is neither. For trustees and top management at health care delivery systems, negative publicity about medical

David Classen, M.D., is vice-president in the performance improvement service, First Consulting Group, Long Beach, California. He can be reached at dclassen@fcg.com.

errors puts the issue of patient safety at the top of the priority list, regardless of the numbers. In many ways the IOM report merely put on the map an issue that all health care delivery systems have been addressing for years: quality. That issue and the associated one of evidence-based medicine have rightly taken center stage for health care in the information age.

Evidence-based medicine systematically uses the best current information in patient care, integrating an individual clinician's expertise with the best available clinical evidence from research. It can be practiced either by the individual clinician or institutionally through the development of protocols.

Missing the Point

"Arguing about the number of medical errors misses the point," declares Phil Mosca, M.D., chair of Integris Southwest Medical Center's board in Oklahoma City and a trustee of Integris Health, the medical center's parent organization. "The important thing is that publication of the IOM report marked the first time the mainstream press has acknowledged there may be patient safety issues on a national scale."

Mosca, a practicing urologist who also chairs the quality committee at Integris Southwest, says health care has long been aware of the prevalence of medical errors. "It's not news to us in the clinical world. Somebody in Washington finally heard the cries," he says. Even though such attention is overdue, he thinks the Clinton administration has overreacted by advocating a national reporting system that goes too far in identifying individual practitioners and their errors. Mosca wants to use only aggregate data in a national reporting system and wants to put greater emphasis on developing a nonpunitive culture of health care safety.

Enter trustees, who are ultimately responsible for patient safety because they credential physicians and approve all policies and procedures related to safety and risk. With the mounting scrutiny of the IOM report, boards are increasingly asking what their organizations are doing about patient safety. In many cases, they breathe sighs of relief. But there are also new initiatives from groups like the Joint Commission on Accreditation of Healthcare Organizations (JCAHO) that require a thoughtful response from health care organizations.

Trustees can be especially helpful through active participation in committees like the one Mosca chairs that oversee quality and risk and regularly report back to the board. A diverse background is a plus—it's perhaps even more important when overseeing something as specialized as clinical quality. "It's wonderful for me to have lay people on these committees because of how differently they view things from physicians trained to see in a uniform way. Sometimes even the most naive clinical questions from a nonclinician can shed light on how to resolve a complex issue," Mosca says.

Who Knew?

Different perspectives will be needed even more as health care providers try to let go of their traditional expert-based culture in favor of a nonpunitive one that encourages error admissions.

"Patient safety is a legitimate issue regardless of the precise numbers. Too many patients die or are harmed by medical error," says Kevin Wardell, executive vice president for operations at the University of Texas M.D. Anderson Cancer Center in Houston. "Historically, the response to error reporting at all levels—medical staff, management, and boards—has been punitive and that has significantly reduced our ability to make things safer," he says.

This rush-to-blame reaction flies in the face of the actual cause of most medical errors: rarely if ever are they the result of a single action or individual but, rather, of compounding chains of errors that escape detection, according to Wardell and most other experts. "As both a manager and a board member, I can say that we've probably never really known what errors were out there," says Wardell.

That shouldn't come as a surprise considering that, as recently as 10 years ago, medical staff kept a lid on all discussions of errors within the secrecy of mortality and morbidity committees. "You could never go back and address system errors," says Wardell, adding that one of the best things to come out of the IOM report's publicity is the launching of national initiatives such as JCAHO's Sentinel Events Policy.

Three Strikes in Texas

"If we can convince our staff, nurses, and doctors that we can address these [errors] in a nonpunitive manner, we can greatly reduce the prevalence of errors," Wardell says. Sometimes that takes local legislative action. For example, Texas requires that any nurse reported three times for an error be subject to losing his or her license. In an effort to change the "three strikes" law and build a nonpunitive culture of safety in the state, M.D. Anderson has helped form the Texas Forum, a statewide education and lobbying coalition consisting of delivery systems and doctors.

Eliminating health care's traditional culture of blame isn't easy, says Jerod Loeb, Ph.D., vice president for research and performance measurement at JCAHO. He acknowledges that even the most sophisticated delivery organizations with highly automated pharmaceutical order entry systems still make mistakes and sometimes degenerate into witch-hunts.

"You can't mandate culture change. It must be conveyed by leadership that it is safe" to admit error; and that will require a "sea change" in the industry, says Loeb.

That sea change will involve trustees at the helm who recognize that reporting a medical error doesn't mean the level of care has necessarily deteriorated. What may need to occur is a culture change that allows people to feel more comfortable reporting errors. "Trustees shouldn't be looking for body counts," warns Loeb.

Sentinel Events

Indeed, when the Centers for Disease Control and Prevention compile data on hospital-acquired infections, the institutions that report zero are often the ones with the poorest infection rates. Organizations with higher incidences tend to be better at controlling hospital-acquired infections. That kind of reverse logic could trip up an uninitiated trustee or executive. "There are a lot of thorny issues that need to be understood by governance boards," notes Loeb.

JCAHO takes no stance on the issue of whether reporting medical errors should be mandatory so long as protections exist for people to come forward with information without fear of recrimination. It's the processes in place that ultimately need correction, asserts Loeb.

In that vein, JCAHO's patient safety efforts take a two-pronged approach. The first prong is the agency's sentinel events policy, which covers events at an institution that result in a patient's unanticipated death or major, permanent loss of function not related to the patient's condition. Sentinel events include such occurrences as suicide; infant abduction, or giving an infant to the wrong family; rape; giving the wrong blood type to a patient; and surgery on the wrong patient or wrong body part.

JCAHO considers such events "reviewable" but does not mandate their reporting. If, however, the commission becomes aware of a sentinel event by way of a telephone call from a patient or employee or a newspaper report, the agency requires the provider organization to submit a root-cause analysis report and an action plan to correct the problem.

Running with the Oryx

The commission also sponsors a program called ORYX, which requires hospitals to have systems in place to track data related to as many as six clinical performance measures in five areas:

• Heart failure
• Acute myocardial infarction (heart attack)
• Community-acquired pneumonia
• Pregnancy and related conditions
• Surgical procedures and complications

At this point, organizations have a choice as to performance measures; they will have to meet standardized reporting measures for specific areas beginning in 2002. JCAHO has approved about 220 different measurement systems on the market for this purpose.

Other accrediting groups are also getting into the patient safety act. The Washington, D.C.–based National Committee for Quality Assurance (NCQA), which accredits health plans, modified its accreditation program to accommodate the need to reduce medical errors and improve patient safety. Initial guidelines for 2001 encourage health plans to establish a high-level team to study and measure the issue of medical errors and make improvements to patient safety.

"This is new territory, so we didn't set ironclad requirements," notes Brian Schilling, an NCQA spokesman, who adds that the agency will phase in expanded requirements in 2002. NCQA-accredited health plans already must meet standards in such related areas as clinical performance, practitioner credentialing, coordination of care, and utilization management.

Worse Before It Gets Better

Things may look worse in the short run as organizations move to a more open reporting culture, warns a legal expert in patient safety. "If you take on the patient safety issue, you have to do so in the public interest and with the recognition that you've been doing some things wrong," asserts William M. Sage, M.D., J.D., an associate professor at Columbia University Law School in New York. "That gets missed in this debate."

Hospital counsel needs to realize that cooperation with a patient safety program may increase the risk of malpractice litigation. "Everyone is saying that we need stronger legal protection if we generate this type of information. But that is starting in the wrong place. It doesn't mean you do stupid things or become passive in putting out information. But you do have to bite the bullet and take the risk. If you get too obsessed with the legal risks, then it is no longer in the public interest but becomes driven by special interests," says Sage. "The same thing can be said for the public relations side. If you look for errors, you will find them. You may look worse in the short run, but people who are involved in patient safety initiatives must be willing to take a few lumps."

Questions Trustees Should Ask Themselves

1. Should improving patient safety be included in the organization's mission statement?
2. Does the organization have an overall approach to patient safety?
3. How can the organization create a culture of safety?
4. Should the organization create a position of chief safety officer in the executive leadership group?
5. What initiatives should the organization immediately undertake to assess how safe its patient care environment is?

Source: First Consulting Group, Long Beach, California.

Raising the Legal Stakes

The legal stakes of increased medical error reporting in general mean that the information an organization digs up can be used by current or potential litigants. "It's a practical risk," says Sage, who agrees with the need for a federal statute that protects the use of information related to medical errors. Passage of such a law is not likely soon, however, Sage acknowledges.

However, once a culture of safety takes hold and reporting becomes integral to a health care system, there's no way to predict whether litigation will rise or fall. "You can't make a projection any more than you can say HMOs will save money. But this is something well worth doing," Sage says.

Focusing solely on quality improvement has unfortunately led to neglecting another issue—compensation for those who have been injured. "If we think about a systems approach to patient safety, then we need to think about a systems approach to compensation for injuries from medical errors. That's a major part of the discussion we're not having," Sage argues, agreeing with the IOM report's conclusion that if the industry moves to no-fault institutional liability—meaning that the institution is to blame and not any individual—then the system should pay for errors.

Transcending Competitive Advantage

Board members may still need to fully realize that they must come to understand the thorny issues surrounding patient safety and provide leadership to address them. A case in point: JCAHO's Loeb recalls that in a show of hands at an important patient safety meeting in Dallas last summer, just a handful of the 700 attendees represented governing boards of health care delivery systems.

"There needs to be awareness of the fact that trustees can provide the leadership for change," he says, noting that patient safety is such an important topic that Premier and Voluntary Hospitals of America, normally two cutthroat competitors, joined forces on the issue last summer. "This is an issue that transcends competitive advantage," says Loeb

Sage believes trustees are both alert and well equipped to provide leadership in patient safety. "For a board member who runs a manufacturing business or works for General Motors, this issue should be immediately appealing. If there is a death on the shop floor, it's a huge deal. These companies are responsible for thousands of lives," he says.

"The bottleneck [to free flow of error reporting] is at the physician level, and it's not the physicians' fault" because the hospital culture and our system of clinical care do not promote such reporting. "The saddest part is that there are relatively few physicians involved in patient safety initiatives," adds Sage. One of the difficult challenges for trustees is that they may not be in the best position to broker between doctors and patient safety advocates because of their traditional distance from the clinical arena and lack of close relationahips with most practicing physicians. The lesson: trustees should get more involved with physicians. One place to start is the quality committee.

Increasing Scrutiny

Health care boards must adopt a broader view of quality that goes beyond the detection and prevention of errors to address the need for the practice of evidence-based medicine. The focus on errors is just the beginning, but the fact that errors exist at all should provide the most important information we need. One fact is clear: Only a nonpunitive environment safe for reporting errors will lead to accurate documentation and eventual elimination of those errors.

Trustees should keep in mind the words Carl Lotus Becker wrote in 1935 in *Progress and Power:* ". . . fact-finding is more effective than fault-finding."

PART EIGHT

Strategic Planning

Putting Your
Financially Based Strategic
Plan into Action

By James E. Grobmyer

When developed within the context of fiscal and operational accountability, strategic plans can detail how an organization will make—rather than spend—money. In fact, the only way for organizations to avoid leaving themselves open to risks is through implementation of a financially based strategic plan.

To ensure the proper development of such a plan, health care organizations should follow seven specific steps.

1. Conduct a Capital Assessment

Before boards and senior managers can begin the planning process, they need to assess the organization's capital position. Because shifting to new products, services, or markets will require an infusion of capital, the budget will define the organization's strategic direction. However, that does not take the cost of capital into consideration. The assessment will point out how much capital the organization needs, but accessing that capital will come at

James E. Grobmyer is president of Grobmyer Associates, St. Petersburg, Florida. He can be reached at (800) 525-3480.

a cost—that is, the opportunity costs of using operating income on one project versus another or through the issuance of bonds, for example.

Properly administered, a capital assessment will answer these questions:

- What is our debt capacity?
- What is our creditworthiness—for example, how does our organization compare with A-rated bond standards?
- How much money do we have available to fund recurring needs (normal capital replacement), new projects, and diversification initiatives?
- How aggressive can we be with new strategic developments based on our past and projected income from operations? Can we absorb new strategy implementation costs and/or fund strategic initiatives until they are profitable?
- Can strategies be funded from operations, or will it be necessary to use foundation monies, raise new money, obtain loans, or issue bonds?
- Can strategies be implemented independently, or will we need to affiliate or select partners to help access capital?

The end product of the capital assessment should be a capital position summary that details for the board the organization's credit analysis, debt capacity, and capital requirements.

2. Conduct an Environmental Assessment

Historically, this is the phase in which strategic planners begin their most substantial work. But this work is often flawed because most strategic plans include a plethora of data that point out changes in primary and secondary markets, patient migration patterns, and payer mix without explaining why these changes are occurring.

The environmental assessment should answer the following questions:

- What specific product lines in the organization are gaining or losing market share?
- Is the organization losing market share because of competition or from such internal causes as too few beds or staff to meet demand, lack of physician support, or high patient dissatisfaction?

- What is the financial impact of changes in volumes, payer mix, or service mix?
- What does the organization need to accomplish in order to reverse declines in profitable service lines?
- What opportunities exist to expand or contract existing service lines?
- What new programs or services are possible?
- What are the competitive strengths and weaknesses that would aid or hinder the organization's ability to expand existing markets or create new ones?

3. Develop Strategic Initiatives

At this point in the process, the strategic plan should look like a laundry list of the most realistic strategies the organization should pursue. In other words, the board and senior management should have an understanding of what strategic opportunities are the most plausible and what capital is available to fund those opportunities.

However, there is still not enough information available to make informed decisions about the final plan. Therefore, organizations should proceed to the next step before identifying the specific strategies needed for each option.

4. Develop a Business Case for Each Strategy

Business case development defines the strategic, operational, and financial assumptions that are required to assess each strategy adequately. As a starting point, the business case should identify how new business will be generated, a conservative estimate of revenue, and operational expenses associated with implementing the strategy. Good business cases also include an in-depth analysis of the following for each project:

- Capital requirements
- Profit margin
- Net present value
- Average payback period
- Weighted cost of capital
- Internal rate of return (used to help evaluate the net present value of competing projects with unequal revenue streams—for example, which strategy contributes to positive cash flow sooner)

In addition, the business case should identify the risk(s) associated with each project. These can be calculated using stand-alone risk, which determines the uncertainty inherent in the project's cash flows; corporate risk, which reflects the project's impact on the organization's total cash flow; and/or market risk.

It's important to remember that the probability for success is not the same for each project. How much risk an organization can, or should, assume depends largely on its capital and market positions, profitability, and the risk profile of other strategies being implemented.

When the board and senior management are evaluating competing strategies, they should base their selections on "asset allocation modeling"—similar to their personal investment strategy—with a healthy mix of high-, medium-, and low-risk projects. Asset allocation is a way to weight investments in a portfolio in order to try to meet a specific objective. For most individual investors, their investment objective is influenced by their age, time frame, and risk-tolerance threshold. Through investment diversification, an investor increases the potential for achieving his/her objectives and actually lowers risk.

When comparing projects, think of them as representing different asset classes, with expansion of existing product lines a low risk, and new lines of business as a higher risk. Of course, the time involved before a strategy becomes profitable also affects its overall risk.

The technique used to evaluate competing projects is not as important as accurate financial modeling. The board should ensure that the organization is equipped with the necessary resources—both technical and human—to conduct this important exercise.

5. Create a Strategy Team

Team members who evaluate each business case and corresponding analysis should include the organization's CEO, CFO, COO, vice president of strategic planning, and trustees. The team's role is to test the validity of assumptions and integrate and prioritize business strategies with the organization's capital and environmental positions.

Whether the strategy team should include physicians depends on the objectivity of your physician leaders and their ability to make decisions for the good of the entire organization. If it is important to the organization to have a physician on the strategy team, the best choice is a board member who has already received board stewardship training and understands the confidential nature of this process.

6. Implement the Plan

Each strategy's implementation should include a team member who can champion the effort by taking responsibility for status updates to the board and senior management as well as troubleshooting when problems arise; identifying changes in assumptions over time; and reporting progress toward meeting the project's strategic, financial, and operational objectives.

For example, if one of the strategies is to increase women's services by starting a breast cancer center, the director of radiology or ob/gyn might be an appropriate strategy leader.

7. Strategic Planning Cautions

While implementing a financially based strategic plan, there are several issues health care organizations should guard against to ensure success:

- *Unrealistic business case assumptions:* Although it's true that no one can predict the future, conservative assumptions about volumes, revenues, and timing are always preferred over aggressive projections. Remember: if a project seems too good to be true, it probably is.
- *Failure to annually reevaluate all business case assumptions and financial projections:* It's ironic that hospital execs and boards make budgets annually, but they typically conduct strategic planning only every three to five years. Financially based strategic planning requires annual reviews of environmental assumptions, internal operations, and the organization's overarching financial position. As situations change, so must the business cases that supported each strategic initiative. For example, if revenue assumptions for expanding an inpatient unit were made prior to the federal Balanced Budget Amendment, the project may look much more favorable than it really would be.

- *An unwillingness to abandon losing strategies:* If dramatic changes in the operating environment have had a negative impact on business case assumptions, organizations should abandon losing strategies. This is difficult for most organizations, because project champions will justify viability by such rationales as meeting a community need or increasing customer awareness of the hospital and its services, which do not take into consideration the impact on capital. The benefit of financially based strategic planning, however, is that it is rooted in numbers and facts. Resources are simply too limited to waste on nonrevenue-producing initiatives, regardless of compelling arguments to the contrary.
- *Lack of modeling rigor:* Some organizations do not have the resources to model and analyze the financial implications of each strategic initiative. If adequate financial modeling expertise and decision support are not available internally, there are numerous consulting firms that can guide an organization through this process.
- *Lack of buy-in from top leadership:* The planning process can be subverted if leaders do not adhere to the same kind of analysis for each strategy.
- *Failure to maintain a commitment to the plan during financial downturns:* Although it's easy to shy away from initiatives that require financial outlays during times of financial stress, leaders that do so are setting themselves up for even more financial problems—they will continue the negative revenue spiral by underfunding future sources of revenue.

Even though implementing a financially based strategic plan means adding a layer of complexity to an already complex process, hospital boards that do so will be better stewards of their respective organization's assets.

The Challenge
of Financially Based
Strategic Planning

By James E. Grobmyer

Most hospitals have strategic plans. In fact, many have standing or ad hoc strategic planning committees of the board, which at first blush implies that the strategic process and subsequent document receive the greatest attention. Yet despite significant effort spent on their development, most hospital strategic plans are critically flawed.

The reason is straightforward: they are not developed within the context of fiscal or operational accountability. Typically, strategic plans are created without the analysis or data required to truly guide an organization's future.

What's Wrong with Strategic Planning?

Strategic planning is often conducted in isolation, without the necessary fiscal checks and balances. Despite the appearance of inclusiveness—that is, the involvement of "interdisciplinary" committees with support from a myriad of survey data and research—the right

James E. Grobmyer is president of Grobmyer Associates, St. Petersburg, Florida. He can be reached at (800) 525-3480.

people aren't at the planning table and the right questions aren't being asked. Such questions include:

- How much is this plan costing us?
- What returns are we getting on our investment?
- Can we afford to implement this plan?

Hospitals get into trouble when they don't quantify their strategic direction. Chief financial officers and vice presidents of strategic planning speak different languages and often have different objectives. For example, many CFOs have been trying to cut costs at the same time strategic planners have been developing programs to generate business. If one believes you need to spend money to make money, the reason for the disconnect is readily apparent.

This disconnect can be traced to the highest level in the organization—the board of trustees. Many boards have finance committees and strategic planning committees that view their roles as separate and distinct when, in fact, they should be working together as stewards of the organization's capital.

It is common for strategic planning committees to focus externally on the organization's market and competitors. While that's a good starting point, organizations also need to integrate that information into their financial position, their operating realities, and their risk/return threshold.

Failure to integrate these concepts may result in a strategic plan that emphasizes market share, community needs, brand positioning, and mission effectiveness but stops short of determining what the organization needs to be doing today to remain fiscally viable. Current resources are too limited to invest in strategies that aren't expected to provide a reasonable return.

A New View of Strategic Planning

A properly developed strategic plan should describe how an organization is going to make money rather than how it is going to spend it. This is a philosophical shift that not-for-profit strategic planners have to make.

A good example was the strategy of the not-too-distant past when health care organizations raced to become integrated delivery systems, requiring expensive information system investment, physician practice purchase, managed care plan development, and so on.

The rationale for integration was to increase market share and gain control by owning all elements along the health care continuum. The problem, however, was that in many instances this strategy was an end that did not justify the means—the incremental revenues from offering a full spectrum of health care services didn't cover the expenses of integration.

A number of organizations didn't recover from failed integration and went broke, whereas others have spent the past several years divesting themselves of the very entities they originally sought to own. Had those organizations viewed their integration strategy from the perspective of how it was going to make money, they would have quickly seen that the expenses involved far outweighed the potential revenues (see the chart below).

The strategic plan and capital plan are synergistic. That is, an organization's strategy will depend on how much capital it has available.

The board should initiate the strategic planning process by first developing a realistic picture of the organization's capital position, which is a direct outgrowth of the prior year's financial performance. This is another reason why the finance and strategic planning committees need to work hand-in-hand.

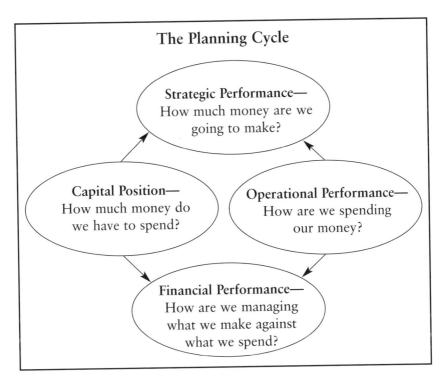

In some instances, boards should have significant overlap between these two committees. In others, they should do away with a separate strategic planning committee altogether and make strategy development a full board activity.

A strategic plan should explain how an organization is going to allocate resources and what return it expects on its investment. Just like the budgeting process, strategic plans should be reviewed and adjusted annually.

In today's environment, organizations cannot conduct strategic planning every three years or so. Even plans with multiple-year projects need to be revisited annually and the assumptions that factored into the original planning updated. The direction of the strategic plan will depend on the organization's past financial performance and corresponding capital position (see below). If the bottom line is healthy, more risks can be taken. Conversely, if the organization is facing a cash crunch, the board needs to "stick to its knitting."

Strategic Strategies			
Financial Performance*	Risk Threshold	Strategic Plan Mode	Typical Strategies
<3% operating margin	Low risk	Preservation mode	• Protect market share • "Stick to your knitting"—Concentrate on existing "cash cows"/ profitable product lines • Use extreme caution and rigor when deploying strategies that expend capital • Divest money losers
>3% operating margin	Moderate to higher risk	Growth mode	• Expand market share • Pump up under-performing product lines that have potential • Develop new programs/ product lines • Divest money losers

*Average adequate operating margins will vary, depending on the size of the hospital.

The Risks of Failing to Do Financially Based Strategic Planning

Organizations that don't conduct financially based strategic planning leave themselves open to several risks:

- Development of a plan they can't afford to implement. It is common in turnaround situations to discover that the organization did not understand the long-term impact of its strategy on its cash flow. Hospitals that drain cash without adequate "restocking" will quickly get into trouble.
- Financial failure. Hospitals that do not embrace financially based strategic planning aren't as successful as those that do because they don't have a way to demand accountability for performance. In these organizations, completing the deal or implementing the strategy becomes the end game, rather than holding executives accountable for the deal's financial success.
- Missed opportunities to establish priorities for competing projects based on sound financial projections. Setting priorities on projects can end up becoming a popularity contest when it should be based on quantifiable financial variables, such as the project's internal rate of return, payback period, and future earnings. Comparing financial projections to actual results also gives board members and executives an unbiased way to evaluate the success or failure of each strategy. That way, intangible or political reasons for strategic initiatives, such as increasing community awareness or eliminating competition, become secondary to the strategy's profitability and sustainability.
- Supporting losing strategies. Sometimes hospitals continue to support a financially failing project because they don't have the data to evaluate it and therefore don't know it's failing. That's why it's so important to include financial and operational projections and assumptions for each strategy and agree up front that those will be the benchmarks by which the project will be measured.
- Weakened competitive position. We frequently see organizations having knee-jerk reactions to competition because they do not have a clear, objective way to evaluate a competitor's actions, nor can they point to their own strategies with any confidence of their staying power.

Despite adding another layer to an already complex process, hospital boards that embrace financially based strategic planning will be better stewards of their organization's assets, and the organizations will ultimately sustain long-term financial health.

Strategic Planning and the Board: The Responsibility to Plan the Future

By Dan Beckham

A health care board has three primary responsibilities: financial oversight, hiring and evaluating the CEO, and strategic planning. The discipline of strategic planning and the trustee's role relative to it are less defined and understood than the first two responsibilities. Although nearly every not-for-profit board will have committees dedicated to finance and executive evaluation, it is much less likely that it will have a strategic planning committee. And when it does, that committee's role may be ambiguous.

Strategic planning involves the allocation of scarce resources to a hospital's best opportunities. It is a process whose output defines what those best opportunities are and how to pursue them. For an analogy, think of making bread: The plan is the bread. The strategic planning process is the act of combining ingredients, letting the dough rise, setting the correct temperature in the oven, and baking the bread. The organization's CEO is the baker. And the trustees own the bakery.

Dan Beckham is president of The Beckham Company, Whitefish Bay, Wisconsin. He can be reached at (414) 963–8935.

Strategic plans take many shapes, but the best share these key characteristics:

- They are focused. There is one mission, one vision, and a handful of driving strategies.
- They enjoy wide ownership among key stakeholders.
- They embody solid strategies based on sound principles.
- They can be implemented and monitored effectively.
- They are well communicated and understood throughout the organization.

What Is the Role of the Board and the CEO?

The board chair or the vice chair should lead the strategic planning committee. As the organization's primary strategist, the CEO should ensure the development of strategic direction and, through leadership of the management team, drive effective implementation. The CEO is responsible for setting forth issues and making recommendations relevant to strategic direction. Indeed, a responsible board will demand that its CEO assume this role.

When it comes to strategic planning, CEOs should participate on the committee as leaders, educators, and challengers. But they can't play these roles and at the same time also chair the strategic planning committee. Leading the committee requires a level of neutrality, but CEOs are usually too close to the action to be viewed as neutral. On the other hand, a board chair, who understands how to keep members focused, balanced, and moving ahead, is probably well positioned to lead an effective strategic planning committee. Vice chairs can also play this role, and the experience often provides valuable experience for moving into the chair position.

Trustee involvement, perspective, and guidance are key to the integrity of a strategic planning process in a not-for-profit organization. Communities are a fabric woven from interrelationships, and many trustees are well woven into that fabric. They often sense changes in community dynamics long before anyone else in the hospital does. Generally, trustees are visible and respected members of their communities. Some bring Fortune 500 corporate experience, some understand the regional retail environment extremely well, and others are connected through a multitude of service or social organizations.

A hospital is, at its core, a service organization but one with many of the same challenges that face trustees who run local banks and manufacturing plants. Because many board members believe that their experiences and perspectives are not relevant to the health care environment, they remain quiet. When they do, they eliminate a rich source of insight. Many health care organizations are starved for ideas and perspectives outside health care. Absent such perspectives, health care professionals often become insular and increasingly parochial. Assertive trustees can inject their varied experiences into strategic planning discussions, helping to create an environment for innovative thinking.

Trustees should not hesitate to offer intuitive ideas that lack quantitative validation. Some of the most important variables in a marketplace may be difficult, perhaps even impossible, to quantify.

It is appropriate for board members to act as a devil's advocate by challenging the CEO, and they should feel comfortable doing so. The CEO, in turn, should also be willing to participate in healthy give-and-take with the board. Every assumption should be challenged; every recommendation should be tested against alternatives.

It's the board's responsibility to put the strategic plan through a rigorous test. During the 1990s, cookie-cutter strategies were widely adopted by many hospitals and health systems. Some typical results included the cobbling together of large hospital systems, massive discounts for health plans, and thousands of physicians being placed on the payroll. The cost of those decisions, which often failed, can be measured in billions of dollars.

Who Should Be on the Planning Committee?

An appropriate mix of participants on the strategic planning committee might include:

- Four nonphysician trustees
- Three to four physicians (who may or may not be trustees)
- Up to five members of executive management (including the CEO, who serves as a voting member)

Physicians should be represented on every critical committee of the hospital board as voting members, and they certainly should be represented on the strategic planning committee. The work they do as well as their relationships with patients, other physicians, and nurses is so central that no hospital can afford not to have their perspective well represented. Some boards choose to avoid or limit the number of physician trustees on the committee because of concerns about conflict of interest. In truth, physicians usually have no more conflicts of interest than do any members of the management team. And no one else can bring the physician's perspective to the strategic conversation.

Of course, it's important to remember that the physician perspective is not monolithic. Physician attitudes vary widely based on age, specialty, and practice situation. Care should be taken to include both specialists and primary care doctors. Furthermore, the committee needs the perspectives of community-based physicians and hospital-based doctors (for example, pathologists and radiologists) as well as a balance of younger and older physicians.

In addition to the CEO, other executive management team members who should be included on the strategic planning committee include the chief financial officer, the chief operating officer, the chief nursing officer, and the chief marketing officer. Each of these managers generally should participate on an ex officio basis.

When it comes to the selection of members for the strategic planning committee, a mix of financial, operations, marketing, and community experience is desirable. Although physicians may embody this experience, their greatest value derives from their involvement in clinical affairs and medical staff relationships. In our experience, a healthy mix of experience and perspective makes for a dynamic, balanced, and productive committee.

The strategic planning committee has important work to do, and it must comprise people who are committed to making progress and obtaining results through productive give and take. The chair of the strategic planning committee in consultation with the president of the medical staff and the CEO should select the committee members. The board chair should appoint the planning committee chair.

What Takes Place Inside and Outside the Committee?

Ultimately, the strategic plan must be a group effort. That's why group dynamics are important. The strategic planning committee, when working properly, becomes a cohesive group. Critical issues, the substance of a vision statement, and the evaluation of strategic options all result from intensive conversations in which participants roll up their sleeves and speak not only from the head but also from the heart.

Because such candor can make strategic planning committee members feel vulnerable, it's important to keep the specific content of those conversations within the committee. Absent the context of the conversations, outsiders who were not at the planning meetings can easily misconstrue a statement or give it more emphasis than it deserves. Members of the strategic planning committee can also feel betrayed if they learn that their statements have been shared outside committee sessions. Such perceived betrayal can have a deadening effect on the honesty and candor of the committee's subsequent strategic conversations. Further, members of a strategic planning committee are unlikely to "own" conversations or decisions in which they didn't participate. Ad hoc deliberations that splinter off from the committee as a whole can be viewed as attempts to unfairly influence and manipulate outcomes. So deliberations should be limited to the committee as a whole.

The emerging strategic plan should be shared regularly with stakeholders outside the committee, particularly physicians and managers. There are good reasons for this: The perception of "smoke-filled rooms" can make nonparticipants suspicious and undermine the planning process. That's why committee members should be encouraged to test key aspects of the emerging plan with others outside the committee's planning sessions. These conversations can be helpful in developing ideas and initiatives that may have received insufficient attention during committee sessions. And such discussions also provide an opportunity to float ideas as trial balloons.

As consultants, we design "update sessions" into the process so that at important points representatives of the strategic planning committee can share progress with key stakeholders (for example, other board members, physicians, and managers) for feedback. This constructive feedback can then be used in subsequent strategic planning committee deliberations. The result is a strategic plan stakeholders are more likely to support because of the opportunities they've had to contribute to it.

Strategic planning committee members and the CEO should also hold one-on-one conversations. Such conversations may allow the CEO to give the committee a deeper explanation of critical issues, or they may give experienced trustees an opportunity to mentor their CEO on strategic questions.

What Kind of Education Do Planning Committee Members Need?

The workings of a modern hospital are confusing and intimidating to many trustees. With good reason, management expert Peter Drucker has called the American hospital the most complex of all enterprises. Hospital language can be overwhelmingly arcane and esoteric. The interrelationships of people who work in the hospital are complex. The politics are tortured. That's why management should clearly explain topics where language, technology, and complexity may stun lay board members into silence. The technical language of hospitals and medicine can become a significant barrier toward understanding strategic issues and the subsequent development of strategic direction. Trustees who don't understand a critical issue should speak up and request an explanation in plain English.

Physician trustees can also be baffled by management topics. Most physicians have had little management training, and its language can be as befuddling to them as a discussion of diagnostic techniques might be for nonphysicians. Without some education and rationale, physicians may simply check out of conversations they don't understand or reject them as irrelevant to what they (and the hospital) do. Physicians, of course, can be equally baffling in their use of technical language and jargon. Because management operates at the interface of medicine and governance, it's incumbent upon the executive staff to serve as active translators and to anticipate when explanations are likely to be necessary.

Ongoing board education is critical to building the comfort and knowledge of trustees, but such education cannot be expected to deal comprehensively with all the barriers to participation that language creates. Only a sensitive CEO and assertive trustees can address this challenge effectively by dealing with it continuously.

Experienced trustees may find it appropriate to conduct some education on their own to help enrich the strategic planning process. For example, one trustee invited the hospital's executives and physician leaders to tour one of his factories to get a better sense of how he had applied advanced management techniques to manufacturing. Another trustee, whose company had engaged one of the country's top business strategists to help with corporate planning, invited this expert to address fellow hospital trustees, the hospital's management team, and the medical staff—with powerful results.

Likewise, some medical staffs have offered to let lay trustees "shadow" them in their offices, in the operating room, and in the emergency department. (See "If You Knew What I Know," in the April 1996 issue of *Trustee*. The article can be accessed from our Web site's archives at www.trusteemag.com.) Such shadowing programs allow lay trustees to move more quickly up the learning curve while simultaneously creating valuable levels of empathy and comradery.

How Do You Conduct Strategic Planning?

Despite the wide variety of approaches to developing a strategic plan, they invariably start with a strategic assessment of the organization. This assessment comes from analyzing available data, such as that describing financial performance and market share. These quantitative data are then combined with qualitative information derived from personal interviews with people who have a meaningful perspective on the hospital and those it serves. This assessment provides the basis for strategy development.

When we conduct strategic planning sessions, they typically last four hours and are held on weekday evenings. Weekends are tough times to give up, and mornings usually represent time physicians dedicate to surgery and hospital rounds. The rest of the day is dedicated to office hours and patients. Meetings should be agenda driven but with a major portion of each session dedicated to disciplined discussion. There may be four to six of these sessions throughout the process. As much as possible, each meeting should end with a tangible result. The following is a typical sequence and subsequent results of the strategic planning process we have employed:

- *Kickoff:* Explain project process, timing, and roles.
- *Issues:* A situation assessment, which has been distributed in advance, forms the basis for committee members to identify critical strategic issues.
- *Vision:* A preliminary vision statement is developed, reviewed, refined, and tentatively approved.

- *Strategic direction:* Within the context of the strategic issues and the vision, the committee recommends, evaluates, refines, and approves a set of driving strategies.
- *Implementation:* Preliminary tactical action plans are developed and approved. The committee determines mechanisms for monitoring, measuring, and adjusting the strategic plan.

As suggested previously, we highly recommend that the strategic planning committee make interim reports to key stakeholders, such as the medical and nursing staff, during the development of the plan. Preliminary thinking can thus be tested and feedback provided for consideration. Such interim reporting, combined with earnest efforts to incorporate the feedback, will contribute immeasurably to the quality of ownership stakeholders have in the final plan.

On average, the strategic planning processes we have facilitated lasted about four to six months. This may seem like a long time, but it is about the minimum necessary to effectively collect information, develop an assessment, and conduct planning sessions. Taking this time gives people a chance to digest elements of the plan and react. It also provides time for the process to demonstrate its integrity. Building trust is a critical by-product to a solid strategic planning process.

The chair of the strategic planning committee, in consultation with the CEO, should decide whether to engage a consultant to help develop the strategic plan. A consultant can play at least eight key roles:

1. Design the process
2. Facilitate the meetings
3. Provide education (particularly related to principles of strategy)
4. Conduct personal interviews with key stakeholders, including physicians, managers, trustees, and community leaders
5. Review and interpret data
6. Make recommendations
7. Challenge accepted thinking
8. Maintain neutrality

The consultant should serve as a complementary adjunct to the CEO's role as chief strategist. Like trustee leadership within the strategic planning committee, involving a good consultant can free up the CEO to more actively participate and drive strategy development. And, typically, an outside consultant will be free of any vested interests.

Organizations that successfully undertake their own strategic planning process without a consultant typically rely on an internal staff member to fill the roles described above. The choice to hire a consultant may rest on the critical determination of whether an internal staff member exists who can credibly assume a neutral role in strategic planning.

What Are the Pitfalls?

There are many pitfalls to avoid in pursuing a meaningful strategic planning process. The following four are the most deadly:

- *Internal focus.* An organization that has suffered mismanagement or internal strife may understandably focus its attention inward, but the planning committee and the CEO must recognize that the most important influences on the organization's future lie outside its walls. Although the first priority set forth in a strategic plan may rightly be "to improve budgeting," no patient is going to pay a penny for a hospital's budget. Patients buy results, and if competitors are doing a better job delivering those results, the marketplace will leave the internally focused hospital behind.
- *Politics as usual.* An entrenched power structure that is already viewed with suspicion by physicians and staff will do nothing to alleviate those suspicions by anointing itself as the strategic planning committee. That's why it's important to reflect a balance of perspectives and interests in the committee's composition.
- *Wasting people's time.* It should not take three four-hour meetings to develop a vision statement. Although the most tolerant participants in the planning process may indulge such use of their time, others will quickly write off the process as unproductive. (This will prove particularly true with physicians.) The committee chair must tell members who tend toward long-windedness when it's time to move on. But there is a fine line between making steady progress and making people feel as if they're being rushed through critical decisions. The chair must walk this line.

- *Nitpicking and wallowing in detail.* Strategic planning is something you do from 30,000 feet, not 30. Much time can be wasted debating decimal points. In the long run, it's not going to matter if one of the market share projections is off by a half of a percent. Those who find data errors should be thanked for their vigilance. Then the process should push ahead.

Besides being sensitive to them, the committee chair can often avoid these pitfalls by setting some ground rules at the onset—look outside the organization; involve key stakeholders; enforce a five-minute speaking rule; and don't nitpick.

How Do We Move to Implementation?

When it's time to move the strategic plan out of committee to the full board for approval, it makes sense to "run it up the flagpole" a couple of times to make sure it will be saluted. A presentation to the medical staff is critical. Feedback should be invited and noted. Do the same thing with the hospital's management team, including nursing leadership. If a diligent effort has been made during the development of the plan to share it, there should not be many surprises in terms of feedback.

Generally, it's best for someone from the strategic planning committee or the CEO to make these presentations. A consultant should speak only following introductions by the committee chair and/or the CEO. It can be particularly powerful when several members of the planning committee make a joint presentation.

During and after developing the strategic plan, communication is key. Once the plan is tested and approved by the full board, every member of the strategic planning committee should be comfortable advocating it.

Communication should also extend beyond the organization to community groups, such as the Rotary Club and the chamber of commerce. To facilitate this, a scripted audiovisual presentation should be developed and provided to each member of the strategic planning committee. Brochures describing the plan should also be distributed to community groups.

The role of the strategic planning committee and the board obviously doesn't end with board approval and communication. Trustees should be "enforcers" of the strategic plan. We know trustees who carry a copy of the plan to every board meeting and other critical sessions to help ensure that the plan aligns with initiatives managers and medical staff leaders suggest.

The board is responsible for monitoring effective implementation of the strategic plan and for requesting modifications when performance lags. Indeed, the best strategic planning processes are not isolated events that occur every few years, but are designed to be continuously updated. While mission and values are usually regarded as immutable, a vision and strategies must change with the times.

Once a strategy is substantially accomplished, it should be replaced. If a strategy appears to be off target, the mistake should be acknowledged and a new strategy developed. As the environment changes, so should your strategies. Management should apprise the board of significant changes in the environment, and the CEO should recommend modifications where appropriate.

Every board agenda should include an update on the strategic plan. And every critical capital decision should be made in the context of the strategic plan. It's the board's job to ensure that all major decisions embody such strategic integrity.

Strategic Planning: Going Beyond the Basics

By Stuart Friedman
and Andrew Draper

As trustees and executives search for answers to hospital financial problems, many are enticed to return to the simplicity of the past. But for many hospitals and systems, a realistic and sustainable solution requires a more careful assessment of the organizational strategy and the organization itself. A majority of hospitals' fiscal troubles are directly attributable to the following fundamental changes in the operating environment:

- *Declining reimbursement.* The Balanced Budget Act of 1997 and subsequent amendments have substantially reduced total reimbursement for most institutions. Recent "give-backs" have softened the blow, but the impact is still significant. Furthermore, managed care rates are moving closer toward Medicare reimbursement rates in many markets after a decade of forming the price floor.
- *Cost escalation.* In 1999, it was Y2K. In 2000 and 2001, it is HIPAA. At a time when customers are demanding lower costs,

Stuart Friedman is vice president and partner, and Andrew Draper is a consultant, at Tiber Group, a Chicago-based health care industry management consulting firm. They can be reached at (312) 609-9900.

most hospitals continue to face significant operating cost inflation. Recent initiatives, such as the Institute of Medicine's report on medical errors and the formation of The Leapfrog Group by leading employers, will continue to press providers to make substantial technology investments.

- *New competition.* Thwarted by declining physician incomes, deregulation, and access to new capital markets, traditional providers are facing unprecedented competition from physicians and new market entrants such as HealthSouth (surgery centers) and MedCath (heart hospitals). In the long term, biotechnology firms will displace traditional inpatient care; and Internet firms will look to take the mantle of "health status manager" from health systems.
- *The fall of the gatekeeper.* Hospitals aggressively formed integrated delivery networks (IDNs) in the 1990s on the assumption that health plans would use capitation for regional systems and that the primary care physician would serve as the system's fulcrum. As a result, health systems expended substantial energy to control managed care enrollees, particularly through acquiring physician practices and creating a full continuum of care. But over the last several years, consumers, employers, insurers, and even regulators have dismantled this approach in favor of patient freedom of choice.
- *More demanding and informed consumers.* Changing demographics, greater access to information, and increasing consumer cost concerns through employer cost sharing have combined to create more demanding consumers. As in other industries that have seen this shift (e.g., banking), the basis for competition is increasingly focused on superior services. Enabled by greater choice, patients will seek the providers that best meet their needs rather than passively accepting health care decisions.

Why the Downturn?

As a result of these environmental phenomena, health care organizations pursued an unprecedented number of new strategies in the 1990s and entered a variety of nontraditional businesses. At the same time, all segments of the health care industry became more competitive, and patients rejected "one-stop shopping"—a key to IDNs.

For some systems, this strategy may not have been overly ambitious, but their situation was plagued by ineffective implementation. In many cases the integration strategies of the 1990s were adopted with:

- The wrong intentions (more control instead of "a better mousetrap")
- Minimal attention to the details of how products would be integrated
- Minimal management expertise in new business lines
- Vague and inappropriate long-term evaluative criteria
- Limited implementation accountability

Taken in isolation, these issues set the stage for inaction and poor results. Exacerbating the situation, these integration activities created a complex maze of organizations, relationships, and incentives that demanded substantial management competencies and capital resources. Worse yet, in their efforts to build the best full-service system with limited capital and management, systems often underinvested in their core product—the hospital.

Fallout from failed strategy and implementation, combined with environmental changes, has been widespread. Hospital financial performance is at its lowest level in recent history. Last year, bond downgrades by Moody's exceeded upgrades by a ratio of 38 to 2, and median hospital operating margins decreased to 0.51% in 1999—the lowest ever.

Return to Fundamentals

For many organizations, the natural response to recent difficulties is a return to their core services. This often includes:

- Rebuilding employee morale and operational efficiency
- Shedding new businesses, such as physician practices or managed care companies
- Refocusing on limited geographic markets
- Dismantling various hospital and physician joint ventures

A return to fundamentals is critical. Under any environmental conditions, a focused and disciplined organization will be well positioned to deliver a strong product. Furthermore, it appeals to physicians, clinical staff, management teams, and sponsors in its simplicity, straightforwardness, and consistency with historical legacy and intended community roles.

However, real and anticipated changes in the marketplace precipitated both the move toward vertical integration and the backlash push for fundamentals. Those same factors also suggest that, for many organizations, a back-to-basics approach will not be sufficient. Consider the following implications.

Case Study #1

The Situation:

A fully integrated health system based in a small city is experiencing a substantial postmerger financial decline.

Analysis Results:

- Contrary to reported financial statements, losses were attributable to poor health plan performance and physician productivity and turnover.
- Tremendous hospital overcapacity and price competition limited the benefits of owning a managed care organization.
- The employed group of physicians remained the only positive point of differentiation in a crowded market but at the cost of independent physician relationships.
- Ultimately, the merger strategy was valid but implementation was ineffective.

The Transformation Plan:

- Deemphasize health plan strategy; turn the operations around or divest.
- Divest underperforming physician departments, energize the remaining doctors, and gain the respect of independent doctors in the community.
- Focus the hospital on core services.

Results:

- Reduced size, role, and losses of the health plan
- Improved morale and financial performance among employed physicians
- Increased independent physician volume in selected services

As the industry matures and competition increases, growth opportunities will be precious and required for future reinvestment. For some systems, the wholesale dismantling associated with a back-to-basics approach may inadvertently and unalterably compromise potential sources of growth. Examples of these lost opportunities include wholesale divestiture of employed physicians, abandonment of underperforming regional satellites, and dismantling of strategically valuable partnerships.

As consumers and employers raise the bar on quality and patient satisfaction, the level of care that was delivered in the past will not suffice. Calls for outcomes measurement and enhancement will increase. Breakthroughs in clinical and information technology will emerge. And the drive for more efficient communication and faster, more accurate diagnoses (ironically, the promise of integrated care) will increase.

Increased demand for customized products and service amenities that improve patients' psychosocial health care experience will add to hospitals' challenges and opportunities. Women's health, cancer, and orthopedic programs are already finding that their "core business" must include traditionally unconventional services, such as over-the-counter products (for example, those for skin care) and complementary therapies.

Scale will finally become an advantage. As costs and required investments rise, as reimbursement remains flat, and as hospitals become smaller, economics will once again drive consolidation. More important, economies of expertise and a more active and free purchaser will once again favor those organizations that possess and leverage higher volumes. This will not necessarily mean the return of the medical center franchise on tertiary care. Instead, it will drive clinical collaboration among hospitals and the use of technology, such as telemedicine, in a way that will concurrently increase access with scale.

As a result of misguided investments and poor operating performance, balance sheets are weaker than in previous eras. Furthermore, there is growing sentiment that the provider sector lacks capable management for the changing skill set, whereas start-ups and e-commerce entice a younger generation. In addition, such long-standing issues as the nursing shortage will not be easily reversed.

Case Study #2

The Situation:

The entrance of single-specialty inpatient and outpatient centers has an increasingly negative effect on an urban, tertiary medical center located in a traditional two-hospital market.

Analysis Results:

- Its historic strategy of becoming the market leader is unrealistic given the medical center's limited access to a key managed care contract in the near term, but it's a sustainable position nonetheless.
- There is minimal hospital differentiation other than the carve-outs. Both the medical center and its competitor provide a full array of services.
- Financial woes in several service lines are exposed by substantial declines in open-heart surgery volume.
- Physicians are seeking carve-outs in other profitable service lines.
- The medical center has minimal access to outside capital.

The Transformation Plan:

- Shift away from full-service mentality. Make service line divestitures and strategic partnerships in underperforming products to cut losses and free up capital.
- Make substantial investment in two to three key programs.
- Joint venture with the key single-specialty physician group in the market.
- Develop a branding strategy to begin differentiation, and gain access to more managed care lives.

Results:

- Gradual improvement in medical center profitability
- Successful partnership with a large physician specialty group
- Significantly improved employee morale

Strategic focus will be essential. As performance expectations rise, resources remain limited, and scale becomes critical, it will be virtually impossible for most institutions to continue to provide all services to all people at a level of quality acceptable to the market. Systems will need to reevaluate underperforming services in order to sustain their success in more profitable niches.

"In today's environment of declining revenues, the importance of strong operational execution cannot be overstated," says John Lucas, M.D., CEO of St. Vincent's Hospital in Santa Fe and a former trustee of St. Louis–based Ascension Health. "At the least, a hospital's clinical and administrative operations must be the most efficient in the market. However, delivering the right mix of services to meet financial targets and focus execution efforts is equally important. It is helpful if the entire organization is structured so that operational resources can be focused on and maximized."

A return to fundamentals will no doubt help pave the way to bottom-line improvement in the short term. But long-term success will require active resolution of more strategic issues. Ultimately, three key questions will help illuminate the best path: Why did we fail? What alternatives still exist? How do we implement them?

Why Did We Fail?

Transformation begins with understanding the reasons for recent problems. First, diagnose the source of poor performance. For some organizations, poor performance is often related to macrolevel issues such as corporate culture or accountability. For others, the issues are more limited. An assessment along the vertical continuum will reveal problems in businesses, such as physician practices and managed care, as well as test the strategic value of investments. A horizontal assessment turns the organization on its side, isolating the performance, requirements, and contribution of the service line portfolio.

Second, check your relevancy in the market. In a changing environment, the role of the hospital and the ability to sustain its services should change, particularly when the market rewards superiority. A candid assessment of market capacity, competitors' positioning, and the role of your institution will provide a foundation for future direction.

Isolate bad strategy from bad implementation. The result of these analyses will shed light on what worked, what failed, and why. This helps focus the strategic planning discussion on "what's next?" Which investments, wise in their time, are now unproductive? What initiatives deserve more patience and discipline? This analysis often leads to a more enlightened and realistic view of the organization. Some key market scenarios might include these:

- A health plan that had been responsible for historical system growth begins to inappropriately drive health system strategy and substantially weaken the system's provider component.
- The source of problems for a traditionally strong "brand name" hospital is not due, as historically believed, to access to managed care enrollees but to an undifferentiated product that consumers no longer demand.
- Financial losses for a health system's employed physicians are falsely attributed to macrolevel cultural issues driven mainly by a number of underperforming departments. In fact, the group is the hospital's greatest asset. Rather than full divestiture, a right-sizing is in order.
- The loss of open-heart market share to a carve-out firm exposes a variety of historically unprofitable service lines that are the real cause of organizational deficiencies.
- A series of ineffective tactical decisions in several service line joint ventures leaves the hospital with limited core strengths and poor physician loyalty in an oversupplied market. A fundamental reassessment of future viability is needed.

What Alternatives Still Exist?

Test your options. Depending on the degree of market evolution and the nature of current issues, patience and discipline to "stay the course" may be a viable option. More likely, some directional changes in composition and focus will be in order. In some organizations, the remaining strengths may not provide a sufficient foundation to rebuild the organization.

"Our system [hospital, health plan, and multispecialty clinic] was at the point where we needed to restructure our strategic direction to improve financial performance," says Gary Kaatz, president and

CEO of Rockford (Illinois) Health System. "We knew that working harder on execution alone was not going to substantially improve our position in the market. Therefore, restructuring and analysis enabled us to better understand and manage our relationships in the community, particularly with physicians. Additionally, the process has reenergized the board's focus with accountable results."

Define an achievable vision. Where does the organization want to be? What role is desired? How important and viable is the current sponsorship model (for example, independence, system participation, joint operating agreements)? The board's wisdom and leadership will be challenged by a sober assessment of these difficult questions.

Face up to the tough choices and challenges. As many have learned, the market no longer tolerates avoiding or rationalizing conflict. The role of underperforming "loss leader" programs must be resolved. "Squeaky wheel" physicians or management staff must be confronted or co-opted. Discipline will prove to be an organizational competency that could make all the difference to success.

How Do We Implement Our Strategy This Time?

In many cases, strong implementation of the wrong strategy might still outperform the poorly executed perfect strategy. In fact, a strategy isn't valid unless you can implement it. The sources of poor execution are varied but start with complexity, management depth, and accountability. It helps if key stakeholders can embrace the system's direction enthusiastically.

Prioritization is a key to success. Organizations must consider the market urgency, required resources, and key interdependencies linked to desired actions. Particularly when trying to regain credibility with physicians, some "quick wins" might lay the groundwork for more difficult and contentious challenges ahead.

To the extent that resources are limited and/or urgent action is needed on several fronts, organizations should test potential alliances. In many cases, multiple, small, targeted alliances can outperform the broader affiliations of the past. They can add capital, a specific clinical or management expertise, or the chance to adopt new technologies early on.

Management accountability must also be in place. Boards must hold their teams to tangible and quantifiable targets and use incentives and sanctions where necessary. At the same time, trustees will need to loyally support management when inevitable staff and physician resistance is encountered. In fact, accountability begins with management and trustees setting the example.

The New Legacy

The integrated delivery network was often an easy sell to trustees because it was positive and optimistic and had a very desirable end point. The nature of the new strategic transformation process will be much different. For example:

- It may be less optimistic.
- It might make the organization smaller in the near term.
- It will be difficult to execute.
- It will upset at least one sacred cow and key constituency.
- It will be risky.

This process may be more than what the typical voluntary hospital board bargained for, and at face value these strategies may be less dramatic and ambitious than previous board initiatives. However, the fact that they will address strategic problems and help the hospital fulfill its mission should energize the board.

Management should be able to execute the back-to-basics turnaround. They must be held accountable to measurable results. The board must plot the future course of the organization. The new legacy is creating meaningful and sustainable change that will fulfill the continuing mission.

Is Strategic Planning Relevant Anymore?

By Alan M. Zuckerman

Many executives and trustees have said they no longer believe that strategic planning in the health care industry is relevant or useful. They argue that:

- The dizzying pace of change makes long-range planning an all-but-outmoded concept.
- The foreseeable future is now, at most, 12 to 18 months versus the 5 to 10 years it used to be—an inadequate time frame for strategic planning.
- Many of today's health care systems are so large that conducting participative strategic planning is too cumbersome and slow and will fall apart from its own weight before it produces any positive results.
- The number and diversity of opportunities available to health care organizations are so great that the real planning challenge is how to sort through these opportunities on a day-to-day basis.

Alan M. Zuckerman is director of Health Strategies & Solutions, Inc., Philadelphia. He can be reached at (215) 636-3500, ext. 106.

- Focused planning, on product lines for example, is more appropriate for systems because it is tangible, manageable, and more easily implemented.

All of these arguments seem plausible on the surface, but it is precisely because of our dynamic environment that strategic planning is more relevant now than ever. How can leaders sort through issues and problems outside the strategic context of mission, vision, and values? How can the health care organization of today be proactive if its leaders don't clearly understand where their organization is going?

Perhaps some of the confusion about the current relevance of strategic planning is due to an outdated notion of what strategic planning is and how it should be conducted. Some of the main differences between the old process and the newer process are described more fully below.

Old versus New

There are seven major differences between the way yesterday's and today's health care organizations practice the strategic planning process:

1. *Assumptions about the future.* In the old strategic planning process, one visualizes a future state and builds strategies around this perspective. In the new process, one develops a number of potential scenarios, recognizing that the future is hardly clear and that diverse scenarios are possible.

   These multiple scenarios are used by the board and management to develop a composite future scenario, either by estimating the probable likelihood of each or by determining common elements or underlying factors that are then combined into one scenario. Contingency planning may also be used to account for potentially diverse futures.

2. *Forecasting methods.* Old strategic planning almost exclusively employs linear extrapolation to project future conditions. New strategic planning may include linear extrapolation, but it also uses a variety of other methods, recognizing that future conditions are often realized through a series of zigs and zags rather

than in a more straightforward fashion. Also, the growing understanding of how multiple factors affect a future condition greatly decreases the likelihood that following a linear path will necessarily be the best way to deal with that condition.

3. *Competitive analysis.* Old strategic planning, which assumes a fairly static environment, is characterized by limited competitive analysis and thus focuses on analyzing past and occasionally current competitive strategies. New strategic planning recognizes today's and tomorrow's more dynamic environment and analyzes current and potential future competitors. The multitude of potential competitive strategies and initiatives also reinforces the need for contingency planning.

4. *Competitive environment.* One assumption in old strategic planning is that there isn't much competition, largely because of the increasing demands of consumers and the relative balance between supply and demand. This situation is one that might be summarized as the "increasing pie" marketplace. In contrast, too many providers and an oversupply of services characterize today's and tomorrow's environment. The marketplace is restructuring in most areas, with a shifting or decreasing "pie." Fierce competition is typical and is expected to become more commonplace in the future.

5. *Basis for strategies.* In old strategic planning, the overwhelming majority of strategies and initiatives come from internal organizational constituents' needs. In contrast, the majority of new strategic planning initiatives reflect marketplace needs, recognizing internal capabilities and desires. Externally driven strategies and initiatives are clearly more responsive to today's and tomorrow's market realities.

6. *Planning process.* Often, old strategic planning processes were somewhat lengthy and relatively leisurely in pace. Also, although a general process was followed, detours and tangents were not uncommon during strategic plan development. An 8- to 12-month time frame for plan development was fairly standard. New strategic planning is faster paced and adheres more rigorously to a specified process. A 4- to 6-month time frame is fairly standard for strategic planning today.

7. *Plan development frequency.* Strategic planning was viewed as a periodic event in the the past; the board and management devel-

oped a plan about every five years with little organizational planning in the interim. Today's strategic planning is an ongoing process. A full strategic plan may be prepared every three years with regular environmental analyses and updating. Quarterly plan review and modification is common, as is a semiannual or annual leadership retreat for updating and revising the plan.

Implications for Leaders

Every organization has an implicit strategy even if the leadership group does not define it in a conscious, deliberate manner or through consensus. The implicit strategy is manifested in the organization's actions and inactions, although it may not be clear what path the organization is actually following.

An organization could still be lucky enough to survive without an articulated strategy, but it's likely to miss opportunities that could have strengthened it and be much more likely to fall prey to financial disaster or even closure.

Most certainly, leaders will be confused about "why we're doing that," and an abundance of their time will be wasted debating choices already made or about to be made.

The question is not whether health care strategic planning is relevant anymore but rather how to conduct it so that it is useful for the 21st century. Under the old strategic planning approach, its relevance is undoubtedly questionable. But the new strategic planning model has adapted to current market realities and should be a critical board and management tool for health care organizations of all sizes.

Growing Into Your Future

By Sandra Elliott

During the last decade, hospitals and health systems have been filling board seats with highly experienced business people. These boards have a more narrowly focused agenda, concentrating extensively on strategic planning and reflecting a growing hunger for business lessons already learned by other industries.

But trustee successes in other corporate sectors have not transferred easily into the health care world.

"Health system boards still live in the past," says Ann Coats, board chair of the Peninsula Regional Medical Center in Salisbury, Maryland. "Board thinking often reflects the realities of the '70s and '80s, when we need to be thinking in terms of 2010."

Part of the problem stems from the perception that the health care environment is unlike the "real business world." Many people believe that although health care providers have some control over expenses, unlike other industries they have little or no control over revenues.

"In health care, we seem to feel we are exempt from the basic competitive forces of business," says Robert Fanning, president and

Sandra Elliott is president and CEO of Growth Inc., Barnegat, New Jersey. She can be reached at (609) 607-0629.

CEO of Northeast Health Systems in Beverly, Massachusetts. "I sometimes feel like I am the only one worried about it. I watch to see if the ambulances are going to turn right or left—to come to us or go to the competitor."

Health care leaders are not accustomed to watching the competition. But every day, niche players with specialties in wound care, physical therapy, incontinence, surgery, radiology, women's care, and outpatient cancer treatment are springing up to erode hospital business centers. The past decade has brought a shift in the health care industry toward consumerism. People now choose and direct who provides their health care, and they vote with their feet.

The challenge is to ensure that health care organizations change, using technological advances and shifts in consumerism in a way that captures market position and financial reward.

Meeting this challenge requires a new leadership approach at the board, executive, and product line level. That does not mean board members must learn the intricate details of day-to-day operations, but they should ask management:

- What are we doing to replace lost revenue?
- What new businesses do we need to develop?
- Why are patient volumes going down, and what will we do about that?

When dealing with declining volumes and revenues, board members need to make it clear that the better alternative to cutting expenses is to develop strategies that rapidly grow volumes and revenues. Board members must find out if the organization is trying to create more value for the organization and for the community. They need to discover what services patients want and how the organization can capture that business by developing those services locally.

Board members can provide the most value to their organization by asking management:

- Is there an aggressive plan to increase sales in the next two quarters?
- How was our performance last quarter compared with projections?
- Are returns as aggressive as stated?

- Is the company planning to aggressively thwart a new competitor or market force?

Push for Results-Oriented Growth

More than a one-time shot, growth is an ongoing use of well-thought-out, disciplined strategies designed to increase revenue.

Health care organizations are familiar with long-term expense reduction plans. Similarly, sustained revenue growth requires a plan with structure and methodology. There needs to be a definitive start date, weekly outcomes, and a concrete date for implementation.

Griffin Hospital of Derby, Connecticut, began using a disciplined growth strategy, The Model for Growth™, in May 1998, and the next year grew its lab business by 70 percent. In addition, the emergency department reduced its "convenient care" turn-around time from 72 minutes to 38 minutes and increased its volume by 6 percent.

Bill Powanda, vice president of support services at the organization, says that the biggest challenge for hospitals is to create a business mentality. "Department and service line leaders have to understand that they have to develop a business plan for expanding existing services or developing new services. The Model for Growth gave us the tools and the discipline to do that."

"The devil is in the details" should be the credo for regular tracking and monitoring and may require that future incentive compensation programs are focused on results and not merely activity. The box on the next page contains questions to ask senior execs in order to keep on top of a growth strategy.

Become the Pied Pipers of Culture

Successful companies such as Staples learned a valuable lesson from IBM—you don't rest on your laurels and wait for the competition to go away. Successful companies see the future and anticipate the impact it will have on their business. They have the hunger to get business and to deliver services better than their competitors. They proactively offer what customers want and deliver it in the way customers prefer. In other words, they have the strong, driving entrepreneurial spirit necessary to continue to succeed in today's markets.

Your Growth Strategy: Questions to Ask Your CEO

- Which services have increased volume and revenues more than 5 percent during the past year? Which have not?
- What steps, if any, are being taken to grow the latter?
- Is there any structure to develop growth strategies for each key clinical service line?
- What has changed about our competitors to concern us? How are we responding?
- What competitive advantages do our competitors have and how will we respond?
- Where are our opportunities for growth? How are we capitalizing on those opportunities?

Peninsula Regional Medical Center is also using a new, structured process for growing revenues. The organization's COO, Bill Snapp, believes leadership must model the new behaviors. "First and foremost, from the board level down," he says, "we must show energy, passion, and interest in the development and implementation of growth strategies. We need to continue, from a governance and executive perspective, to 'live it' and to constructively reshape this organization by openly discouraging the old way of doing things."

Board members can do this by familiarizing themselves with revenue growth stories from other industries and applying those lessons to their health care organization whenever the opportunity arises, always emphasizing that business basics are business basics, no matter what the business. For example:

- Hershey Foods added a low-fat label to York Peppermint Patties to take advantage of fat-conscious customers. Because the candy had only three grams of fat, already meeting low-fat food requirements, Hershey didn't have to make any other changes to the product.
- Cadbury-Schweppes entered a joint venture with Coca-Cola to create a $1 billion United Kingdom bottling enterprise, partnering with Hershey, Perrier, and Kraft to grow revenue.

Boards can also change their culture by offering positive feedback, promotions, and financial compensation based on how well department and service line leaders identify opportunities to grow and capitalize on innovation.

Peninsula's Snapp acknowledges that his organization is not much different from the "thundering herd" when it comes to dealing with meeting the challenges of day-to-day operations. "Our department and service line leaders still spend a lot of time putting out fires," he says. But he is noticing that they are starting to spend more time planning than just minding the store. "They are starting to realize that the world is not as fixed as it used to be and they must be more fluid to fit in."

How can a board tell if its management team is looking ahead or merely putting out fires? Try asking:

- Has the hospital market share eroded because competitors are providing services never offered before?
- Has the competition intensified over the past two years?
- Have more resource-rich competitors entered the market?

If the answers are "yes" to these questions, the board may need to think about how to create an environment where people are not afraid to take risks and make mistakes.

"If there's one thing I've learned from mistakes," says Jack Welch, CEO of General Electric, "it's that it's better to act too quickly than it is to wait too long. You've got to pursue business opportunities where they exist, not just where you're comfortable doing business."

Trustees have a responsibility to use their business skills and experience to lead health care organizations out of the comfort zone and into the future.

Put Yourself in the Picture: Planning by Strategy Development

By David Miller
and John Hill

Some things in health care never change. Take strategic planning, which many executives still approach the same way they did 20 years ago. Ongoing processes for strategy development and evaluation are often nonexistent. The result, all too often, is a plan that is linear in nature and not as flexible as it needs to be.

In looking at the process of strategy development, there are seven key barriers to effective planning:

Barrier 1: Assuming You Know the Future

Too often, strategies are based on a single view of the future. This view may be linear in nature—that is, believing that the future will be an extension of the past or the present. It may assume that all customers will want integrated systems or that the United States will have national health care reform.

Scenarios are the most helpful way to deal with an uncertain environment. These descriptions of possible futures are useful as

David Miller is a partner in D.W. Miller & Co., Louisville, Kentucky, and John Hill is a partner in PSA Consulting Group, Louisville.

windows through which executives can view proposed strategies. They foster discussions that help decision makers assign varying degrees of likelihood to different scenarios.

Barrier 2: Copying Industry Successes

From staff model HMOs to TQM to physician integration and integrated delivery systems, the health care field often shows a herd mentality.

Part of this has to do with risk management—it is better to be wrong with everyone else than to be wrong and alone. Part of it is assuming that what happens in Southern California or Minnesota will surely happen in Virginia or Ohio. And part of the problem is board education programs that focus on "hot" new trends.

Learning from what other people do well is not inherently bad— it's only bad if applied without proper analysis, thought, and review. When looking for answers is substituted for critical thinking, the end result is often failure.

The recent christening of integration as the strategy of choice is one example of this. It has worked well in some situations, but more often it's led to steep losses from physician practices and managed care ventures. It has often provided no advantage in the marketplace. The use of scenarios would have provided the different perspectives needed to more adequately evaluate this strategy.

Barrier 3: Not Differentiating Your Organization

Hospitals are often faced with a significant dilemma. Despite their best efforts, they are selling a commodity. They cannot control prices in a market where many hospitals look alike and successful managed care networks can be constructed while excluding many organizations.

To a degree, being unable to control prices relates to the supply of hospital beds. But even in badly overbedded communities, some are able to command higher prices. How? These organizations are uniquely positioned in the minds of consumers and insurers. They may have superior location, be a children's hospital, be a leader in heart care, or be known as a center of excellence.

Michael Porter, the Harvard Business School strategy guru, defines strategy as differentiation. In a 1996 article, he asserted that the essence of strategy is choosing to perform activities differently than competitors do—a difference that is valued by the marketplace and can be preserved.

To do this, organizations must be willing to make trade-offs. They must focus resources and management attention on building their key strengths. Then they must develop and reinforce their brand to communicate these priorities to the market. This approach is risky. But so is remaining a generic hospital.

Barrier 4: Strategy as Reaction

All too often, strategy is reactive. Strategies are often driven by factors that, while important, should not be drivers. Key among these is political pressure. This is particularly true in community-owned not-for-profit hospitals, as many constituencies demand input into the process. This is unavoidable and not necessarily bad. But without a board educated in strategy development, it can be an inappropriate driver.

A second reactive approach is dependence on experts. Again, experts have their place, but they cannot be substituted for clear thought and analysis. The use of consultants must be tempered with the understanding that the management team will be held accountable for any failures.

At the same time, opportunities should be evaluated carefully. Analysis should evaluate a venture not just as a stand-alone business but also how it may affect the organization's strategy and the provision of its core business.

Barrier 5: Limiting Innovation

Innovation and strategy are generally not linked in the health care industry. Most organizations don't focus on innovation but, rather, depend on creative people within the organization to innovate for the entire organization.

Part of the problem is that health care executives are not trained to foster innovation. Meetings on innovation often deteriorate into critiques of each new idea. And innovation, of course, involves risks. Untried strategies can fail, injuring the organization and its leaders.

Educating a board to support innovation is difficult, but it is the key to developing transformational strategies. Those strategies will be necessary if organizations are to succeed (instead of just survive) over the long haul.

One key is to be very selective in evaluating innovations. Pilot programs should be encouraged before major commitments are made. In addition, organizations should be careful not to get too far removed from their strengths.

Barrier 6: Financial Disconnect

One limiting factor to strategy development is the leadership's failure to tie it to the financial plan. Organizational visions are proclaimed and goals articulated, but only limited financial analysis is completed.

Every strategic plan should incorporate this critical step. A financial baseline must be developed and the new strategies quantified. Capital plans should be completed and income statements projected.

In doing this, the philosophy behind the scenarios must also be used. Although the plan will reflect the goal, financial planning must account for the fact that plans tend to be optimistic. Boards must understand not only the financial impact of achieving all goals but the financial implications of partially achieving them.

Barrier 7: Strategy Development as an Event

Perhaps the most limiting philosophy for strategy development is viewing it as an event. A consultant is engaged, a board retreats, a management team writes it all down, a notebook is created. There is nothing inherently bad about these steps, but they must be supplemented by other actions that support successful strategy development.

In total quality management (TQM) there is the simple philosophy of plan, do, check, act. The first step is to plan your actions in detail to help ensure they are appropriate and executed well. Implementation follows, then results are checked through measurement. Finally, action is taken to correct any deficiencies. It is these last two steps that health care executives often omit in strategic planning.

Checking should take place at two levels. Level one, the most obvious, is asking whether the strategy and its supporting actions are achieving the results that were expected.

A second level of checking relates to checking the underlying assumptions used in the planning process. What are the underlying assumptions of each scenario? The environment will give you clues as to which worldview is developing, what scenario is unfolding. This can be incredibly valuable as executives and boards decide how plans must be adjusted.

Conclusions

Historically, strategic planning has received mixed reaction from health care executives. When it works, it has provided value by focusing the organization and fostering discussions among its various stakeholders.

By guarding against the seven barriers listed above, executives can vastly increase the effectiveness of such a process. Risks can be reduced, boards can be better educated, and the effectiveness of management actions can be increased.

Strategic Planning
by the Board

By James E. Orlikoff
and Mary K. Totten

Strategic planning is one of the most critical responsibilities for trustees. But experience shows that it is also a task that they tend to perform the least effectively. Why? Because the board frequently focuses on, and attempts to perpetuate, the past rather than facilitating strategic thinking and action about the future.

That's why board members and other health care organization leaders should realize this simple truth: The health care system is undergoing rapid, sweeping changes that will affect everyone involved in it—hospitals, physicians, providers, purchasers, the government, communities, and patients.

Furthermore, health care delivery is being reformed by such forces as informed and aggressive payers and employers; the rapid growth of managed care and at-risk capitation; the increasing availability of quality data; reductions in Medicare payments; and the linking of health care delivery and financing systems. Change is also being spurred by the movement away from inpatient acute care, the increasing emphasis on wellness and illness prevention, the move-

James E. Orlikoff is president of Orlikoff & Associates,. Inc., Chicago.
Mary K. Totten is president of Totten & Associates, Oak Park, Illinois.

ment toward healthy communities, and the growth and acceptance of alternative medicine.

Each of these changes in significant; together, they are revolutionary. Effective health care leaders realize that these changes are happening now, not in the distant future. Thus, health care leaders must act now.

In this environment, a failure to plan is surely a plan to fail.

What Is Strategic Planning?

Strategic planning is the process of determining what an organization should do, as well as when and how it should do it. That's why effective strategic planning involves strategic thinking, strategic decision making, and strategic action. Strategic planning has been defined as "the process of building a vision and assembling the means to carry it out" (Dabne G. Park, Jr., *Strategic Planning and the Nonprofit Board*) and "an organized way of applying common sense and judgment to your hospital's decision-making process." (Norman H. McMillan, *Planning for Survival*).

Although these definitions seem to describe a simple, straightforward process, effective strategic planning involves a series of complex steps. Among other things, the process requires soul-searching, hard work, thinking ahead and assessing the environment, anticipating many alternative futures and choosing one, diagnosing problems, determining solutions, choosing a course of action and having the courage to commit to and implement that course, monitoring the implementation of the plan, and keeping the plan dynamic so that it responds to the changing environment and the changing needs of the organization.

One of the major components of a meaningful strategic plan is an organizational vision—a sense of where the organization is heading and what it hopes to achieve. In fact, strategic planning engages the organization in a systematic process of determining what the organization is going to be and how it will get there. "Strategic planning is worthless unless there is first a strategic vision," says futurist John Naisbitt. With the vision as the basis, the strategic planning process can then focus on how best to achieve it in light of projected environmental changes.

Strategic Planning: Questions for Discussion

A strategic planning process helps you to answer a set of critical questions, such as those presented below. Please consider and answer the following questions. You may do this individually and then discuss your answers with the board as a whole.

1. What is our organization's purpose or mission?
2. What is our vision for the organization's future?
3. Whom do we serve today?
4. Who are our stakeholders?
5. Whom should we serve tomorrow?
6. Which services do/should we provide?
7. What tools can we use to measure our performance?
8. How can we change our priorities if conditions change?

Strategic Planning Development/ Improvement Exercises

A common problem with many strategic planning processes arises from organizational denial: the inability or refusal of the board and other leaders to recognize the most critical issue, whether external or internal, confronting the organization. As a result, many strategic plans identify and address dozens of minor issues but fail to address the one or two absolutely crucial ones. In other words, many plans nibble at the toes of the giant rather than striking at his heart.

The entire board should discuss and agree on answers to the following questions:

1. What are the three most critical issues facing your organization?
2. What are the greatest strengths your organization can draw on to address these issues?
3. What are the greatest weaknesses your organization must change/ overcome to address these issues?
4. What are the likely consequences of not implementing changes to address these issues:
    • For the hospital?
    • For the physicians?
    • For the community?

The Strategic Planning Process

Determining where to focus the finite resources of your organization is a complex task and often one that is unique to each organization. Consequently, the strategic planning process is not a set formula that each organization's board can easily follow. Each board must establish and oversee its own strategic planning process.

Nevertheless, there are steps and tasks that are common to most strategic planning processes, such as the following:

1. Get organized:
   - Plan to plan.
   - Possibly establish a planning committee.
   - Develop a committee charge, such as:
     —Work products
     —Responsible parties
     —Approvals
     —Timetable
2. Develop or reaffirm the mission statement.
3. Develop or at least revise the vision statement.
4. Gather data and conduct an internal and external environmental assessment.
5. Analyze data: identify strategic issues.
6. Select strategic priorities and develop strategies: make the best use of limited resources to achieve the vision.
7. Develop action plans: alternatives, recommendations, assignments of responsibilities and time frames.
8. Determine performance measures: object criteria, time frames.
9. Approve the strategic plan.
10. Implement the strategic plan.
11. Monitor, evaluate, and update the plan and its performance targets at least annually.

Whichever process you use to develop it, an effective strategic play will have several essential components:

1. A clear vision for the organization
2. Between 4 and 10 primary areas of focus, with goals and objectives for each area

3. Strategies to achieve the goals and objectives
4. Tactics to turn the strategies into action (often contained in action plans)

The Role of the Board

The principal responsibility for strategic planning rests with the board. Although the board does not usually conduct all of the steps involved in the planning process, it does make certain that they get accomplished appropriately. Among the board's responsibilities for strategic planning:

- Ensuring that a planning process is in place
- Assigning responsibility to oversee the process (usually assigned to a strategic planning committee of the board but can be assumed by the board as a whole)
- Making policy decisions on the strategic direction of the organization
- Ensuring that the strategic direction is consistent with the mission and vision, and is appropriate relative to the environment
- Reviewing and approving specific projects and actions to verify that they are consistent with and support the strategic plan
- Monitoring the implementation of the strategic plan and how goals and objectives are being achieved
- Modifying and updating the plan on a regular basis

It's important to remember that strategic plans are not static. Planning involves evaluating and modifying existing plans and constantly developing new ones.

Because of the accelerating pace of change in health care, time horizons of strategic plans have generally been shortened to one to three years rather than the longer time horizons of the past.

Role Clarification Exercise

Following is a series of potential roles that a governing board might be expected to play in the strategic planning process.

Please rank (with 1 being the highest) each role from highest to lowest priority. Each trustee should perform this exercise individually first; then the whole board should collate and discuss the results.

Board Roles

—— Organize, oversee the process

—— Maintain the mission

—— Pursue the vision

—— Contribute community perspective

—— Ask questions

—— Set strategic direction

—— Set goals, priorities

—— Approve the strategic plan

—— Monitor plan implementation

—— Evaluate performance toward plan achievement

—— Maintain institutional viability

—— Track environmental changes

—— Improve community health

—— Oversee tactical implementation

—— Achieve stakeholder buy-on to the plan

—— Communicate the plan

—— Identify the strengths and weakness of the organization

—— Develop goals and objections

—— Examine alternative approaches and solutions

Strategic Planning Case Example

The following case example will help you analyze a market situation and determine the best market position and strategic direction for Our Town General Hospital. This example can be used as part of a board retreat or, if distributed and reviewed in advance, as part of an educational component of a board meeting.

Our Town General Hospital is a 500-bed, not-for-profit community hospital serving a metropolitan area of 300,000 people. Competitors are a 350-bed community hospital, a 220-bed religiously sponsored institution with long-term care and elderly housing, and a 90-bed county-owned facility providing specialized services, including rehabilitation, chemical dependency and women's health programs. Thirty miles away is a well-respected academic medical center with which Our Town General has a teaching affiliation.

Our Town General maintains a primarily local focus and offers a broad range of services, many of which are not well differentiated. It is the most expensive local provider. The community perceives the hospital as delivering good-quality service.

Although the hospital has traditionally focused on inpatient care, it was the first provider in town to diversify into outpatient services, primarily ambulatory surgery. Two years ago, the hospital also entered into a joint venture with a physician group from its medical staff to purchase and operate an MRI unit.

Our Town General's medical staff also has staff appointments at other local hospitals. Referral patterns to the hospital are moderately strong, especially for obstetrical care. Most of the medical staff fall into the 45–65 age group. Discussions are under way with key medical staff leaders about establishing a physician-hospital organization; two of Our Town General's competitors already have established PHOs.

Over the past five years, Our Town General's operating margins have been close to 4 percent. Accounts receivable now run 71 days, down from 85 days five years ago. The physical plant averages 10 years of age.

Like many communities, Our Town General's service area has a growing elderly population. The area has experienced a "baby boomlet" over the past five years, and this trend is expected to increase.

The area's employer profile is slowly changing from a manufacturing to service focus. One of the major employers in town has decided to participate in managed care.

Analysis:

As a board member of Our Town General, you are now participating in the hospital's strategic planning process. Management has told you that if the hospital simply maintains its current focus, this position as local market leader will likely erode and lead to continuing cost increases, reimbursement constraints, and other typical problems.

How would you answer the following questions?

1. What are the three most critical issues facing Our Town General?

2. What are Our Town General's current strengths and weaknesses?
3. What key issues will the hospital face in the future? Note the potential planning implications of each issue you identify.
4. What position should Our Town General seek in the local health care delivery system?
5. Which strategic direction should the hospital adopt and why?
6. Our Town General Hospital's mission statement, approved five years ago, is as follows:

> Our Town General Hospital is a 500-bed, not-for-profit community hospital serving Our Town and adjacent communities. Our Town General provides a broad range of acute care and outpatient services and maintains a teaching focus. Our goal is to be the leading hospital in our market by delivering the highest-quality services as efficiently as possible.

Given the strategic direction you have recommended, rewrite the mission statement to clearly and specifically indicate the hospital's purpose and identity.

Tips for Effective Governance Involvement in Strategic Planning

1. Lead, don't follow. Many health care leaders are "waiting to see what's going to happen." This approach is reactive and unproductive.
2. Involve key stakeholders in the planning process. Stakeholders can include the board, executive management, physician leaders, community representatives, and organizations that are strategic partners with your hospital.
3. Plan, then act. Do not fall prey to the "paralysis of analysis," where the constant state of gathering information and planning precludes action by creating the false sense of security that the board is "doing something."
4. Make certain that the strategic plan has the commitment of the key stakeholders before it is finalized or implemented. As Norman McMillan says: "The 25 percent plan that gets 100 commitment is a winner; the 100 percent plan that gets 25 percent commitment is a loser."

5. Keep the strategies simple, the goals specific, and the objectives measurable.

6. Place the top strategic objectives on the first or second page of every board agenda book (following the mission and vision) to enable the board to coordinate its time and attention with the strategic plan.

7. Develop annual board and board committee objectives and work plans that flow from, and focus on, the strategic plan; integrate them into the board self-evaluation process.

8. Use the strategic plan as a basis for the CEO performance evaluation process: develop specific CEO performance objectives based on measurable goals and objectives in the strategic plan.

9. Make certain that the strategic plan focuses on the *critical* issues confronting your organization, not just the secondary ones.

10. Most health care market conditions will require strategies for cost efficiency, quality improvement and demonstration, integration of physicians, streamlined leadership structures, and establishing or maintaining strategic partnerships with other organizations. Does your plan address these issues?

A Self-Assessment Questionnaire

Instructions: The following brief survey addresses the board's key roles and responsibilities in oversight of, and involvement in, the strategic planning process. It can be used as a stand-alone survey or as part of an overall board self-evaluation process. Each trustee should independently and anonymously rate the board's performance on each of the following questions.

Then compile and analyze all the responses of the board and discuss them with the entire board. Pay particular attention to questions with significant variation in responses (where some trustees rate board performance high and some rate it low) and those with predominantly negative responses. The discussion should result in the formation of a board action plan to increase the effectiveness of its oversight and involvement in strategic planning.

1. The board takes a leadership role in organizing and overseeing the strategic planning process.

☐ Strongly Agree   ☐ Agree
☐ Somewhat Disagree   ☐ Disagree

2. The board approves a strategic plan and ensures it is consistent with the organization's mission.

   ☐ Strongly Agree   ☐ Agree
   ☐ Somewhat Disagree   ☐ Disagree

3. The board ensures that community perspectives and issues are addressed in the planning process.

   ☐ Strongly Agree   ☐ Agree
   ☐ Somewhat Disagree   ☐ Disagree

4. Management, the medical staff, key clinical and administrative staff, community leaders and representatives, and other advisors, as appropriate, participate in our planning process.

   ☐ Strongly Agree   ☐ Agree
   ☐ Somewhat Disagree   ☐ Disagree

5. The board questions planning data and assumptions and deliberates alternative strategies during our strategic planning process.

   ☐ Strongly Agree   ☐ Agree
   ☐ Somewhat Disagree   ☐ Disagree

6. The board sets a strategic direction for strategic plan development.

   ☐ Strongly Agree   ☐ Agree
   ☐ Somewhat Disagree   ☐ Disagree

7. The board monitors implementation of the strategic plan and evaluates accomplishment of plan goals and objectives at least annually.

   ☐ Strongly Agree   ☐ Agree
   ☐ Somewhat Disagree   ☐ Disagree

8. The board periodically reviews, discusses, and, if necessary, amends the strategic plan to ensure that it remains current and relevant.

   ☐ Strongly Agree   ☐ Agree
   ☐ Somewhat Disagree   ☐ Disagree

9. The board monitors the organization's programs and activities to ensure that they are consistent with the strategic plan

   ☐ Strongly Agree   ☐ Agree
   ☐ Somewhat Disagree   ☐ Disagree

10. Our board takes corrective action when necessary to ensure compliance with the mission and the strategic plan.

    ☐ Strongly Agree   ☐ Agree
    ☐ Somewhat Disagree   ☐ Disagree

Conclusion

The purpose of strategic planning is not only to position the organization for the future but, in a very real sense, to create the future for the organization. For the board to effectively oversee such a process, it must break the bonds of the past to envision the future. This is why Arie P. De Geus says: "The real purpose of effective planning is not to make plans but to change the microcosm, the mental models that decision makers carry in their heads" (*Planning as Learning*). Finally, remember that "the output of planning is not a plan; the output is action!" (John Abendshien, *A Guide to the Board's Role in Strategic Business Planning*).

Balance of Power:
Encouraging Physicians
to Help Set
the Strategic Plan

By Laurie Larson

It's every parent's worst nightmare. Trust a teen with the keys to the car for one quick errand—and he never comes back. Or he does, with the police officer who witnessed the reckless fender bender that totaled the car. That's the kind of chill that runs through many hospital administrators' blood when they think of allowing physicians to have a bigger say in strategic planning.

"Hospital [administrators] unintentionally infantalize physicians," because they tend to focus only on their own work, says Robert Harrington, cofounder of Cambridge Management Group (CMG), Cambridge, Massachusetts. CMG counsels health care systems on governance and management, including introducing ways to give physicians more strategic say. In a conversation with Harrington, based on a presentation he made at the VHA Leadership Conference in Chicago, he shares his views of the physician's evolving importance in strategic planning.

Although he may be exaggerating somewhat, it has been his experience that management often thinks physicians are "enemies, smart

---

Laurie Larson is *Trustee*'s associate editor.

children, or a toxic substance to be contained by management, who consider themselves the adults." Not surprisingly, the "smart children" don't appreciate being thought of as such, and thus physicians are usually "suspicious of [hospital] administration," Harrington says. "I tell physicians, 'the CEO isn't your dad or Santa Claus or a demon,'" but, he adds, "physicians tell me, 'If you want to get doctors together, ask us [as a group] how things should work overall—just us.' There's nothing wrong with inviting physicians on boards and committees, but [the discussion tends to be] hospitalcentric."

Whose Show Is It Anyway?

The truth is that physicians have always been in charge, Harrington says, as their behavior drives 80 percent of hospital revenue. In addition to determining where patients will seek primary and specialty care, they control referrals and, to a great extent, quality of care. Also, because physicians are taking huge chunks of hospitals' most lucrative service lines, such as imaging and ambulatory surgery, and creating "niche" facilities (see "Hospitals Feeling 'Niched to Death,'" in the June 2002 issue of *Trustee*), they can seriously hurt hospitals' bottom line.

"Most hospital profits are made through ambulatory services—hospitals lose money on inpatients for the most part," Harrington says. As declining reimbursements cut more deeply into their own incomes, physicians are increasingly starting their own speciality services. They know where the money is to be made—and they can make better use of their own time as a result. "At the moment, 60 to 70 percent of [hospitals'] revenue comes through ambulatory services, and the rest comes from surgery, which can often be done outside the hospital," Harrington says.

Physicians' desire to move such services to an office setting is not motivated by profit alone, however, Harrington says. "Hospitals are not efficient organizations. They do not handle bundles of activity consistently; they are messy and chaotic. With doctors' incomes under increasing pressure, they are asking, 'How can I make better use of my time?'" Moving services to a specific outpatient setting provides efficiency and economy, while appealing to patients who would prefer an office setting over a hospital one, he says.

So if they want to call their building a true hospital, administrators and trustees must learn to reestablish better connections with physicians. The solution: Get physicians to take more responsibility by sharing the considerations, regulatory headaches—and the books—with which administration struggles. By providing physicians with management's side of the hospital equation, "physicians can immediately see how fragile the picture is," Harrington says.

A structure that many health systems are finding helps create this dialogue is a medical advisory panel (MAP)—a group of physicians meeting among themselves, armed with administrative knowledge to set strategic direction, and bringing their recommendations back to management. But there is skepticism on both sides about starting a MAP.

"The first step is based on trust," Harrington says. "Physicians are competitive, data-driven people, and they do excellent work if they care about something. Once management finds out that physicians really want to help, and once physicians see that this is not a consultant's game for management's benefit, the work can begin."

Here's how it's working at three different hospitals.

Bridgeport Hospital

Bridgeport (Connecticut) Hospital brought Harrington in a year and a half ago to establish a MAP as part of its five-year strategic plan, Destination 2005. The MAP's goal has been to define the organization's clinical programming and move from an administratively driven relationship with physicians to a clinically driven one.

The 350-bed community teaching facility affiliated with the Yale School of Medicine, like many hospitals, has been facing financial constraints, the need for upgraded facilities, and a "silo" atmosphere of poor communication and fragmented procedures. Frustrated by these conditions, medical staff would often go around their department chairs to complain to senior management, feeling powerless and ignored. CEO Robert Trefry and Bruce McDonald, M.D., senior vice president of medical affairs, thought the Cambridge Management Group could help if physicians and middle managers could be convinced.

"I told the department chairs that we were going to turn over strategic planning to the community physicians, and it took two meetings to sell it to them—some of them were angry," McDonald says. "I wanted to convince them it was a process that works and that we would get new leaders out of it." Indeed, MAP members have since joined the board and the medical executive committee, bringing with them a much greater understanding of administrative issues.

The first task was to select the panel's cochairs, and McDonald asked department chairs for their input. "We really reinforced the primacy of the department chairs, asking them to use their resources to help solve the problems and reassuring them that we were not taking their authority away from them," he says. By design, however, no department chairs actually sat on the MAP, although they had authority to approve MAP recommendations.

In choosing the 11 panel members, Cochair Michael Ivy, who runs the surgical ICU, sought a mix of young and senior physicians, those in private practice and on staff, and primary care practitioners as well as subspecialists.

"We looked for different personalities too, choosing some confrontational people, because they . . . ask the hard questions," Ivy says. "But we didn't choose those with ego issues who would conflict with each other. We looked for those who were committed to the hospital."

Panel members began by asking themselves, "How should we invest our resources over the next five years? What should the hospital look like by then?" They went through a six-month process of weekly meetings to answer those questions, beginning with comprehensive education on hospital finance, managed care, nurse staffing, planning and marketing, and information systems. This "grounding in the basics" was essential for useful deliberation and recommendations, Senior Vice President McDonald says.

"Our physicians had no concept before of reimbursement mechanisms, how items get [included] on [patients'] bills," he says. "They are much more collaborative now. They understand how difficult it is to recruit staff—they thought we were withholding our help, but now they know we weren't." Based on their deeper understanding of these and other issues, the MAP looked at ways to better use existing resources—making patient satisfaction the overriding goal and process, rather than outcomes, the focus.

As a result, the MAP reorganized clinical areas, moving from a departmental approach to a service line one organized into eight clinical program teams: diagnostic services, emergency services, the Heart Institute, internal medicine, pediatrics, psychiatry, surgery and anesthesia, and women and maternity.

Each new service line prepared a white paper based on meetings among all medical staff and department chairs in that area, determining how they would reorganize their work flow and what resources they needed to do so. They had a month to put the white papers together, and each service line sent a representative to present its paper to the MAP.

McDonald helped coordinate the meetings and he, Trefry, and other leaders were allowed to attend but not comment.

Trefry says he knew it was important that he mainly "stay away" from the MAP's work, not always a comfortable feeling, he admits. "If you're in the room, it's hard for them. They need the freedom to not look to me for guidance and the space to gather their own recommendations. It demonstrates that you have faith in them."

"As much as you might want to manage the process, you shouldn't," agrees Dorothy Bellhouse, Bridgeport's senior vice president for planning and marketing. "You have to give physicians the information they need and let them run [the committee]." That stepping back is precisely what made physicians believe in the MAP, she adds. "There were no preconceived ideas of where things would end up. [Physicians realized] 'this is not administration telling us what to do, but instead they're really asking us what we think.'"

The MAP then pored over the white papers for six months to synthesize all their ideas and come up with goals centered around four areas: organizational health (that is, creating a satisfying work environment to keep and draw employees), quality and process improvement, volume and market share growth, and financial health.

These goals have resulted in several initiatives, including a stronger focus on outpatient care; a new wellness center; minimally invasive care, such as complementary medicine; coordinated diagnostic evaluations; and a technology task force. Work in all service lines is supervised by clinical program teams, comprising the clinical chair, staff director, and a senior management staff member.

"They [the clinical program teams] have the responsibility and the authority to move the strategy along however it relates to their team," Bellhouse says. Each team reports to the CEO every four to eight weeks and to the MAP three times a year, marking their progress toward the Destination 2005 goals. She has noticed relationships growing between the formerly suspicious department chairs and the MAP physicians and a greater ease on the senior management side.

"We've found MAP to be very valuable," Trefry says. We have a strong base of support [for strategy development] among the medical staff instead of resistance. They see the overall logic of the plan—it has been developed by colleagues they respect."

There have been some surprises along the way. For example, some departments had no idea what new procedures or areas of expertise other departments had. Now in the auditorium used for physician meetings, a film "scroll" projects the latest clinical news from each department on the wall. There are more internal referrals as a result. Ivy says the MAP hopes to go through the evaluation process again in two years to assess how far it's come and what the panel needs to do next. "The most valuable thing about [MAP] is getting everyone to sit down together," Ivy says. "The point, really, is the discussion."

Albemarle Hospital

Not every facility needs to start so formally, however. Albemarle Hospital in Elizabeth City, North Carolina, is using what it calls its "physician relations committee," a new board committee, to rebuild its relationship with physicians. The 286-bed hospital had gone through an extensive restructuring, moving from county ownership to becoming its own hospital authority over the two prior years, and physician relations had deteriorated as a result.

To reconnect and brainstorm the hospital's future direction, Trustee Ernest Sutton proposed forming the committee as one of his first actions after becoming board chair a year ago.

"Physicians are unique in themselves. We want to hear their voice, and this is a formal way—a communication network—to talk about their concerns. It's an ongoing resource for them . . . and it keeps lines open so they can hear our issues too," Sutton says.

He appointed four board members to the committee, including one physician. The committee became active, working hand in hand with the medical executive committee, which acts as a "hub" to focus its efforts, Sutton says. The committee meets monthly, chaired by former Board Chair and Trustee Phil Donahue, and he considers it an excellent move after the change in ownership.

"It was a controversial changeover," Donahue says. "Physician recruitment and retention fell away. Our purpose, from the management and board perspective, was to find out what physicians' concerns were and deal with them in an [honest] manner, asking what the hospital could do for them, developing a team approach."

The new group met with the strategic planning committee to contribute its thoughts to future planning. Now, at each meeting all participants discuss whatever current clinical or management concerns they have, as well as what skills and procedures are obsolete or need to be improved and which ones should be enhanced. The emphasis throughout is on good general communication and education on both sides. As chair, Donahue presents a report to the full board after each meeting.

"What I like about how we've handled this is that it seems logical," Donahue says. "Six months into it, doctors are more open, they're sharing their experiences with us. . . . I have to say we've gone from being 'seat-of-our-pants' to having a well-thought-out plan in place."

As an example of the difference in culture, Donahue says the administration decided it needed to replace the hospital-based anesthesiology department, whose contract was up for renewal, with a group that offered a better price for its services. That's where he says the committee "really paid off. Five years ago, the doctors would have been all over us, demanding that we reverse our decision," Donahue says. "But the CEO kept them informed as to why and how we were making the change, and there was not a big outcry against it. That may be a good sign."

Although she came on board last November when the committee had already been decided upon, new CEO Sharon Tanner had worked with similar groups in previous administrative positions and fully supports the committee's contributions.

"Physicians need to be at the table," Tanner says. "The more information you give them, the more support you get. It's been a very positive, collaborative experience." In addition, the "frontline" information physicians have shared has been invaluable, she affirms.

For example, an apparent staff shortage was actually the result of too many people calling in sick, physicians informed them. This is still a problem but one to be handled completely differently. "You find out the real issues, not the rumors," she says. "You give [physicians] the facts and you improve the process."

Eventually, Sutton sees physicians becoming more directly involved in strategic planning, with improved communication and education as the first steps toward that goal. He plans to issue a self-evaluation [survey] to the group to see how well the committee thinks it is working and how it could be more effective. All along, trust has been the cornerstone.

"It's preemptive—before [situations] become problems," Sutton says. "We do better business when we talk to each other."

North Colorado Medical Center

Three years ago, relations between physicians and management at North Colorado Medical Center in Greeley had deteriorated so badly that physicians were writing letters to the newspaper and going to the board asking for a vote of no-confidence in the CEO. That CEO was set to retire and his replacement, Jon Sewell, brought in Robert Harrington, who had supervised MAP creations in three previous hospitals.

In hearing physicians' versions of hospital problems, Sewell says they were "outrageous, festering versions of the truth. When stories sound this way, there is no channel of accurate information, . . . doctors felt a lack of input and control over their practice. When there's no connection, if there's a problem, you think it's because of the other guy." John Miller, an assistant administrator over clinical services, agrees, calling MAPs "just-in-time learning."

"Doctors are really small business owners, tied to their income streams; whereas hospitals have more cash flow and are more corporate," Miller says. "It's easy to lose sight of the fragile reimbursement situation that physicians face. They have been impacted by technology, reimbursement, patient expectations . . . so they are falling behind . . . and then by the time [administration] sees this, the walls have gotten so high, it's hard to get to an open dialogue."

Harrington began by meeting with physicians in small groups, asking them first how they wanted their practice to evolve, and secondly, how they wanted the medical center to evolve. As skeptical as they were, Sewell says doctors had to participate because of how vocal they had been about their unhappiness.

Sewell identified the most widely respected physicians in the medical center and asked 2 of them to cochair the MAP. Those leaders then chose 10 to 15 more physicians that they respected for the panel. "At the end of the day, doctors follow those they respect clinically," Sewell says. Surgeon Michael Peetz, M.D., was one of those asked to join the panel.

"At first I said I was too busy, but other [colleagues] said they would do it if I did it . . . and I decided if I was going to practice here for another 10 to 15 years, I needed to get involved in my destiny," he says. His current position as assistant administrator of medical staff grew out of the MAP, as he helped to sort out conflicts. For example, a proposed day surgery center that would have taken business away from the hospital is now a joint venture, something he and the MAP worked out.

To give the panel the operations information it lacked, Sewell says administrators spent 16 hours covering accounting, regulatory issues, marketing, and demographics—what he calls "Hospital 101. . . . Most doctors haven't a clue [about operations]. They don't understand the seemingly dumb decisions that administrators make."

Physicians met and discussed their needs by department, and by January 2000, they were ready to present the MAP with white papers centered around service lines, as Bridgeport Hospital did, analyzing and planning what their future work methods and services would look like. The MAP spent 12 weeks hearing 26 presentations based on the papers. Of importance, considerable time was left at the end of each presentation for questions and discussion between MAP members and physicians designated to present papers from their departments. The MAP then distilled its conclusions down to what the "body of the medical staff thinks we should do," Sewell says.

Of their recommendations, he says "10 were cultural issues before we got to financial requests"—how staff treated each other, fairness in outside contracts, and other issues. Further, he says, the MAP's conclusions "very nicely aligned with the strategic plan." The administrative team (Sewell, Miller, and three other assistant administrators) laid out all 326 recommendations in a spreadsheet format and presented them to the MAP and the medical executive committee. Miller says between 70 and 80 percent of the recommendations have been addressed, and about that same percentage were concerned with issues driven by relationships rather than finance. Sewell says many recommendations were taken on the basis of the reports only, as they involved easy changes that could be made quickly. This, in turn, created immediate goodwill and went a long way toward building trust and better communication.

Changes resulting from the MAP's work have focused around three key initiatives: developing a new cardiovascular center; coordinated diagnostics; and customer (i.e., staff) satisfaction.

"Physicians stepped back and realized that they had to treat employees better, build morale, and become an employer of choice," Miller says. "They also wanted to do peer review and hold themselves more accountable for their own behavior—it was a real awakening. They realized, 'We've got to keep our quality people. We are driving these people away.'"

MAPs do not always continue once they have met their strategic planning goals, but North Colorado decided to maintain its panel. They now meet monthly, and Sewell has invited all departments to revisit their recommendations from three years ago and see what they think now.

"I make no decisions without the medical advisory panel," Sewell says. "I always ask, 'Will it play well with the medical staff?' That impact is crucial to me." He adds that the self-discipline to ask that question may be the hardest change for a CEO or a board to make.

Leadership First

"The key to [MAP] success is a personally and professionally secure CEO," Harrington says. "He or she must understand how profoundly this business is changing—and boards need to be able to [accept] a new paradigm." Trustees may actually find it easier than their CEOs to do so, however, because they may have learned similar lessons in their own industry, realizing that the best way to fix problems in any business is to talk to those on the front lines who are creating the product or service.

"Management needs to realize that they were never really in control anyway," Harrington says. "You have to say, 'Here's the situation. How do we create a better margin with you?' Share information and you will reach the same desired outcomes."

North Colorado's Peetz adds, "Physicians are bright people and you cannot filter the information you give them. Show them how difficult it is to manage a hospital. Done well, MAPs restore communications that are being severed right and left in today's economy. When doctors are treated like equal partners, they will respond very well."

Index

Hospital trustees *(continued)*
    looking outside neighborhood for,
        6–7
    mentoring, 164–165
    patient safety and, 284, 348, 364,
        367
    performance evaluation, 166–169
    physician, 390
    preparing new, 74–82
    providing data for, 192–201
    qualified candidates for, 4
    quality of care and, 278–288
    quality quiz for, 277
    recruiting tips for, 6
    responsibilities of, 9
    selection of, 162
    in strategic planning, 414
    teaching moments for, 189–191
    techniques for recruiting, 3–10
    time demands on, 5, 8, 9
    tips for development of, 169–171
    underutilized, 178
    unspoken agreements between
        management and, 154
Human capital, 208

I

Iatrogenic illnesses, 276
Indicator report, 192–201
Information. *See also* Data
    making decisions based on objec-
        tive, 261, 263
    qualitative, 391
    sharing between CEO and board,
        122–123
    trustee need for financial, 251–252
Information technology (IT)
    in balancing health care needs,
        264–270
    capacity and, 268–269
    infrastructure, 269, 270
    investing in, 240–241
Innovation, educating a board to sup-
    port, 417–418
Inpatient surgery per 100 admissions,
    200

Institute for Diversity in Health Man-
    agement (IFD), 27–28
Institute for Safe Medical Practice,
    354
Institute of Medicine (IOM) reports,
    273, 278, 307, 317, 327–328,
    343, 351, 352, 362–363, 363
Integrated delivery networks (IDNs),
    255
    aggressive implementation of a
        high-growth, 253
    need for strategic planning and,
        397
Integrity in board-CEO relations,
    124–125
Interview
    of board candidates, 24–25
    one-on-one, 164
Investment management policy,
    173–174
Investment management practices,
    217–218, 220, 221

J

Joint Commission on Accreditation of
    Healthcare Organizations
    (JCAHO), 105, 354
    ORYX program of, 366–367
    patient safety standards of, 100,
        318, 328, 333–334, 345, 349,
        360, 363, 365–366
    performance measures of, 280
    quality standards of, 275
    self-evaluations and, 100
    Sentinel Events Policy of, 365–366
Just-in-time learning, 438

L

Law of Triviality, 66, 69
Leaders, 144
    competition and, 411
    diversity of, in hospitals, 27–36
    implications for, in strategic plan-
        ning, 409
    strategies for, in patient safety,
        356–358